LARYNGOLOGY

CLINICAL REFERENCE GUIDE

LARYNGOLOGY

CLINICAL REFERENCE GUIDE

Justin Ross, DO
Haig Panossian, MD
Mary J. Hawkshaw, RN, BSN, CORLN
Robert T. Sataloff, MD, DMA, FACS

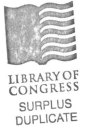

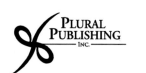

PLURAL
PUBLISHING
INC.

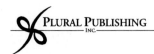

5521 Ruffin Road
San Diego, CA 92123

e-mail: information@pluralpublishing.com
Website: https://www.pluralpublishing.com

NOTICE TO THE READER
Care has been taken to confirm the accuracy of the indications, procedures, drug dosages, and
diagnosis and remediation protocols presented in this book and to ensure that they conform
to the practices of the general medical and health services communities. However, the authors,
editors, and publisher are not responsible for errors or omissions or for any consequences from
application of the information in this book and make no warranty, expressed or implied, with
respect to the currency, completeness, or accuracy of the contents of the publication. The
diagnostic and remediation protocols and the medications described do not necessarily have
specific approval by the Food and Drug administration for use in the disorders and/or diseases
and dosages for which they are recommended. Application of this information in a particular situation remains the professional responsibility of the practitioner. Because standards of
practice and usage change, it is the responsibility of the practitioner to keep abreast of revised
recommendations, dosages, and procedures.

Library of Congress Cataloging-in-Publication Data:
Names: Ross, Justin, DO author. | Panossian, Haig, author. | Hawkshaw, Mary,
    author. | Sataloff, Robert Thayer, author.
Title: Laryngology : clinical reference guide / Justin Ross, Haig Panossian,
    Mary J. Hawkshaw, Robert T. Sataloff.
Description: San Diego, CA : Plural Publishing, [2020] | Includes
    bibliographical references and index.]
Identifiers: LCCN 2019017790| ISBN 9781635501407 (alk. paper) | ISBN]
    1635501407 (alk. paper)
Subjects: | MESH: Otorhinolaryngologic Diseases | Laryngeal Diseases |
    Otolaryngology | Handbook
Classification: LCC RF46 | NLM WV 39 | DDC 617.5/1--dc23
LC record available at https://lccn.loc.gov/2019017790

CONTENTS

Section VII. Pediatric Laryngology

Section VIII. Surgery

Section IX. Swallowing Disorders

Section X. Therapy

PREFACE

As with the other books in this series, *Laryngology: Clinical Reference Guide* is written in bullet point format to provide information conveniently and quickly. Although this is not a 2,000-page laryngology textbook, we have tried to keep the content comprehensive if not complete, including all of the important and practical information necessary to guide clinical thinking and care.

Chapter 1 reviews the evolution of laryngology from the pre-Grecian period to the state-of-the-art. Chapters 2 and 3 provide a clinically relevant review of laryngeal embryology, anatomy and physiology. Chapter 4 on the history and physical examination is supplemented by Chapter 5 on the clinical voice laboratory (including techniques for objective voice assessment) and Chapter 6 on laryngeal electromyography (an important extension of the physical examination). Chapter 7 reviews many of the infectious and inflammatory disorders of the larynx; and Chapter 8 provides information on structural abnormalities. Vocal fold scar is presented in considerable detail in Chapter 9, and information on scar is supplemented by Chapter 10 on vocal fold injury and wound healing, an outstanding chapter by Susan L. Thibeault. Chapters 11 through 14 provide a wealth of practical information on laryngotracheal trauma, glottic and subglottic stenosis, and tracheal stenosis, focusing on both diagnosis and current concepts in treatment. Chapters 15 and 16 review benign and premalignant lesions of the larynx, and laryngeal cancer.

The section on neurolaryngology summarizes current thinking on laryngeal neurophysiology, vocal fold paresis and paralysis, laryngeal dystonias, and other neurological disorders that affect the larynx (voice, swallowing and airway) in Chapters 17 through 20.

The lengthy section on laryngeal manifestations of systemic diseases is particularly valuable. Chapter 21 discusses the effects of aging on the larynx and voice. Chapters 22 and 23 summarize laryngopharyngeal reflux and thyroid disorders. Autoimmune diseases, allergy, respiratory dysfunction, and cough and the unified airway are covered thoroughly in Chapters 24 through 27. Chapter 28 provides the latest information on care of transgender and gender non-conforming patients; Chapter 29 reviews psychological aspects of voice disorders; and the effects of medication in laryngology are discussed in Chapter 30. Chapter 31 is a comprehensive overview of pediatric otolaryngology. Voice surgery (with lasers and traditional instruments), and other airway surgery is detailed in Chapters 32 through 34. Chapters 35 and 36 review diagnosis and treatment of dysphagia, and of structural disorders of the esophagus. Voice and swallowing therapy are reviewed in Chapters 37 and 38. The book also includes useful appendices on tracheotomy tube sizing, and cricothyrotomy and tracheotomy technique.

The authors enjoyed crystalizing current thinking in laryngology and hope that our readers will find this clinical reference guide useful and enjoyable.

ABOUT THE EDITORS

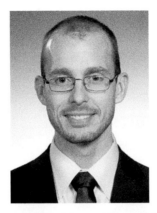

Justin Ross, DO is an Otolaryngology resident at Philadelphia College of Osteopathic Medicine in collaboration with Dr. Robert Sataloff at Drexel University College of Medicine. He was raised in southern York County, PA and completed his Bachelor of Science in Biology at York College of Pennsylvania. He is the author of several peer-reviewed publications and book chapters, and has now co-edited one book. Dr. Ross' research interests include treatment of vocal fold scar and the link between hearing loss and dysphonia.

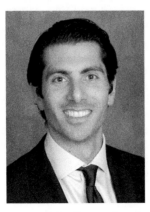

Haig Panossian, MD attended college and medical school at Boston University. He then completed his otolaryngology residency at the Icahn

School of Medicine at Mount Sinai. Dr. Panossian completed his fellowship in Laryngology under the direction of Dr. Robert T. Sataloff at the Drexel University College of Medicine, where Dr. Panossian is Assistant Professor of Otolaryngology-Head and Neck Surgery. He also is currently in private practice in Westlake Village, California.

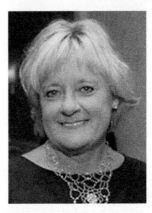

Mary J. Hawkshaw, BSN, RN, CORLN, is a Research Professor of Otolaryngology-Head and Neck Surgery at Drexel University College of Medicine. She has been associated with Dr. Robert Sataloff, Philadelphia Ear, Nose & Throat Associates and the American Institute for Voice & Ear Research (AIVER) since 1986. She has served as Secretary/Treasurer of AIVER since 1988 and was named Executive Director of AIVER in January 2000. She has served on the Board of Directors of the Voice Foundation since 1990. Ms. Hawkshaw graduated from Shadyside Hospital School of Nursing in Pittsburgh, Pennsylvania and received a Bachelor of Science degree in Nursing from Thomas Jefferson University in Philadelphia. In collaboration with Dr. Sataloff, she has co-authored more than 180 articles, 102 book chapters, and 14 textbooks. She is on the Editorial Board of the Journal of Voice, the Ear, Nose and Throat Journal, and the Journal of the Society of Otorhinolaryngology and Head-Neck Nurses (SOHN). She has been an active member of the Society of Otorhinolaryngology and Head-Neck Nurses since 1998. She is recognized nationally and internationally for her extensive involvement in the sub-specialty of care of the professional voice.

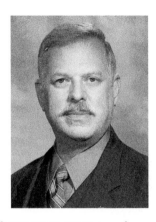

Robert T. Sataloff, MD, DMA, FACS, is professor and chairman in the Department of Otolaryngology-Head and Neck Surgery and senior associate dean for Clinical Academic Specialties at Drexel University College of Medicine. He is also adjunct professor in the Department of Otolaryngology-Head and Neck Surgery at Thomas Jefferson University and Temple University; as well as on the faculty of the Academy of Vocal Arts. Dr. Sataloff is a professional singer and singing teacher and has conducted the Thomas Jefferson University Choir for over four decades. He holds an undergraduate degree in Music Theory and Composition from Haverford College, medical degree from Jefferson Medical College, Thomas Jefferson University, and doctor of musical arts in voice performance from Combs College of Music. He completed his residency in otolaryngology-head and neck surgery and fellowship in otology, neurotology and skull base surgery at the University of Michigan. Dr. Sataloff is chairman of the boards of directors of the Voice Foundation and the American Institute for Voice and Ear Research. He is editor-in-chief of the *Journal of Voice* and *Ear, Nose, and Throat Journal,* associate editor of the *Journal of Singing,* and on the editorial boards of numerous otolaryngology journals. He has written more than 1,000 publications, including 65 books. His medical practice is limited to care of the professional voice and otology/neurotology/skull base surgery.

CONTRIBUTORS

Asyia Ahmad, MD, MPH
Professor of Medicine
Chief, Division of
    Gastroenterology
Director, Motility Laboratory
Drexel University College of
    Medicine
Philadelphia, Pennsylvania
Chapter 36

Ghiath Alnouri, MD
Laryngology Fellow
Department of Laryngology
Drexel University College
    of Medicine/Hahnemann
    Hospital
Philadelphia, Pennsylvania
Chapter 30

Kenneth W. Altman, MD, PhD
Professor and Vice Chair for
    Clinical Affairs
Bobby R. Alford Department of
    Otolaryngology
Baylor College of Medicine
Houston, Texas
Chapter 27

Tess T. Andrews, MS, CCC-SLP
Speech-Language Pathologist
UC Davis Department of
    Otolaryngology
Sacramento, California
Chapter 38

Austin T. Baker, BS
Medical Student
Texas College of Osteopathic
    Medicine
University of North Texas Health
    Science Center

Fort Worth, Texas
Chapter 25

Ayman Bodair, MD
Department of Medicine
Walter Reed National Military
    Medical Center
Bethesda, Maryland
Chapter 3

Jacob Burdett, DO
Resident Physician
Department of Otolaryngology-
    Head and Neck Surgery
Philadelphia College of
    Osteopathic Medicine
Hahnemann University Hospital
Philadelphia, Pennsylvania
Chapter 24

Nicholas C. Cameron, BS
Medical Student
Touro College of Osteopathic
    Medicine
Middletown, New York
Chapter 23

**Deborah Caputo Rosen,
PhD, RN**
Clinical Psychologist
Private Practice
Ardmore, Pennsylvania
Chapter 29

Bhavishya S. Clark, MD
Resident Physician
Department of Otolaryngology
University of Southern California
Los Angeles, California
Chapter 13

Jason E. Cohn, DO
Resident Physician
Department of Otolaryngology-
  Head and Neck Surgery
Philadelphia College of
  Osteopathic Medicine
Hahnemann University Hospital
Philadelphia, Pennsylvania
Chapter 24

Jaime E. Moore, MD
Assistant Professor
Department of Otolaryngology-
  Head and Neck Surgery
Adjunct Professor
Department of Music
Virginia Commonwealth
  University
Richmond, Virginia
Chapter 9

Marissa Evarts, DO
Resident Physician
Department of Otolaryngology-
  Head and Neck Surgery
Philadelphia College of
  Osteopathic Medicine
Hahnemann University Hospital
Philadelphia, Pennsylvania
Chapters 30 and 31

**Christopher E. Fundakowski,
MD, FACS**
Associate Professor of
  Otolaryngology-Head and
  Neck Surgery
Thomas Jefferson University
Philadelphia, Pennsylvania
Chapter 16

Jared M. Goldfarb, MD
Resident Physician
Department of Otolaryngology-
  Head and Neck Surgery
Thomas Jefferson University
  Hospital

Philadelphia, Pennsylvania
Chapters 12 and 14

**Jonathan Aaron Harounian,
MD**
Resident Physician
Department of Otolaryngology-
  Head and Neck Surgery
Lewis Katz School of Medicine at
  Temple University
Philadelphia, Pennsylvania
Chapter 35

**Mary J. Hawkshaw, RN, BSN,
CORLN**
Research Professor
Department of Otolaryngology-
  Head and Neck Surgery
Drexel University College of
  Medicine
Philadelphia, Pennsylvania
*Chapters 1, 2, 3, 4, 5, 6, 7, 8, 15,
17, 18, 20, 22, 23, 24, 26, 28, 30,
31, 33, and 34*

**Yolanda D. Heman-Ackah, MD,
MS, FACS**
Director
Philadelphia Voice Center
Clinical Professor
Drexel University College of
  Medicine
Adjunct Associate Professor
Thomas Jefferson University
Bala Cynwyd, Pennsylvania and
  Philadelphia, Pennsylvania
Chapter 11

Nausheen Jamal, MD
Associate Dean of Graduate
  Medical Education / DIO
Chief, Division of
  Otolaryngology-Head and
  Neck Surgery
University of Texas Rio Grande
  Valley School of Medicine

Edinburg, Texas
Chapter 35

Aaron J. Jaworek, MD
Laryngology and Care of the
    Professional Voice
Specialty Physician Associates,
    Bethlehem, Pennsylvania
St. Luke's University Health
    Network School of Medicine
Clinical Assistant Professor
Drexel University College of
    Medicine
Philadelphia, Pennsylvania
Chapter 19

Michael M. Johns, MD
Director
USC Voice Center
Division Director, Laryngology
Professor
USC Caruso Department of
    Otolaryngology-Head and
    Neck Surgery
University of Southern California
Los Angeles, California
Chapter 13

Karen M. Kost, MD, FRCS
Professor of Otolaryngology-Head
    and Neck Surgery
Director of the Voice and
    Swallowing Laboratory
McGill University
Montreal, Québec, Canada
Chapter 21

David J. Lafferty, DO
Resident Physician
Department of Otolaryngology-
    Head and Neck Surgery
Philadelphia College of
    Osteopathic Medicine
Hahnemann University Hospital
Philadelphia, Pennsylvania
Chapter 31

Andrew E. Lee, MD
Resident Physician
Department of Medicine
Hahnemann University Hospital
Philadelphia, Pennsylvania
Chapter 36

**Brian J. McKinnon, MD, MBA,
MPH, FACS**
Associate Professor and Vice
    Chair
Department of Otolaryngology-
    Head and Neck Surgery
Associate Professor
Department of Neurosurgery
Drexel University College of
    Medicine
Philadelphia, Pennsylvania
Chapter 25

Sarah Christine Nyirjesy, BA
Medical Student
Drexel University College of
    Medicine
Philadelphia, Pennsylvania
Chapter 25

Sammy Othman, BA
Medical Student
Drexel University College of
    Medicine
Philadelphia, Pennsylvania
Chapter 7

Haig Panossian, MD
Assistant Professor
Department of Otolaryngology-
    Head & Neck Surgery
Drexel University College of
    Medicine
Philadelphia, PA
Director, Division of Laryngology
C/V ENT Surgical Group
Westlake Village, CA
*Chapters 2, 5, 6, 15, 26, 32,
and 33*

Paul M. Papajohn, DO
Resident Physician
Department of Otolaryngology-
   Head and Neck Surgery
Philadelphia College of
   Osteopathic Medicine
Hahnemann University Hospital
Philadelphia, Pennsylvania
Chapter 23

Luke J. Pasick, BS
Medical Student
Drexel University College of
   Medicine
Philadelphia, Pennsylvania
Chapter 16

**Bridget A. Rose, MM, MS,
CCC-SLP**
Senior Speech Language Pathologist
Singing Voice Specialist
Philadelphia Ear, Nose and Throat
   Associates
Philadelphia, Pennsylvania
Chapter 37

Justin Ross, DO
Resident Physician
Department of Otolaryngology-
   Head and Neck Surgery
Philadelphia College of
   Osteopathic Medicine
Hahnemann University Hospital
Philadelphia, Pennsylvania
*Chapters 1, 3, 4, 7, 8, 12, 13, 17,
18, 19, 20, 21, 22, 28, and 31*

**Robert T. Sataloff, MD, DMA,
FACS**
Professor and Chairman
Department of Otolaryngology-
   Head and Neck Surgery
Senior Associate Dean for Clinical
   Academic Specialties
Drexel University College of
   Medicine

Conductor
Thomas Jefferson University
   Choir
Adjunct Professor
Department of Otolaryngology-
   Head and Neck Surgery
Sydney Kimmel Medical College
Thomas Jefferson University
Philadelphia, Pennsylvania
*Chapters 1, 2, 3, 4, 5, 6, 7, 8, 15,
17, 18, 20, 22, 23, 24, 26, 28, 30,
31, 33, and 34*

Jennifer M. Schwartz, DO
Resident Physician
Department of Medicine
Drexel University College of
   Medicine
Philadelphia, Pennsylvania
Chapter 36

Harleen Sethi, DO
Resident Physician
Department of Otolaryngology-
   Head and Neck Surgery
Philadelphia College of
   Osteopathic Medicine
Hahnemann University Hospital
Philadelphia, Pennsylvania
Chapter 34

Rupali N. Shah, MD
Associate Professor of
   Otolaryngology
Department of Otolaryngology,
   Division of Voice and
   Swallowing Disorders
The University of North Carolina
   at Chapel Hill
Chapel Hill, North Carolina
Chapter 27

Joseph R. Spiegel, MD
Professor
Department of Otolaryngology-
   Head and Neck Surgery

Co-Director
Jefferson Voice and Swallowing
  Center
Thomas Jefferson University
Philadelphia, Pennsylvania
Chapters 12 and 14

Kevin Tie, BS
Medical Student
University of North Carolina
  School of Medicine
Chapel Hill, North Carolina
Chapter 27

**Susan L. Thibeault, PhD,
CCC-SLP**
Professor
Department of Surgery, Division
  of Otolaryngology-Head and
  Neck Surgery
School of Medicine and Public
  Health
University of Wisconsin-Madison
Madison, Wisconsin
Chapter 10

Katherine L. Tsavaris, MD
Resident Physician
Department of Medicine

Hahnemann University Hospital/
  Drexel University
Philadelphia, Pennsylvania
Chapter 36

Arthur Uyesugi, MD
Resident Physician
Virginia Commonwealth University
Richmond, Virginia
Chapter 9

Travis Weinsheim, DO
Resident Physician
Department of Otolaryngology-
  Head and Neck Surgery
Philadelphia College of
  Osteopathic Medicine
Hahnemann University Hospital
Philadelphia, Pennsylvania
Chapter 16

Peak Woo, MD, FACS
Clinical Professor
Department of Otolaryngology-
  Head and Neck Surgery
Icahn School of Medicine at
  Mount Sinai
New York, New York
Chapter 32

To Our Families

SECTION

History of Laryngology

CHAPTER

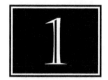

History of Laryngology

Justin Ross, Mary J. Hawkshaw, and Robert T. Sataloff

PRE-GRECIAN CIVILIZATIONS

- most ailments thought to be divine punishment for sin or wrongdoing
- most Egyptian gods had an association with health
- the goddess Isis was the patron deity of healing, and her physician Thoth was the repository of all medical knowledge to the gods
- Asclepios was the primary god of healing, and son of Apollo
- Asclepios' oldest son was Machaon, god of surgery, and his other son was Podalirios, god of medicine; his daughters Hygieia and Panacea were the goddesses of public health and therapy, respectively
- Imhotep was the son of the god Ptah, and the most famous Egyptian physician; he was later deified and combined with Asclepios
- Egyptians believed lungs contained magic powers, frequently wore protective amulets
- <u>2900 BC</u>: King Aha created a monument to an unknown healer who might have performed a tracheotomy or other neck surgery
- <u>2500 BC</u>: Sekhet'eanack, physician to pharaoh Sahura "cured the king's nostril"
- <u>2000 BC</u>: Babylonian god Nabu ruled over all science; the demon Namtary caused throat disease

GREEK AND ROMAN CIVILIZATIONS

- medicine was defined by the efforts of philosophers
- Hippocrates (fifth century BC) composed the *Corpus Hippocraticum*
    1. defined the vocal qualities of clarity, hoarseness, shrillness, and others
    2. believed lungs and trachea contributed to voice production, and lips and tongue were involved in articulation
- Aristotle speculated voice was produced by airflow through the larynx and trachea; vocalization inspired by the soul, and that process was located in the heart and lungs
- Greek medical practices heavily influenced the work of Roman physicians as Rome came to dominate Greek culture
    1. *De Morbis Chronicis* by Caelius Aurelianus devoted a chapter to hoarseness, and in *De Acutis Morbis*, he refers to Hippocrates' treatment of dysphonia by a practice similar to intubation
    2. Claudius Galen (131–220 AD), physician to Emperor Marcus Aurelius, was the founder of laryngology; described three major cartilages and six paired muscles of the larynx, and identified it as the organ responsible for voice production

MIDDLE AGES

- the disciple Luke was known as "The Beloved Physician"
- Christian physician St. Blaise was reportedly proficient in tracheotomy, and he became famous treating children with respiratory difficulties; Blessing of the Throats performed on February third in all Catholic churches
- the first picture of the larynx and trachea was created by an unknown Italian artist in the sixth century
- the majority of medical advancement during the Middle Ages arose from Arab physicians in the middle east, primarily Baghdad, Cordova, and Cairo
- the writings of Arab physicians were primarily based on those of Galen
- Rhazes the Experienced (850–923) is considered one of the great Muslim physicians
  1. wrote 237 books, but the most important was the *Continens* in which he discussed maladies of the voice
  2. believed changes in voice were related to pathologies of the larynx, respiratory system, and brain, and advocated treatment with vocal training and respiratory exercises
- in the 10th century, Arab physician Haly Abass wrote *Liber Regius*, a medical tome including a concise description of the larynx, and voice production as a function of the passage of air through a closed glottis
- Avicenna the Persian (980–1037) is considered the most famous Arab physician; wrote over 100 books including the *Quanun,* which includes a chapter dedicated to voice
- Abul Quasinu of Cordova (936–1013) described laryngotomy and was responsible for the revival of surgical cautery in the region
- Maimonides (1135–1204) was the most famous physician in Cairo, and personally attended the caliph Saladin
- within Western Europe, Mondino de Luzzi (1275–1327) was considered the greatest anatomist of his age, and based his work primarily on Galen
- any discrepancy with Galen's work was considered a fault with the anatomist or the cadaver
- European physicians Johannes von Ketham and Johann Peyligk in 1493 and 1499, respectively, believed the voice originated from an artery that connected heart to throat

RENAISSANCE TO LATE 19TH CENTURY

- modern medical care began in the Renaissance, pioneered by Leonardo da Vinci
    1. da Vinci authored *Quaderni d' Anatomia* (1500), in which he included drawings of the larynx and assigned articulation to upper airway structures—this tome was lost until 1784, when it was discovered in an English royal house
    2. he also produced tones from a larynx by squeezing a goose's lungs, described the difference between waves and vibrations, and postulated on the waveform of a string
- Andreas Vesalius (1514–1565) was a professor of anatomy at the University of Padua, and authored *De Humani Coroporis Fabrica* (1543), in which he disputed Galen's account of the laryngeal framework
- Gabriele Fallopio (1523–1563), also a professor at the University of Padua, is responsible for naming the cricoid cartilage
- Bartolomeus Eustachius (1520–1574), a professor at the University of Rome, authored the *Tabulae Anatomicae* (1552), a tome of anatomy accurate to nature that was lost until 1714
- Hieronymus Fabricius ab Aquapendente (1537–1619), also a professor at the University of Padua, authored several books on the larynx, and postulated that the vocal folds create voice
- Julius Casserius (1561–1616) succeeded Hieronymus at Padua, and also wrote several anatomical texts on voice and hearing, including *De Vocis Auditusque Organis*
- Caspar Bauhinus (1550–1624), professor at the University of Basel in Switzerland, authored *Theatricum Anatomicum* where he described the extrinsic and intrinsic laryngeal muscles as they are known today
- Thomas Willis (1621–1675), of the University of Oxford, was the first to describe the origin of the superior laryngeal nerve in his book *Cerebri Anatome Nervorumque Descriptio et Usus*
- French architect and anatomist Claude Perrault (1613–1688) described laryngeal musculature as responsible for variations in the voice
- French physician Dennis Dodart (1634–1707) described the larynx as the only organ responsible for voice production
- Giandomenico Santorini (1681–1737) first described the corniculate cartilages, otherwise known as the Cartilages of Santorini
- Giovanni Batista Morgagni (1682–1771), a professor at the University of Padua, authored *De Sedibus et Causis Morborum*, and described laryngeal anatomy and pathology in a more complete manner than his predecessors

1. responsible for identifying the laryngeal ventricles as the source of mucus production for the vocal folds
2. structure was named Morgagni's sinus or the ventricles of Morgagni

- Antoine Ferrein (1693–1769), a professor of anatomy at University of Montpellier, described the vocal folds as strings through which sound is produced by vibratory motion
- Albrecht von Haller (1708–1777) was a professor of physiology and anatomy in Germany who described the relation of vocal resonance to the nose, throat, and paranasal sinuses in his book *Elementa Physiologiae*
- Heinrich August Wrisberg (1739–1808) first described the laryngeal cuneiform cartilages
- Philipp Bozzini (1773–1809) was a German physician credited with invention of the earliest endoscope, which he named a light conductor or Lichleiter
- Francois Magendie (1783–1855) first described vibration and movement of the vocal folds in vivo, and later in relation to nervous injury, but was mistaken about the function of superior and recurrent laryngeal nerves
- Robert Willis (1800–1875), a British professor of applied mechanics at Cambridge, was the first to describe rotation of the arytenoids on the cricoarytenoid joint, and the correct function of the laryngeal muscles and nerves
- Jacob Henle (1809–1855), a professor of anatomy in Zurich, was the first to characterize laryngeal epithelium as squamous and ciliated
- French scientist Claude Bernard (1813–1878) was the first to demonstrate the abductor and adductor functions of the recurrent laryngeal nerve
- French neurosurgeon Pierre Paul Broca (1824–1880) was the first to identify the speech center in the brain
- in 1839, German physiologist Johannes Muller (1801–1858) devised the myoelastic theory of phonation that posited that voice is produced by vibrations generated from air passing through passive vocal folds
- German physiologist Hermann von Helmholtz (1821–1894) made pioneering contributions on the acoustics of sound; his work served as a basis for future research in the field
- Manuel Garcia (1805–1906) was a renowned voice teacher, catering to nobility and world-class singers alike; he is responsible for first observing phonation in a living subject via dental mirror in 1854
- neurologist Ludwig Türck (1810–1868) and physiologist Johann Nepomuk Czermak (1828–1873) were responsible for development and initial descriptions of laryngeal mirror utilization in medicine

- shortly after its invention, UK physician Sir Morell Mackenzie (1837–1892) learned laryngoscopy from Czermak, and subsequently authored several texts on diseases of the larynx
    1. so great was Mackenzie's renown, that in the summer of 1887, he was consulted in the treatment of Crown Prince Frederick of Prussia whose personal physicians believed that he had laryngeal cancer. Following several negative biopsies, Mackenzie proclaimed him cancer free, but the condition worsened, and required eventual tracheotomy. Frederick died on June 15, 1888, and Mackenzie languished in relative obscurity until his death 4 years later
- in 1878, German physician Max Joseph Oertel (1835–1897) was the first to perform laryngeal stroboscopy, using gaslight prior to the invention of electricity
- German physician Gustav Killian (1860–1921) performed the first bronchoscopy in 1876 with an esophagoscope; in 1897, his colleagues developed the rigid bronchoscope
- Theodore Billroth (1829–1894) performed the first total laryngectomy in 1873
- the laryngectomy was refined by Themistocles Gluck (1853–1942), who developed the tracheostoma; Gluck also combined lymph node dissection with laryngectomy which resulted in improved patient outcomes

20TH CENTURY TO PRESENT

- Chevalier Jackson (1865–1968) was a renowned Philadelphia physician responsible for the development of endoscopy of the upper aerodigestive tract using hollow tubes and distal lighting; during his career he removed over 2000 foreign bodies using endoscopy and popularized the use of endoscopy in common practice
- in 1911, Wilhelm Brünnings performed the first injection medialization laryngoplasty using paraffin
- in 1913, anesthesiologist Henry Janeway (1873–1921) of Bellevue Hospital in New York invented a laryngoscope with a light source at the distal tip powered by batteries in the handle, which was specifically for tracheal intubation
- Japanese laryngologist Minoru Hirano (1937–2017) is credited with first describing the multilayered structure of the true vocal folds in 1975
- ultrahigh-speed photography of vocal fold movement was developed in the 1950s by Hans van Leden, MD, ScD, and G. Paul Moore, PhD

- Wilbur James Gould founded the Voice Foundation in 1969, and the Foundation's Interdisciplinary Symposium on Care of the Professional Voice in 1972
- Japanese laryngologist Minoru Hirano (1932–2017) is credited with first describing the multilayered structure of the true vocal folds in 1975.
- Philadelphia physician Robert T. Sataloff (1949–) published the first modern article, chapter, and book on clinical care of professional singers, and developed various surgical techniques including fat injection laryngoplasty, fat implantation, microflap, and mini-microflap, among others

SECTION

Embryology, Anatomy, and Physiology

CHAPTER

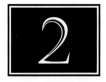

Embryology and Development of the Larynx

Haig Panossian, Mary J. Hawkshaw, and Robert T. Sataloff

STAGES AND STRUCTURES
OF DEVELOPMENT

Histology-Based Theories of Development

- early descriptions of development theorized by His in 1885
- **Respiratory primordium (RP):** an outpouching of the cephalic portion of the pharynx which gives rise to lungs and bronchi
- theorized that tracheoesophageal (TE) separation was an ascending process initiated by groove posterior to RP separating foregut into ventral trachea and dorsal esophagus
- led to decreased distance between floor of pharyngeal pouch (IV) and RP over time
- Zaw-Tun (1982) developed alternative theory based on study of Carnegie and Shatner collections of human embryos
- **Primitive laryngopharynx (PLPh):** segment of foregut that separates pharyngeal floor (at level of pharyngeal pouch IV) from RP
- PLPh lengthens (descending process) as embryo matures and distance between pharyngeal pouch IV and RP remains constant
- PLPh becomes supraglottis
- primitive pharyngeal floor develops into glottis

Carnegie Stages 11 Through 14
(According to Zaw-Tun's Theory)

- hepatic primordium (HP) and RP are both within the septum transversum (ST)
- rapid proliferation of HP causes foregut to lengthen and RP to separate from HP
- separation of RP allows it to dilate and bifurcate into lung buds
- as RP descends from pharyngeal floor, gives rise to funnel-shaped structure
    1. cephalic end becomes infraglottis; caudal end becomes trachea, bronchi and lungs
- concurrently, foregut segment develops into esophagus, stomach, and cephalic half of duodenum
- **Laryngeal inlet:** median slit in pharyngeal floor in Stage 13 (described by Arey in 1965)
- proliferation of pharyngeal mesoderm and arteries of fourth branchial arch lead to arytenoid swellings lateral to entrance of slit
- growth of median epiglottic swelling derived from hypobranchial eminence causes slit to become a T-shaped laryngeal outlet
- transverse pouch of the T descends along epithelial lamina to form laryngeal cecum (see later section, Stages 15–18)

- recanalization of epithelial lamina forms supraglottis (see later section, Stages 19–23)
- controversy regarding interpretation of median slit:
  1. Kallius (1897) and Frazer (1910) reported it represented the cephalic portion of the trachea/glottis
  2. Zaw-Tun demonstrated that it was entrance to PLPh and hence the entrance to supraglottis

Computer Model-Based Theories of Development

- Henick et al (1993) used computer-generated 3-dimensional studies of mouse embryos
- led to discovery of several additional structures but largely supported Zaw-Tun's theories, with the following additional details

Stages 12 Through 14

- **Respiratory diverticulum (RD):** ventral outpouching of foregut lumen that extends into RP
- originates at primitive pharyngeal floor—eventually becomes glottis
- cephalic portion of RD becomes infraglottis
- RD gives rise to bilateral projections known as bronchopulmonary buds
  1. tethered to superior aspect of septum transversum so are drawn caudally as foregut lengthens
  2. develop into lower respiratory tract
  3. carina develops from caudal aspect of RD
- foregut lengthens in cephalocaudal plane as heart and hepatic primordium proliferate on opposing surfaces of septum transversum
  1. gives rise to developing trachea and esophagus
  2. vascular compromise to developing esophagus or trachea can lead to developmental anomalies
- **Laryngeal mesodermal anlage:** triangular-shaped proliferation
  1. develops into laryngeal cartilages and muscles
- elevation of median pharyngeal floor leads to arytenoid swellings at level of fourth pharyngeal pouch

Stages 15 Through 18

- **Epithelial lamina:** formed as ventral aspect of PLPh compressed
- temporarily obliterates PLPh in ventral to dorsal direction
- obliteration incomplete, spares dorsal pharyngoglottic duct (PhGD) and ventral laryngeal cecum

- PhGD is last remnant of patent communication between hypopharynx and infraglottis
- **Laryngeal cecum**: triangular-shaped lumen that originates at ventral aspect of arytenoid swellings
  1. progresses caudally along ventral aspect of PLPh until reaches level of glottis in stage 18

Stages 19 Through 23

- epithelial lamina begins to recanalize from dorsocephalad to ventrocaudal direction
  1. forms the laryngeal vestibule and supraglottis
- Stage 21: laryngeal cecum becomes the two laryngeal ventricles
- Stage 23: glottis is last portion of PLPh to recanalize
  1. stenosis if process incomplete

Development of Laryngeal Cartilages and Muscle

- **Third pharyngeal arch:**
  1. stylopharyngeus muscle
  2. common and internal carotid arteries
  3. body and greater cornu of hyoid bone
  4. glossopharyngeal nerve
- **Fourth pharyngeal arch:**
  1. inferior pharyngeal constrictor, cricothyroid, and cricopharyngeus muscles
  2. subclavian artery (on right) and aorta (on left)
  3. thyroid cartilage, cuneiform cartilages
  4. superior laryngeal nerve; jugular and nodose ganglia
- **Sixth pharyngeal arch:**
  1. all intrinsic muscles of larynx (except cricothyroid)
  2. pulmonary artery (on right) and ductus arteriosus (on left)
  3. cricoid, arytenoid, and corniculate cartilages, trachea
  4. recurrent laryngeal nerve (left remains with ductus arteriosus, while right moves cranially and laterally in association with subclavian artery as the right homologue of the sixth arch disappears)
- **Extrinsic muscles develop from epicardial ridge:**
  1. superficial layer develops into sternohyoid and omohyoid muscles
  2. deep layer attaches to oblique line of thyroid cartilage as sternothyroid and thyrohyoid muscles

DEVELOPMENTAL ANOMALIES

Esophageal and Tracheal Anomalies

Esophageal Atresia

- present in ~8% of infants with TE anomalies
- <u>Sx</u>: increased salivation requiring frequent suctioning, pulmonary triad of coughing, choking, and cyanosis as saliva overflows from blind pouch of esophagus into airway
- aspiration greater in infants with associated TE fistula and direct airway connection

Tracheoesophageal Fistulae (Figure 2–1)

- esophageal atresia with distal TE fistula (~85% of affected infants)
- <u>Sx</u>: gastric distention as air ingested with each breath, respiratory symptoms result from direct aspiration of mix of air and stomach contents as well as decreased diaphragmatic excursion
- TE H-fistula without atresia (~8%)
- proximal TE fistula with atresia (~1%)
- proximal and distal TE fistulae with atresia (~1%)

Tracheal Anomalies

- not associated with laryngeal or pulmonary abnormalities because vascular insult limited to developing trachea
- tracheal agenesis/atresia
- tracheal stenosis with complete tracheal rings
    1. concentric circular tracheal cartilage with loss of posterior membranous trachea

Supraglottic and Glottic Atresia

- incomplete recanalization of PLPh can lead to supraglottic and glottic atresias
    1. <u>Type I</u>: complete supraglottic stenosis
    2. <u>Type II</u>: partial supraglottic stenosis, where communication between supraglottis and infraglottis maintained through patent pharyngoglottic duct
    3. <u>Type III</u>: glottic web
- associated subglottic stenosis in types I and II due to prevention of development of infraglottic region

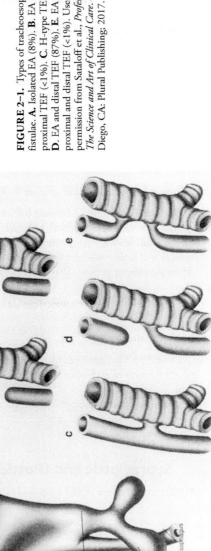

FIGURE 2–1. Types of tracheoesophageal fistulae. **A.** Isolated EA (8%). **B.** EA and proximal TEF (<1%). **C.** H-type TEF (4%). **D.** EA and distal TEF (87%). **E.** EA with proximal and distal TEF (<1%). Used with permission from Sataloff et al., *Professional Voice: The Science and Art of Clinical Care.* 4th ed. San Diego, CA: Plural Publishing; 2017.

Laryngeal Clefts

Benjamin and Inglis Classification

- Type I: interarytenoid area
- Type II: partial cricoid
- Type III: total cricoid, remains above the thoracic inlet
- Type IV: laryngotracheoesophageal cleft

POSTNATAL DEVELOPMENT

Laryngeal Position

- at birth, thyroid cartilage and hyoid bone are attached
- in infancy, epiglottis is bulky and omega shaped, larynx is at level of C3 and C4
- descends to level of C6 by age 5, then C7 between ages of 15 and 20
- descent continues in adulthood, causing vocal tract to lengthen and average voice pitch to lower

Vocal Folds

- in infancy, membranous and cartilaginous portions equal in length
- by adulthood, membranous portion accounts for approximately three-fifths of total vocal fold length
- 12 to 17 mm in adult female, 17 to 23 mm in adult male

Laryngeal Skeleton

- separates and ossification begins slowly
- hyoid bone: ossifies by 2 years of age
- thyroid and cricoid cartilages: ossify in early 20s
- arytenoid cartilages: ossify in late 30s
- entire laryngeal skeleton ossified by age 65 except for cuneiform and corniculate cartilages

CHAPTER

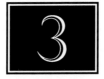

Anatomy and Physiology

Justin Ross, Ayman Bodair, Mary J. Hawkshaw, and Robert T. Sataloff

LARYNGEAL ANATOMY (Figure 3–1)

Laryngeal Subunits

- **Anatomic subunits:** skeleton (cartilages, ligaments, membranes), mucosa, musculature, and related neurovascular structures

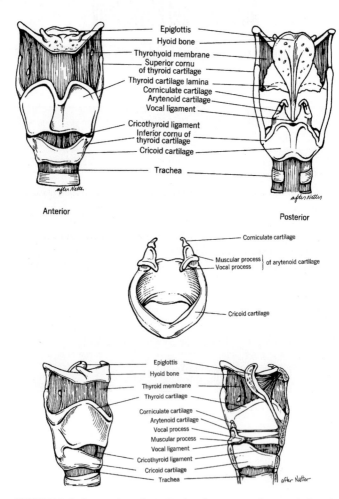

FIGURE 3–1. Laryngeal cartilages. Used with permission from Sataloff et al., *Professional Voice: The Science and Art of Clinical Care.* 4th ed. San Diego, CA: Plural Publishing; 2017.

1. **Supraglottis**: extends from tip of epiglottis to lateral walls of laryngeal ventricles (ventricle of Morgagni); includes paired aryepiglottic, ventricular folds, and saccule of Hilton (anterior-superior aspect of the laryngeal ventricle)
2. **Glottis**: extends from floor of laryngeal ventricles to inferior aspect of the true vocal folds
3. **Subglottis**: extends from the squamocolumnar epithelial junction inferior to the true vocal folds (~5 mm below vibratory margin) to inferior border of cricoid

Laryngeal Skeleton

- Major structural components: thyroid, cricoid, and paired arytenoids
- Laryngeal suspensory mechanism: thyrohyoid, cricothyroid, and cricotracheal membrane and ligaments, stylohyoid and thyroepiglottic ligaments, pharyngeal constrictor muscles

Thyroid Cartilage

- shield-like hyaline cartilage with gender-specific anterior angulation, posteriorly arranged superior cornu and inferior cornu
- Anterior angulation: ~120° in women, ~90° in men; most pronounced at the thyroid prominence (more projected in men)
- **Superior cornu**: connected to the hyoid via thyrohyoid ligament
- **Inferior cornu**: articulates with posterolateral cricoid; diarthrodial synovial joint
- Muscular insertions: thyrohyoid, sternothyroid, and inferior constrictors attach at the oblique line; palatopharyngeus and stylopharyngeus attach posteriorly
- **Montgomery's aperture**: small absence of inner perichondrium between thyroid notch and the inferior border; attachment point of Broyle's ligament and anterior commissure tendon

Cricoid Cartilage

- circumferential signet-ring shaped hyaline cartilage, with greatest height posteriorly (~30 mm), and a narrow anterior arch of only a few millimeters
- anterior arch more susceptible to iatrogenic fracture due to late ossification
- Luminal cross-sectional diameter: narrowest anteriorly; varies between gender (average 11.6 mm in women, and 15 mm in men)
- Tracheal cross-sectional diameter: >9.9 mm in women, >12 mm in men

Arytenoid Cartilages

- pyramidal hyaline cartilages (vocal process and apex are fibroelastic)
- <u>Components</u>: muscular process, vocal process and apex, body, concave inferior articular surface (cricoarytenoid joint)
- ossification of hyaline portions begins at age 20
- arytenoid asymmetry is common, but without clinical significance
- **Cricoarytenoid joint**: synovial joint allowing rocking and gliding motion of arytenoids on cricoid cartilage

Hyoid Bone

- ossified by age 2
- attaches to suprahyoid (mylohyoid, geniohyoid, hyoglossus) and infrahyoid (sternohyoid, omohyoid) musculature, and to the thyroid cartilage via thyrohyoid membrane

Epiglottis

- leaf-shaped fibroelastic cartilage with an inferior petiole that attaches just inferior to the thyroid notch via the thyroepiglottic ligament, and anterosuperiorly to the hyoid via the hyoepiglottic ligament
- located inferiorly on the laryngeal surface, the epiglottic tubercle can sometimes obscure view of the anterior commissure
- edema is more common on the lingual than laryngeal surface due to reduced perichondrial adherence
- <u>Boundaries of the pre-epiglottic space</u>: superiorly—vallecular mucosa; anteriorly—thyroid cartilage and thyrohyoid membrane; posteriorly and inferiorly—epiglottis

Other Laryngeal Cartilages

- **Corniculate cartilages (cartilages of Santorini)**: fibroelastic cartilages superior to the arytenoids, which help provide rigidity to the aryepiglottic folds
- **Cuneiform cartilages (cartilages of Wrisberg)**: nonossifying hyaline cartilages found within the aryepiglottic folds, which improve their rigidity
- **Triticeal cartilages**: hyaline cartilages found in the lateral thyrohyoid ligament, which frequently ossify and may be mistaken for foreign bodies on x-ray

Conus Elasticus

- paired triangular fibroelastic membranes

- extend from vocal ligament to the inferior border of cricoid, and posteriorly from the vocal process to the cricoid and thyroid cartilages anteriorly
  - anteriorly constitutes the cricothyroid ligament, and forms part of Broyles' ligament
  - superiorly forms the vocal ligament (intermediate and deep lamina propria)
- **Quadrangular membrane**: paired fibroelastic membranes extending superiorly from the aryepiglottic folds to the vocal process inferiorly, and laterally from thyroid lamina to supraglottic mucosa medially
  - superiorly forms the aryepiglottic ligament
  - inferiorly forms the vestibular ligament

Laryngeal Mucosa

- primarily pseudostratified ciliated columnar epithelium except the true vocal folds
- lubrication is provided by goblet cells (most prevalent in false vocal folds) and seromucinous, tubuloalveolar glands that are found in the saccule and aryepiglottic folds
- **False vocal folds (FVFs)**: only contact with forceful closure (dysphonia plica ventricularis), play important role in aerodynamics by providing downstream air resistance, contain superior fibers of thyroarytenoid muscle
- **True vocal folds (TVFs)**: musculomembranous folds beginning at the anterior commissure, connected to thyroid cartilage via Broyles' ligament, and includes the vocal process and interarytenoid region posteriorly
  1. 60% musculomembranous (anterior to vocal process); 40% cartilaginous (vocal process)
  2. layering of lamina propria (LP) begins at age 4 → complete by end of adolescence
  3. dimensions of TVF and thickness of LP vary based on gender
  4. anterior 55% to 65% of TVF approximates; posterior larynx closes at the supraglottis
  5. blood vessel and collagen/elastin fibers run parallel to the vibratory margin

True Vocal Fold Layers

- **Epithelium**: nonkeratinizing, stratified squamous epithelium
- **Superficial LP (13%)**: contains mucopolysaccharides, hyaluronic acid, decorin, fibronectin, and elastin precursors; responsible for mucosa wave

- **Intermediate LP (51%):** contains elastin fibers (primarily), hyaluronic acid, and fibromodulin
  1. thickens anteriorly and posteriorly (anterior and posterior macula flava) and inserts into Broyles' ligament and vocal process, respectively
  2. the gradual change in stiffness from posterior macula flava to vocal process protects against mechanical damage and dampens vibratory motion
- **Deep LP (35%):** contains collagen fibers (primarily) and fibroblasts
- **Thyroarytenoid/vocalis muscle**
- **TVF Mechanical subunits:** (1) epithelium and superficial LP; (2) intermediate and deep LP (vocal ligament); (3) thyroarytenoid/vocalis muscle

Laryngeal Blood Supply

- External carotid a. → Superior thyroid a. → Superior laryngeal a. (via lateral thyrohyoid membrane)
  1. supply structures superior to cricoid cartilage, including all intrinsic laryngeal muscles except posterior cricoarytenoid m. (PCA)
  2. enters the larynx posterior to lateral thyrohyoid ligaments with internal branch of the superior laryngeal nerve (SLN)
  3. anastomoses with inferior laryngeal a. and contralateral superior laryngeal a.
  4. cricothyroid a. arises distally to supply CT muscle and membrane, extrinsic musculature, and subglottic pharynx
- Subclavian a. → Thyrocervical trunk → Inferior thyroid a. → Inferior laryngeal a.
  1. supply PCA and portions of the ventricles and false vocal folds
  2. may arise directly from subclavian a. on the left
  3. travels with the recurrent laryngeal nerve (RLN) to supply PCA
- Superior laryngeal v. → IJV; Inferior laryngeal v. → Thyrocervical trunk
- the serpentine, parallel orientation and frequent arteriovenous anastomoses of TVF blood vessels enhance vascular patency and resistance to shearing forces
- blood vessels on the vibratory margin are more resistant to shearing forces than those on the superior surface

Laryngeal Lymphatic Drainage

- **Supraglottic:** travel with superior laryngeal a. to bilateral level II and III deep cervical nodes, and prelaryngeal, prethyroid, supraclavicular, pretracheal, and paratracheal nodes
- **Glottic:** no clinically significant drainage

- **Subglottic**: travel with inferior laryngeal a. to ipsilateral level III and IV deep cervical nodes, and subclavian, delphian, pretracheal, paratracheal, and tracheoesophageal nodes

Laryngeal Innervation

Superior Laryngeal Nerve (SLN)

- SLN branches off from the vagus nerve just inferior to nodose ganglion, and divides into internal and external branches at the posterior hyoid bone
- eSLN usually crosses superior thyroid artery and vein <1 cm above or slightly below the superior pole of the thyroid (~85%), entering the posterior cricothyroid membrane near the inferior cornu
- variation in anatomic course of eSLN puts ~75% to 80% of patient at high risk of iatrogenic injury during thyroidectomy
- eSLN contributes to motor and sensory innervation of the vocal folds in >40%
- sensory innervation of the larynx is primarily mediated by the internal branch of SLN (iSLN), and may provide a smaller motor contribution to laryngeal musculature
- iSLN is organized into three anatomic divisions of sensory innervation: (1) Superior—laryngeal surface of epiglottis; (2) Middle—TVF, FVF, AEF; (3) Inferior—arytenoids, upper esophageal sphincter, anterior hypopharynx, portions of subglottis
- thyroepiglottic ligament and cricothyroid joint also derive sensory innervation from iSLN

Recurrent Laryngeal Nerve (RLN)

- both left and right RLN branch off the vagus nerve within the thoracic cavity, looping around the aortic arch and either brachiocephalic or subclavian artery, respectively
- following passage around the great vessels, RLN travels in the tracheoesophageal groove, then dives medially crossing the inferior thyroid artery close to inferior parathyroid, and penetrates the larynx posterolaterally at the cricothyroid joint
- the right RLN is positioned more laterally, and so enters the larynx at a more oblique angle
- nonrecurrent laryngeal nerves branch directly from the vagus in the neck in <1% of individuals, and are most common on the right due to presence of an aberrant right subclavian artery
- RLN usually enters the larynx just inferior and 4 to 5 mm posterior to cricothyroid joint, but may split around it or pass anteriorly (~15%)

- within the larynx, RLN divides into anterior (antRLN) and posterior (postRLN) branches
- <u>Sensory</u>: to spindles of intrinsic muscles and areas distal to the TVF
- <u>Motor</u>: intrinsic laryngeal musculature (*see following*)

Autonomics and Special Senses

- sympathetic innervation arises from the superior cervical ganglion
- parasympathetic innervation originates in the dorsal motor nucleus and travels to the supraglottic larynx via internal branch of superior laryngeal nerve, and to the subglottis via recurrent laryngeal nerve
- postRLN communicates with inferior division of iSLN via ansa Galeni in the region of the interarytenoid muscle; provides motor innervation to tracheal and esophageal musosa, and tracheal smooth muscle
- autonomic dysfunction may be a reflection of the patient's psychoneurologic health

Laryngeal Musculature

Intrinsic Muscles (Figure 3–2)

- skeletal muscles responsible for TVF abduction, adduction, and tension
- innervated by RLN (anterior and posterior branches) and eSLN
    1. <u>antRLN</u>: thyroarytenoid (TA), lateral cricoarytenoid (LCA)
    2. <u>postRLN</u>: posterior cricoarytenoid (PCA), interarytenoid (IA)
    3. <u>eSLN</u>: cricothyroid (CT)
- muscular action on TVF (*see* Figures 3–1 and 3–2)
    1. <u>TA</u>: adducts, lowers, shortens, rounds
    2. <u>LCA</u>: adducts, lowers, elongates, thins
    3. <u>IA</u>: adducts
    4. <u>PCA</u>: abducts, elevates, elongates, thins
    5. <u>CT</u>: lowers, stretches, elongates, thins
- IA is the only unpaired intrinsic laryngeal muscle and has bilateral innervation
- largest muscle is CT, then PCA

Thyroarytenoid Muscle

- extends from the thyroid cartilage anteriorly to the vocal process and fovea oblonga of the arytenoid cartilage
- termed *vocalis* medially and *thyromuscularis* laterally

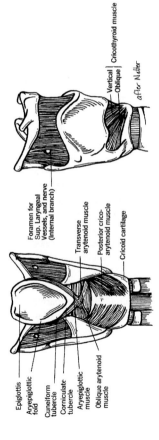

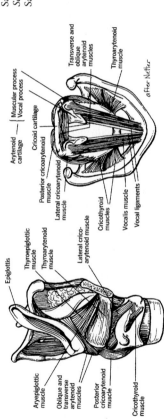

FIGURE 3–2. Intrinsic laryngeal musculature. Used with permission from Sataloff et al., *Professional Voice: The Science and Art of Clinical Care.* 4th ed. San Diego, CA: Plural Publishing; 2017.

- vocalis fine-tunes tension along the vocal fold edge, and provides lateral resistance during vocal fold contact
- thyromuscularis may cause rapid shortening of the vocal fold

Extrinsic Muscles

- strap muscles elevate or depress the larynx relative to their orientation about the hyoid
- responsible for vertical position of larynx and anterior/posterior tilt
- **Suprahyoid muscles (elevators)**: digastric, mylohyoid, geniohyoid, stylohyoid
- **Infrahyoid muscles (depressors)**: thyrohyoid, sternothyroid, sternohyoid, omohyoid
- Innervation:
  1. Mylohyoid nerve (CN V3): anterior belly of digastric, mylohyoid
  2. CN VII: posterior belly of digastric, stylohyoid
  3. C1 via CN XII: geniohyoid, thyrohyoid
  4. Ansa cervicalis (C1 through C3): omohyoid, sternohyoid, sternothyroid

Extralaryngeal Anatomy

- upper airway structures contribute to vocal resonance
- Vocal power: volume and force of air that passes between the vocal folds
  1. Volume: lungs
  2. Active inspiratory force: diaphragm and external intercostal muscle (primary); abdominal musculature, pectoralis major and minor, serratus anterior and posterior, subclavius, sternocleidomastoid, scalenes, latissimus dorsi, and levatores costarum (accessory)
  3. Active expiratory force: abdominal musculature (primary); internal intercostals, transversus thoracis, subcostal muscles, serratus posterior inferior, quadratus lumborum, and latissimus dorsi (accessory)
  4. Passive inspiratory/expiratory force: lungs and ribs
- conditioning of abdominal and back musculature is integral to vocal training; improper posture results in functional impairment

PHONATORY PHYSIOLOGY

- <u>Volitional phonation</u>: cerebral cortex → precentral gyrus (motor cortex) → corticobulbar tract → nucleus ambiguus → laryngeal, thoracic, and abdominal musculature
- extrapyramidal and autonomic nervous systems mediate additional motor refinements
- auditory and tactile feedback improve corrective efforts to match intended sound
- <u>Requirements for phonation</u>:
  1. <u>Power source</u>: lungs
  2. <u>Oscillator</u>: TVF (primary), FVF (secondary)
  3. <u>Resonator</u>: supraglottic larynx, tongue, lips, palate, pharynx, nasal cavity, oral cavity, sinuses
- **Myoelastic-aerodynamic theory**: air from the lungs generates an inferior to superior mucosal wave and a collision-separation cycle (frequency) where air escapes during open phase; the TVF then reapproximate in an inferior to superior direction
- frequency and intensity of TVF contact determined by volume of inspired air, expiratory force, subglottal and supraglottal pressure, and glottal tension
- **Subglottal pressure**: mediated by alveolar pressure less airway resistance and expiratory muscles; impaired by obstructive lung disease (ie, asthma, emphysema)
- sound produced by TVF contains a complete set of harmonic partials—modulated and refined by resonators in the supraglottic vocal tract
- <u>Vocal range classifications</u>: (1) Bass (E2–E4); (2) Baritone (G2–G4); (3) Tenor (B2–B4); (4) Alto (E3–E5); (5) Mezzo-soprano (G3–G5); (6) Soprano (B3–B5)
- <u>Vocal register (low to high)</u>: vocal fry, chest, middle, head voice, falsetto, whistle
- <u>Modal register</u>: optimal TVF vibration via ideal airflow and glottal tension; refers to the continuum of chest, middle, and head voice
- **Vibrato**: voluntary rhythmic alteration of pitch and loudness
  1. pitch alterations mediated primarily by cricothyroid and laryngeal adductors with possible contributions from supraglottic vocal tract
  2. loudness modulated by variations in subglottic pressure, frequency, and vocal tract resonance

ESOPHAGEAL EMBRYOLOGY

- arises from the middle segment of the foregut along with the trachea in the fourth week
- separates from the trachea in the fifth week, failure to fully separate causes tracheoesophageal fistulas
- continues to elongate and assumes final geographic relationship with surrounding organs by seventh week
- branchial arches → striated muscle of esophagus
- splanchnopleuric mesoderm → smooth muscle of esophagus

ESOPHAGEAL ANATOMY

Introduction

- <u>Dimensions</u>: length spans 24 to 34 cm, defined as the distance between the cricoid bone and gastric orifice, 39 to 48 cm when measured clinically from the incisors
- <u>Pathway</u>: descends slightly to the left of midline at C6 → posterior to left main stem bronchus → right of spine at the T6 vertebra → passes through esophageal hiatus left of T12 → stomach
- regions of luminal narrowing
    1. commencement of esophagus due to upper esophageal sphincter (UES) narrowest
    2. area of contact of the aortic arch and left wall of esophagus
    3. area of contact of the left main stem bronchus and left wall of esophagus
    4. at the esophageal hiatus
- <u>Anatomical divisions</u>
    1. <u>Cervical</u>: C8 through T1, ~15 cm
    2. <u>Thoracic</u>: T1 through T10, ~18 to 22 cm
    3. <u>Abdominal</u>: T10 through T12 ~3 to 6 cm

Vasculature

Introduction

- longitudinal arterial anastomosis in the submucosa allow for ligation of esophageal arteries without ischemia
- esophageal tributaries of the left gastric and the azygos vein create a portal systemic anastomosis that can be engorged and hemorrhage in portal hypertension

Cervical

- <u>Arterial supply</u>: thyrocervical trunk → right and left inferior thyroid aa., bronchial aa.
- <u>Venous drainage</u>: inferior thyroid v. → thyrocervical v.

Thoracic

- <u>Arterial supply</u>: thoracic aorta → esophageal aa.
- <u>Venous drainage</u>: azygos and hemiazygos vv. → inferior vena cava

Abdominal

- <u>Arterial supply</u>: left gastric artery, supplemented by left inferior phrenic artery
- <u>Venous drainage</u>: esophageal tributaries to the left gastric vein → portal vein

Lymphatics

- a deep intramural plexus of lymphatic vessels allows for spread of malignant cells bidirectionally in the esophagus submucosa, allowing for esophageal tumors spreading over long distances.
- blockages of the lymphatic plexus during malignancy can lead to reversed lymphatic flow, diminishing the regularity of lymphatic pathways and metastasis predictability
- common lymph drainage sites include deep cervical lymph nodes, tracheobronchial nodes, posterior mediastinal nodes, celiac nodes

Innervation

Motor Innervation

- <u>Cervical</u>: left and right recurrent laryngeal nerves, from the vagus nerve that arises from the efferent fibers of the nucleus ambiguus
- <u>Thoracic and abdominal</u>: vagal afferents; extrinsic control → dorsal motor nucleus; intrinsic control → Auerbach (mesenteric) plexus
- Auerbach plexus located between the circular and longitudinal layers of the muscularis propria and responsible for rhythmic contraction of the esophagus; acts via nicotinic receptors

Sensory Innervation

- controlled by visceral afferents in the sympathetic nerves and parasympathetic vagal fibers

Structural Layers

- <u>Mucosa</u>: (1) nonkeratinized, stratified squamous epithelium; (2) lamina propria; (3) muscularis mucosa; Z-line is the transition zone from squamous (esophageal) to columnar (gastric) epithelium found at the esophagogastric junction (EGJ)
- <u>Submucosa</u>: contains mucous glands; provides lubrication for food bolus
- <u>Muscularis propria</u>: (1) inner circular muscle; (2) outer longitudinal muscle
    1. upper third is striated (skeletal) voluntary muscle; lower third is smooth (visceral) involuntary muscle; middle third is mixed
    2. inner circular layer continuous with cricopharyngeus, inferior pharyngeal constrictor, and LES
    3. outer longitudinal layer originates at lateral aspect of the cricoid cartilage, continuous with cricoesophageal tendons, leaving a weakened tissue gap in the cranial posterior section of the esophagus (Laimer's triangle)
- <u>Adventitia</u>: outermost layer, has no serosa, provides minimal barrier to infection and tumor infiltration

Anchoring Structures

- inferior pharyngeal constrictor
- longitudinal layer origin at the lateral cricoid cartilage
- phrenoesophageal membrane
- posterior gastric ligaments

Upper Esophageal Sphincter

- <u>Function</u>: prevents esophagopharyngeal reflux, prevents entry of air into the esophagus
- <u>Anatomy</u>: major contributor is the cricopharyngeus, proximal contributions from inferior constrictors/thyropharyngeus, and distal contributions from the circular muscles of the upper esophagus
- <u>Motor innervation</u>: pharyngeal, superior laryngeal and recurrent laryngeal nerve branches of the vagus; cell bodies located in the nucleus ambiguus
- <u>Mechanism</u>: strongest contractile force of the UES is anterior-posterior due to anterior attachment to the cricoid cartilage, lateral forces are only 33% of sphincter
- <u>Physiology</u>: (*see* Chapter 36)
- <u>UES resting pressure</u>: significantly variable, ranging from 30 to 142 mm Hg

Lower Esophageal Sphincter

- <u>Function</u>: basal tone prevents gastroesophageal reflux
- <u>Anatomy</u>: composed of all smooth muscle, the LES contains transverse muscle fibers toward the lesser curvature of the stomach and oblique fibers toward the greater curvature that form a collar
- <u>Motor innervation</u>: medullary dorsal motor nucleus → efferent fibers via Vagus Nerve → Myenteric Plexus near the LES
- <u>Mechanism</u>: both physiologic and anatomic aspects contribute to relaxation and tension including of the LES: compression of the esophagus at the diaphragmatic crura, maintenance of resting tone, and contraction of the oblique and transverse fibers in a left posterior, dominant direction
- <u>Physiology</u>: (*see* Chapter 36)
- <u>Normal manometric values</u>:
    1. <u>LES resting pressure</u>: 14.5 to 34 mm Hg or less
    2. <u>LES relaxation pressure</u>: ≤8 mm Hg

Deglutition and Peristalsis (*See* Chapter 35)

SECTION

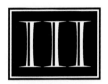

Evaluation and Physical Examination

CHAPTER

Patient History and Physical Examination

Justin Ross, Mary J. Hawkshaw, and Robert T. Sataloff

PATIENT HISTORY

- should include all components of a standard otolaryngologic history: demographics, chief complaint (onset, duration, cause, related symptoms, exacerbating/alleviating factors), unintentional weight loss, allergies, medical and surgical history, tobacco/alcohol/coffee/drug use, family history (eg, head and neck cancers, autoimmune disorders, etc), sexual history (eg, HPV and HIV exposure), current medications
- additional components relevant to professional voice evaluation: voice/instrument training (duration, most recent lessons, current and previous teachers), practice and warm-up patterns, occupation (eg, actor, singer, announcer), work environment, exposure to fogs/smokes, upcoming performances, vocal hygiene (eg, warm-up routine, voice use patterns, noise exposure)
- common laryngologic complaints: hoarseness, breathiness, chronic cough, vocal tremor or spasm, voice fatigue, loss of voice range, sore throat, odynophonia, globus sensation, excess mucus, difficulty breathing, dysphagia/aspiration, odynophagia, others
- **Indications for expedited laryngoscopy**: stridor; respiratory distress; unintended weight loss; recent head, neck, and/or chest surgery; recent intubation; neck mass; head and neck cancer history; tobacco abuse history; laryngeal trauma; professional voice user; absence of red flags but hoarseness >2 weeks

Dysphonia

- altered voice quality reported by a clinician
- ~30% lifetime risk by 65 years
- <u>Risk factors</u>: female, older adults, occupations with heavy voice use (ie, singers, actors, teachers, lawyers, coaches), recent intubation, neck or chest surgery (eg, thyroidectomy, anterior cervical spine approach, carotid endarterectomy, cardiothoracic procedures), steroid inhalers, medications with drying effects
- <u>Etiology</u>: *see* Table 4–1
- treatment is based on etiology, but voice therapy and good vocal hygiene are always prudent

TABLE 4–1. Differential Diagnosis of Dysphonia	
Benign structural lesions	Vocal fold cyst, Pseudocyst, Polyp, Nodule, Scar, Web, Varix, Sulcus, Granuloma, Contact ulcer, Hemorrhage, Reinke's edema, Laryngocele, Saccular cyst, Presbylarynx, Laryngotracheal stenosis
Functional voice disorders	Muscle tension dysphonia, Functional aphonia
Infectious/ inflammatory	Viral laryngitis, Fungal laryngitis, Bacterial laryngitis, Rhinoscleroma, Syphilis, Leprosy, Rhinoscleroma, Tuberculosis, Diphtheria, Laryngopharyngeal reflux, Allergic laryngitis, Prolonged ulcerative laryngitis
Neoplastic	Premalignant lesions, Laryngeal cancer, Laryngeal papillomatosis, Granular cell tumor, Lipoma, Schwannoma, Paraganglioma, Chondrosarcoma, Chondroma
Neurologic	Vocal fold paresis and paralysis, Myasthenia gravis, Spasmodic dysphonia, Laryngeal tremor, Singer's dystonia, Laryngeal manifestations of neurologic conditions (ie, Parkinson's disease, Huntington's disease), Post-polio syndrome, Paradoxical vocal fold motion
Congenital	Laryngomalacia, Anterior glottic web, Laryngeal cleft, Laryngeal hemangioma
Systemic/ autoimmune	Sarcoidosis, Amyloidosis, Granulomatosis with polyangiitis, Relapsing polychondritis, Rheumatoid nodules
Traumatic	External or internal trauma (eg, cartilage fracture, endolaryngeal mucosal injury), Intubation, Arytenoid dislocation/subluxation, Ingestion injury (acidic/caustic), Inhalation injury (smoke/steam)
Endocrine	Hypothyroidism, Hyperthyroidism

- may refer to AAO-HNSF 2018 Clinical Guideline: Evaluation of Hoarseness (Dysphonia)

Common Terms

- **Hoarseness**: change in voice quality noticed by a patient
- **Breathiness**: excessive air loss during phonation
- **Voice fatigue**: loss of endurance, characterized by progressive hoarseness, loss of range, difficulty with passaggio; common in glottic insufficiency and muscle tension dysphonia (MTD)
- **Globus sensation**: feeling of lump or foreign body in the throat
- **Odynophonia**: painful speech or singing

COMMON LARYNGOLOGIC PROBLEMS

Voice Abuse/Misuse

- commonly present with voice fatigue, chronic hoarseness, and loss of soft voice
- may have vocal fold irregularities such as polyps, cysts, nodules, sulcus, scar, ectasia, and varicosity
- frequent time spent in noisy environments increases risk
- common in cheerleaders, conductors/choral directors, singing instructors, teachers
- Tx: voice therapy, and ideally, instruction by a singing specialist, are essential to gain proper technique

Cough (See Chapter 27)

- common chief complaint in the primary care setting
- classified as acute (<4 weeks), subacute (4–8 weeks), and chronic (>8 weeks)
- Etiology:
  1. **Acute**: infectious (cold, bronchitis, pneumonia), allergic rhinitis
  2. **Subacute**: postinfectious, mycoplasma, rarely pertussis
  3. **Chronic**: asthma, laryngopharyngeal reflux (LPR), upper airway cough syndrome (UACS), other chronic pulmonary conditions (ie, chronic obstructive pulmonary disease, chronic bronchitis, bronchiectasis), aspiration, neoplasia, psychogenic, cardiogenic (ie, congestive heart failure), drug-induced (angiotensin-converting enzyme [ACE]-inhibitor commonly), tobacco use, environmental exposure, exercise-induced, cough-variant dystonia, unexplained chronic cough (UCC)
- Dx: history and physical (H&P), flexible and/or rigid laryngoscopy, strobolaryngoscopy, bronchoscopy, pulmonary function testing, therapeutic trials (ie, proton pump inhibitor, Flonase, ACE-inhibitor discontinuation, 24-hour pH-impedance test
- Tx: address underlying condition (eg, LPR, asthma, UACS), antitussives, gabapentin, voice therapy, botulinum toxin (recalcitrant cases and cough-variant dystonia)
- quality of life (QoL) instruments are important adjuncts in evaluation of treatment outcomes:
  1. Age ≥14: Cough-Specific QoL Questionnaire, Leicester Cough Questionnaire
  2. Age <14: Parent Cough-Specific QoL Questionnaire
  3. response to antitussives is not a good outcome measure

Odynophonia

- Etiology: **muscle tension dysphonia (most common)**, acute laryngitis, reflux laryngitis, vocal fold tear or hemorrhage, laryngeal myofascial pain syndrome, laryngeal tendonitis, laryngeal granuloma or ulceration, phonotrauma, external or endolaryngeal trauma (eg, blunt, penetrating, intubation, foreign body, acidic/caustic ingestion), smoke or steam inhalation, neuralgia
- Dx: H&P, flexible laryngoscopy, strobovideolaryngoscopy, speaking/singing posture and support, jaw/tongue/neck tension, palpation of laryngeal structures, with or without computed tomography/magnetic resonance imaging (if indicated)
- normal vibratory mechanics and lack of structural abnormalities may indicate musculoskeletal or neurologic etiology
- **Musculoskeletal odynophonia**: commonly presents as point tenderness during neck exam, superolateral and superoposterior thyroid cartilage and hyoid most common sites, associated with supraglottic hyperfunction, Tx: voice therapy, nonsteroidal anti-inflammatory drug (NSAID), steroid injection
- **Neurologic odynophonia**: neuropathy usually affecting superior laryngeal nerve (SLN) or glossopharyngeal nerve, possible viral etiology (eg, HSV), may be associated with sensory deficits (eg, diminished unilateral gag reflex), SLN typically more superficial discomfort while glossopharyngeal nerve is deeper and difficult to localize, Tx: gabapentin, carbamazepine, amitriptyline

Muscle Tension Dysphonia

- altered voice quality due to excess tension of the paralaryngeal musculature
- results in positional changes of the larynx, altering tension and function of the vocal folds
- can be primary or secondary
- Etiology: recent upper respiratory infection (URI), LPR, vocal fold mass/lesion, paresis, vocal abuse, emotional stress, recent laryngeal trauma, underlying disease (ie, mechanical, neurologic)
- Presentation: dysphonia, palpable neck tenderness, odynophonia, odynophagia
- Voice characteristics: pressed, voice fatigue with breaks, loss of upper pitch range, decreased quality with stress, may have associated hoarseness/roughness
- Dx: H&P, neck palpation, flexible and/or rigid laryngoscopy, strobovideolaryngoscopy, aerodynamic analysis
- circumlaryngeal tenderness on palpation is common

- aerodynamic evaluation commonly shows elevated subglottal pressure with increased adductory force and decreased maximum phonation time
- <u>Laryngoscopic findings</u>: anteroposterior and lateral supraglottic compression, plica ventricularis, often mild glottic gap, soft closure, LPR findings common
- <u>Tx</u>: vocal hygiene, voice therapy, circumlaryngeal massage therapy, management of underlying condition (eg, LPR, URI, allergic rhinitis, etc), surgery rare unless primary cause glottic insufficiency or mass

PHYSICAL EXAMINATION

Introduction

- thorough history often points to etiology, and is an essential adjunct to the physical examination
- evaluation of general and psychosocial condition may have diagnostic utility
- objective analysis of voice function advisable for most patients presenting with dysphonia

General Head and Neck Examination

Appearance

- note age, body habitus (eg, cachectic, morbidly obese, pregnant), level of fatigue, emotional state (eg, depressed, agitated, anhedonic, manic), acute or subacute musculoskeletal injury causing postural changes, or indications of chronic illness (eg, cancer and neurologic, endocrine, or autoimmune disorders)
- associated factors affecting speech, voice, and swallow: diminished upper aerodigestive muscular tone and control, decreased abdominal support, postural changes, loss of true vocal fold ground substance within the superficial lamina propria (SLP), age or systemic illness associated loss of mucosal lubrication

Eye

- assess conjunctiva, sclera, and periorbita
- periorbital venous engorgement, mucosal irritation, erythema, and excess tearing may be indicative of allergy
- subconjunctival pallor may indicate anemia that is associated with esophageal webs (Plummer-Vinson syndrome), neoplasia, chronic illness, malnutrition, debility, and often with MTD

- scleral icterus may indicate hepatic dysfunction related to neoplasia or systemic illness

Ear

- always perform **external ear examination, otoscopy, and Weber and Rinne testing**
- **audiogram** and **tympanogram** helpful since unrecognized sensorineural hearing loss (SNHL) can lead to dysphonia
- slight hearing loss can result in excessive vocal intensity to compensate for inaccurate, self-perceived loss in volume
- SNHL is associated with **diplacusis, distorted pitch perception,** and tinnitus → may increase risk of phonotrauma
- there is a significant but weak correlation between increasing pure tone average of 0.5, 1, 2, and 3 kHz and Voice Handicap Index-10
- dysphonia and hearing loss frequently coprevalent in the elderly; decreases quality of life and increases subjective reports of depression

Nose

- **anterior rhinoscopy** and/or endoscopy should be performed to assess for nasal obstruction, mucosal pallor, erythema, or edema, and septal deviation or perforation
- if chronic rhinosinusitis (CRS) is suspected, **nasal endoscopy** should be performed to assess patency of the **osteomeatal** complex, presence of mucopus and polyposis
- allergic rhinitis often comorbid with related mucosa changes in the upper aerodigestive tract, generates postnasal drip that may increase laryngeal inflammation

Oral Cavity and Oropharynx

- assess oral cavity mucosa and salivary flow, dentition, floor of mouth, tongue, hard and soft palate, tonsils, and posterior pharyngeal wall
- <u>Mucosa</u>: evaluate for ulceration and xerostomia → impaired laryngeal function, dysphagia
- <u>Dentition</u>: absence of anterior teeth (impaired articulation), wear facets (bruxism), erosion of enamel on incisors (excess acid intake, bulimia)
- bruxism associated with temporomandibular joint dysfunction (TMJD) and muscle tension
- <u>Tongue</u>: lateral scalloping and retrusion are common with tongue tension → associated with pressed speech
- <u>Palate</u>: Tori and cleft palate may impair food bolus formation and propulsion in the oral phase of swallowing

- <u>Palatine tonsils</u>: hypertrophy, signs of chronic infection, tonsillolith
- <u>Posterior pharyngeal wall</u>: cobblestoning (allergy), enlarged adenoids
- low-hanging soft palate, large tongue base, and tonsillar hypertrophy predict difficult intubation and obstructive sleep apnea (*see Friedman classification*)

Neck

- assess for length and thickness, range of motion and strength, thyromental distance (thyroid notch to mentum), mass or lymphadenopathy, muscle tension/spasm, thyroid abnormalities, scar, laryngeal tenderness, and crepitus
- evaluate laryngeal position and strap muscles at rest, during conversational speech, and while singing, document tension and tenderness
- prior iatrogenic strap muscle transection may produce dysphonia due to laryngeal tilt
- current or prior tracheotomy may tether trachea to skin, interfering with laryngeal elevation

Cranial Nerves (CNs)

- always examine CN II–XII
- evaluate facial and upper airway sensation, gross hearing, gag reflex, palatal deviation, strength of shoulder shrug, and tongue mobility
- laryngeal sensory testing when indicated
- postviral, infectious neuropathies can involve the SLNs and recurrent laryngeal nerves (RLNs)
- diminished sensation, gag reflex, and palate/tongue control can result in dysphagia in all phases of swallowing

LARYNGEAL EXAMINATION

Laryngeal Mirror

- traditional method for examination of the larynx
- least technology intensive: only requires a dental mirror, light source, and head mirror
- requires substantial practice
- provides accurate assessment of mucosal color
- typically tolerated without topical anesthesia (avoid touching tongue base and posterior pharynx)
- <u>Technique</u>:
    1. have patient assume sniffing position (described later)

2. warm mirror to prevent fogging
3. grasp tongue between thumb and third finger and rotate anteriorly, keeping third finger against teeth to avoid trauma to frenulum
4. insert mirror resting on soft palate
5. examine hypopharyngeal and laryngeal subsites
6. have patient phonate /i/, alternating /i - hi/
- technique pearls are similar to those for rigid endoscopy

Endoscopy

Introduction

- evaluation of the upper airway under continuous or stroboscopic light with flexible or rigid endoscopic instruments
  1. **Flexible**: transnasal evaluation of entire upper airway, permits dynamic voice assessment during phonation, fiber optic or digital (chip-tip), useful for conditions of altered speech (eg, spasmodic dysphonia, vocal tremor, etc), paresis, MTD, others
  2. **Rigid**: transoral performed with 70° or 90° endoscope, provides better resolution, cannot evaluate structures above tongue base, limited to evaluation during sustained or repeated vowel phonation and respiration
- typically performed in office, rigid endoscopy rarely requires general anesthesia except when unable to tolerate otherwise or during surgical procedure
- evaluate nasal cavity, nasopharynx, tongue base, vallecula, pharyngeal walls, piriform sinuses, postcricoid region, epiglottis, arytenoids, aryepiglottic folds, false vocal folds, ventricles, true vocal folds (TVFs), subglottis (if possible)
- TVF evaluation: mass (eg, nodule, cyst, polyp, granuloma, neoplasia), hemorrhage, ectasia, varicosity, paralysis, sulcus, scar, contralateral reactive lesion (CRL), anterior and posterior glottis (web, stenosis), vocal process avulsion, other
- vibratory motion during phonation is imperceptible with continuous light and requires stroboscopy for complete assessment
- Normal fundamental frequency (f0):
  1. Men: 85 to 155 Hz
  2. Women: 165 to 255 Hz

Normal Laryngeal Variants

- Laryngeal skeleton: almost universal variation in size, shape, and symmetry; right cricoarytenoid joint is typically posterior, lateral, and inferior relative to the left; left thyroid lamina typically has a longer AP diameter than the right; when it occurs, arytenoid complex crossover is typically right over left; variable degree and location of angulation of the epiglottis

- despite common asymmetries of the laryngeal skeleton, vocal fold length, width, and thickness are normally symmetric in the absence of pathology
- <u>Glottic closure</u>: more complete and of greater duration in males; females and children often have a posterior glottic chink
- <u>Amplitude</u>: may be reduced in the elderly

Flexible Endoscopy: Technique

- apply topical anesthetic (ie, lidocaine) and vasoconstricting agent (ie, oxymetazoline) as needed
- warm or place defogging solution on lens of laryngoscope
- insert scope into most patent nasal cavity and advance either along the floor or middle meatus
- observe the nasopharynx during phonation (/i/ and /sss/) and/or while playing a musical instrument when appropriate
- evaluate tongue base, glossotonsillar sulcus, vallecula, pharyngeal walls, piriform sinuses, and postcricoid region
- once all laryngeal subsites are in view, perform dynamic voice assessment under continuous light
- advance to area superior to false vocal folds or deeper, and switch to stroboscopic light to complete evaluation (vocal tasks described later in chapter)

Flexible Endoscopy: Technique Pearls

- avoid topical anesthetic if performing evaluation of swallowing or laryngeal sensation
- evaluate nasal cavity for sources of nasal obstruction
- soft palate tremor during sustained /i/ may indicate neurological disorder (ie, essential tremor, pseudobulbar palsy, Parkinson's disease)
- velopharyngeal insufficiency often presents as lateral bubbling and occasionally as a frank gap
- tongue protrusion will allow full assessment of tongue base and vallecula
- tongue base fasciculations or asymmetry may indicate underlying amyotrophic lateral sclerosis
- cheek distention will expose the piriform sinuses
- chin tilt, high-pitched /i/, or ascending glissando can cause the epiglottis to tilt forward

- high-pitched /i/ and inhalational phonation can relax supraglottic hyperfunction
- always perform dynamic voice assessment in the patient's native language as well as English

Dynamic Voice Assessment

- examine vocal folds during respiration → observe for paradoxical TVF motion and myoclonus
- modal, high- and low-pitched /i/ at various intensities
- ascending and descending glissando → evaluation of SLN function
- modal, high- and low-pitched counting from 1 to 10 → observe for resolution of MTD
- alternating /i/ - /hi/ → evaluate abductor and adductor function
- alternating /i/ - sniff → evaluate coordinated adductor and abductor function
- repeated sniff → evaluate abductor function
- repeated /pa/-/ta/-/ka/ → evaluate laryngeal coordination
- count 60 to 69 slowly in one breath → pronounced symptoms in abductor SD
- count 80 to 89 slowly in one breath → pronounced symptoms in adductor SD
- whistle a song (eg, Yankee Doodle)
- sing "Happy Birthday" and/or a piece the patient is currently practicing
- assess for presence of generalized (MTD) versus intermittent (laryngospasm, spasmodic dysphonia, tremor, myoclonus, psychogenic) vocal strain and correlate with examination

Additional Descriptive Terms

- **Plica ventricularis**: approximation of false vocal folds during phonation, suggests severe MTD
- **Cogwheeling**: uncoordinated, jerking movements when transitioning from abduction to adduction, suggests upper motor neuron or extrapyramidal disorder
- **Laryngeal tremor**: rhythmic oscillations of vibratory frequency and intensity, associated most commonly with PD and essential tremor
- **Pseudosulcus**: describes subglottic edema extending the full AP length of the TVF (sulcus ends at vocal process, pseudosulcus does not)

Rigid Endoscopy: Technique

- if gag reflex is limiting exam, spray topical anesthetic (ie, Cetacaine, 4% or 10% lidocaine) on the posterior pharyngeal wall and have the patient swallow
- position the patient with his/her bottom against the back of the chair, back angled slightly forward, elbows on knees, and chin slightly superior (sniffing position)
- grasp tongue just anterior to circumvallate papillae with gauze between thumb and third finger of nondominant hand
- gently rotate anterior or inferior with third finger in firm contact with the teeth
- warm or place soap solution on lens of laryngoscope to reduce fogging
- insert as close to midline as possible and advance while having the patient breathe through the mouth
- advance past tongue base while avoiding the tongue base and posterior pharyngeal wall and without contacting mucosal surfaces with the lens
- observe all laryngeal subsites
- assess all components of Reflux Finding Score (*see* Chapter 22)
- have patient perform vocal tasks under stroboscopic lighting and continuous lighting as indicated

Rigid Endoscopy: Technique Pearls

- <u>Predictors of difficult examination</u>: short, thick neck, small mouth, anterior lingual frenulum, high Mallampati score (large tongue base, low-hanging soft palate, large tonsils), omega-shaped, long, and/or posterior epiglottis
- **avoid forceful tongue traction** and displacement from natural position when possible—patient will usually respond with equally forceful retraction
- to avoid lens smearing in patients with small mouths or superiorly displaced tongue base, rotate the scope slightly (45°–90°) on insertion
- insert the scope slightly lateral to the uvula, and move to midline once the endolarynx is visualized
- additional information can be obtained from placing the scope at an angle resting on the third molar on each side
- avoid contacting the tongue base prior to patient relaxation so to not stimulate gag reflex
- **avoid nasal breathing** as it will cause the tongue to arch superiorly
- sustained /i/ can be used to tilt the epiglottis anteriorly if it is obstructing view of the glottis

- if epiglottis obstructs view of the glottis despite best efforts, can approach with scope laterally and place the tip between the epiglottis and posterior pharyngeal wall, then swing medially
- supraglottic hyperfunction will often partially or fully correct with sustained /i/ or glissando
- gag reflex can be minimized when **eyes are open**, with **continuous slow deep breathing** through the mouth, **sustained vowel phonation** (ie, /i/) and if the **patient has been counseled prior and is sufficiently distracted during the exam**
- can be performed without topical anesthesia if tolerated by patient

Stroboscopy

Principles

- allows the observation of TVF vibratory motion in two ways:
    1. **Stop motion:** captures a "frozen" image by sampling the same phase of motion across successive vibratory cycles (not an option on the most recent equipment)
    2. **Simulated slow motion:** displays apparent motion by strobing at a frequency <f0 across sequential phases of TVF motion during successive vibratory cycles
- **not a true slow-motion evaluation** of vocal fold vibration like high-speed video
- while Talbot's law and the theory of persistence of vision do not specifically pertain to stroboscopy, they are frequently cited explanations of the effect
    1. **Talbot's law:** when different brightnesses or colors are alternated above a particular frequency, flicker will cease, and they will appear as a uniform brightness or color
    2. **Theory of persistence of vision:** visual images will be retained for about 0.2 s after removal of the initial stimulus
- stroboscopy generates real-time representations of vocal fold motion based on two visual phenomenon:
    1. **Flicker-free illumination:** light strobed at >50 Hz is indistinguishable from continuous light
    2. **Perception of apparent motion:** successive images presented at >17 Hz will appear as one figure in continuous motion if the voice is reasonably periodic
- motion is typically simulated at 0.5 to 2 Hz (ie, if f0 is 120 Hz, light is strobed at 118-119.5 Hz)
- simulates the vibratory motion of true vocal folds at a visually perceptible frequency

- **Time aliasing**: apparent reversal of TVF motion when light is strobed at a frequency >f0
- can be performed with flexible or rigid laryngoscopes, but rigid provides greater resolution

Videostroboscopy: Equipment

- requires digital recording equipment, stroboscopic light source, microphone and endoscopes (flexible, rigid, or ideally both)
- microphone placed against the lateral thyroid lamina measures vibratory frequency and is used to determine strobe frequency (synchronous versus asynchronous)

Components of Glottal Assessment

- <u>Amplitude</u>: extent of medial to lateral excursion of the vocal folds during phonation
- <u>Mucosal wave/glottal edge</u>: extent of vocal fold tissue deformation, smoothness and straightness during the vibratory cycle
- <u>Vibratory motion abnormalities</u>: identification of hypodynamic and/or adynamic segments
- <u>Phase symmetry</u>: vibratory symmetry of adjacent vocal folds
- <u>Regularity</u>: periodicity of vibratory cycles
- <u>Glottal gap/closure</u>: shape and strength of glottis during closure
- <u>Supraglottic function</u>: presence/extent of compression in lateral and anterior-posterior (AP) orientations
- <u>Vertical height difference</u>: discrepancies between adjacent vocal folds
- <u>Arytenoid position/movement</u>: vertical and horizontal discrepancies at rest and during motion

Stroboscopic Vocal Tasks

- hold /i/ at modal, high and low pitch at various intensities and examine mucosal wave, amplitude, symmetry and glottal closure (use stop motion for periodicity if available)
- ascending and descending glissando (glide) → decreased longitudinal tension may indicate SLN paresis
- alternating /i-hi-i-hi/ or /i/—sniff → decreased adduction or abduction may indicate RLN or SLN paresis
- forceful sniff ×5 (or more) → decreased abduction may indicate RLN paresis
- assess arytenoid movement during tasks and at rest → unilateral TVF immobility in the presence of absent jostle sign suggests cricoarytenoid joint fixation or arytenoid dislocation

Standardized Methods of Glottal Assessment

- there is no universally accepted evaluation protocol for assessment of vocal fold characteristics and laryngeal mechanics
- lack of broad consensus limits the ability to communicate findings between practitioners and the consistency of those observations
- poor interrater but relatively consistent intrarater reliability
- Most common parameters: extent, location, and shape of glottal gap, amplitude, periodicity, phase symmetry, presence of lesions
- a multitude of grading scales exist to describe each laryngeal parameter (eg, glottal gap, amplitude, etc)
- analog and visual scales may improve interrater reliability (eg, Visual-Vibratory Assessment with Laryngeal Imaging [VALI])

VOCAL FOLD VIBRATORY ABNORMALITIES

Decreased Amplitude

- lateral excursion ~one-third width of the TVF is considered normal
- Causes: reduction of lateral excursion can be physiologic (normal) or pathologic
  1. Physiologic: increased TVF tension during elevation of pitch, decreased subglottal pressure during low-intensity phonation
  2. Pathologic: vocal fold shortening (eg, anterior glottal web), vocal fold stiffness (eg, scar, benign or malignant mass, sulcus vocalis), increased vocal fold bulk (eg, Reinke's edema, polyp, acute laryngitis), vocal fold tension (eg, MTD, adductor spasmodic dysphonia), glottic gap
- unilateral or asymmetric bilateral reduction is typically pathologic
- symmetric bilateral reduction may be physiologic or pathologic (eg, bilateral scar, sulcus vocalis)

Glottic Gap

- allows uncontrolled air leakage through the glottis during phonation in the absence of hyperfunctional compensation
- more air required to produce voice quality and volume approaching unimpaired phonation
- compensatory increase in medial compressive forces via supraglottic hyperfunction results in:
  1. increased vocal fatigue
  2. muscle tension dysphonia
  3. vocal fold injury

- results in soft, breathy voice with decreased maximum phonation time
- gaps visible under continuous light
- stroboscopy allows assessment of small gaps and soft closure
- effect on mucosal wave depends on size of gap → large gap may result in aperiodic vibratory motion which is poorly visualized with stroboscopy
- small posterior gap normal in females and some males
- <u>Causes</u>: reduced TVF mobility (ie, paresis, paralysis, CAJ ankylosis), mass (ie, polyp, cyst, nodule papilloma, carcinoma), bowing (ie, presbylarynx, TVF paresis/paralysis, neuromuscular disease), medial edge defect (eg, prior mass excision or cordotomy, scar, sulcus vocalis)
- etiology determines glottal shape at closure
  1. **Immobility**: complete AP gap, may achieve complete closure at high pitch and sometimes low pitch if isolated RLN lesion due to activation of cricothyroid muscle (SLN); increased medial compressive force by unaffected, contralateral vocal fold often seen in unilateral immobility (may cross midline)
  2. **Mass**: typically anterior and posterior gaps (hourglass shaped), but depends on location and nature of the mass
  3. **Bowing**: spindle-shaped gap, may result from paresis or loss of SLP volume or vocalis muscle bulk
  4. **Defect**: gap associated with structural pathology, sulcus vocalis can cause a central gap that resembles bowing (spindle shaped)

Mucosal Wave Abnormalities

Increased Mucosal Wave

- commonly bilateral and symmetric
- generally results from an inflammation-mediated increase in contents of the superficial LP
- <u>Causes</u>: **Reinke's edema**, polyp, LPR, acute laryngitis
- increased TVF bulk typically lowers f0 and produces a characteristically husky voice
- requires increased subglottic pressure compared with normal for pitch elevation and may have accompanying voice fatigue

Decreased Mucosal Wave

- commonly asymmetric and segmental
- most often results from changes to the epithelium and/or SLP
- <u>Causes</u>: **vocal fold scar**, sulcus, mass (eg, nodule, cyst, papilloma, leukoplakia, carcinoma), iatrogenic (ie, TVF stripping), vocal fold atrophy (ie, presbylarynx)

Symmetry

- assessed by observing both vocal folds simultaneously
- should open with same amplitude (amount of lateral excursion) and phase symmetry (vibratory waves are mirror images)
- phase asymmetry more common in untrained voices
- <u>Causes</u>: differences in vocal fold position, tension, elasticity, viscosity, shape, mass, or other mechanical properties

Aperiodic Motion

- normal periodicity requires balanced control of expiratory force and mechanical characteristics of vocal folds
- assess by locking stroboscope in phase with vocal fold vibration
- <u>Causes</u>: inability to maintain steady expiratory stream of air, inability to sustain steady laryngeal muscle contraction (neuromuscular disease), differences between mechanical properties of vocal folds

Vocal Fold Mass

- benign and malignant laryngeal masses involve the vibratory margin or impair TVF motion or motor function
- vibratory abnormalities and voice changes are relative to mass characteristics

VOICE EXAMINATION

Subjective Assessment (See Chapter 5)

- simple assessment of voice range, timbre, and quality can be performed by most physicians
- thorough evaluation ideally should be performed by a licensed speech-language pathologist
- quality of life assessment tools
- tools used for auditory-perceptual analysis include the following:
  1. **GRBAS** (grade, roughness, breathiness, asthenia, strain) Voice Rating Scale
  2. **CAPE-V** (Consensus Auditory-Perceptual Evaluation of Voice)

Objective Assessment (See Chapter 5)

- multidimensional evaluation of voice quality during sustained vowel phonation and continuous speech using spectrography and voice analysis programs

- <u>Spectrography</u>: visual depiction of acoustic signals as a waveform using time (x-axis), frequency (y-axis), and intensity (z-axis)
- analysis of spectrographic data with voice analysis algorithms provides objective voice measures
- well over 100 voice measures reported in the literature
- validity of most measures is controversial, as the majority correlate poorly with perceptual voice analysis
- commonly includes fundamental frequency (f0), frequency range (physiologic and musical), jitter, shimmer, relative average perturbation, maximum phonation time (MPT), mean flow rate (MFR), cepstral peak prominence (CPP), smoothed CPP, harmonic-to-noise (H/N) ratio, breathiness index
- aerodynamic evaluation also part of a comprehensive voice examination
- laryngeal electromyography (LEMG) may be required to confirm suspected TVF paresis or paralysis, determine affected nerves (SLN versus RLN), distinguish mechanical causes (ie, cricoarytenoid joint fixation) from paresis/paralysis, diagnose laryngeal myasthenia or other neurolaryngologic disorders, diagnose functional disorders or malingering

Aerodynamic Evaluation

- aerodynamic performance measures include subglottal pressure, supraglottal pressure, glottal impedance, airflow volume velocity
- measured by spirometer, pneumatochronograph, or hot-wire anemometer
- <u>Spirometry</u>: pulmonary function testing (PFT) and measurement of phonatory airflow
- <u>PFT measures</u>: tidal volume (TV), functional residual capacity (FRC), inspiratory capacity (IC), total lung capacity (TLC), vital capacity (VC), forced vital capacity (FVC), forced expiratory volume in 1 s and 3 s (FEV1, FEV3), maximal mid-expiratory flow
- <u>Pneumatochronograph</u>: multicomponent device (laminar air resistor, differential pressure transducer, amplifying/recording system) measures airflow and voice; superior evaluation of phonatory aerodynamics (relative to spirometry) due to simultaneous measurement
- <u>Hot-wire anemometer</u>: airflow causes cooling of a hot wire, altering its resistance pattern; airflow velocity measured based on changes in wire resistance
- <u>Flow glottography</u>: evaluates relationship of TVF adductory force and subglottal pressure; may be used for diagnosis and for biofeedback therapy

- <u>Glottal impedance</u>:　cannot measure directly; mean subglottal pressure/MFR
- <u>Phonation quotient (mL/s)</u>:　estimation of flow rate during phonation and a useful measure of vocal efficacy, calculated by VC/MPT

Laryngeal Electromyography (See Chapter 6)

SWALLOWING EVALUATION
(*See* Chapter 35)

- presence of retained food or copious pooling of secretions in pyriform sinuses and vallecula on laryngoscopy indicates dysphagia
- dysphagia may be assessed with transnasal or transoral esophagoscopy, and functional endoscopic evaluation of swallowing without (FEES) or with sensory testing *(FEEST)*
- consider when high clinical suspicion of dysphagia after negative modified barium swallow (MBS), or clinician/patient preference

CHAPTER 1

Laryngeal Electromyography (See Chapter 6)

SWALLOWING EVALUATION

CHAPTER

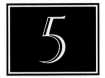

The Clinical Voice Laboratory

Haig Panossian, Mary J. Hawkshaw, and Robert T. Sataloff

THE PURPOSE OF THE CLINICAL VOICE LABORATORY

- a battery of tests that allows reliable, valid, objective assessment of voice function
- clinical diagnosis of voice disorders
- outcome assessment of voice therapy, medical treatment, and laryngeal surgery
- assist in diagnosis of various systemic diseases associated with voice change
- research

CLINICAL ASSESSMENT AND EXAMINATION

Physical Examination Sequence

- clinical use of the voice laboratory is understood best when viewed in the context of total voice-patient management
- patient completes specialized history and quality of life questionnaires
- larynx visualized with mirror
- limited evaluation of the speaking voice and singing voice
- strobovideolaryngoscopy, ideally with speech-language pathologist (SLP) and singing voice specialist (SVS) present
- if not possible, physician provides preliminary impressions and assures that it is medically safe to proceed with rest of examination (voice therapy and singing evaluations may be vocally stressful)
- evaluation continued by the voice technologist, SLP, SVS, sometimes by the acting voice specialist (AVS)

Quality of Life Assessment Tools

- used for baseline at initial assessment and to track effects of interventions
- multiple dysphonia-specific patient-reported outcome measures have been proposed, including the following:
  - Voice Handicap Index (VHI), VHI-10, and Singing VHI-10
  - Voice-Related Quality of Life (V-RQOL)
  - Voice Outcome Survey (VOS)
  - Voice Activity and Participation Profile (VAPP)
  - Voice Symptom Scale (VoiSS)
  - Clinical Auditory-Perceptual Evaluation of Voice (CAPE-V): assessed by raters

- ○ Pediatric Voice Outcome Survey (PVOS)
- ○ Pediatric VHI
- ○ Pediatric V-RQOL

Auditory-Perceptual Evaluation

- increased validity when performed independently by at least 3 examiners (physician, SLP, and SVS)
- **GRBAS Scale (Grade, Roughness, Breathiness, Asthenia, and Strain)**
  1. each component assessed on scale from 0 (normal) to 4 (extreme)
  2. normal voice rating: G0 R0 B0 A0 S0
- **Consensus Auditory Perceptual Evaluation–Voice (CAPE-V):** superior sensitivity and interrater reliability; time-consuming assessment
  1. sustain vowels /a/ and /i/ 3 times each
  2. read 6 specific sentences
  3. converse naturally in response to the question "tell me about your voice problem"
- assessment on 100-mm visual analog line allows for numerical measurement
  1. overall severity
  2. roughness
  3. breathiness
  4. strain
  5. pitch
  6. loudness

Laryngeal Strobovideolaryngoscopy and Visual Assessment

- *see Chapter 4* (Patient History and Physical Examination) for detailed protocol and stroboscopy findings
- flexible laryngoscopy (for evaluation of laryngeal biomechanics and dynamics)
- rigid laryngoscopy with strobovideolaryngoscopy
- assessment of vibratory function with strobovideolaryngoscopy provides information about the leading edge of the vocal fold
- possibly single most important technological advance in diagnostic laryngology
- allows routine, simulated slow motion evaluation of the mucosal cover layer of the leading edge of the vocal fold through illumination of different points on consecutive vocal fold waves that are fused visually

- slow motion effect is created by having stroboscopic light desynchronized with the frequency of vocal fold vibration by approximately 2 Hz
- detection of vibratory asymmetries, structural abnormalities, small masses, submucosal scars, and other conditions that are invisible under ordinary light
- vibratory behavior has normal variations depending on fundamental frequency, intensity, and vocal register (eg, glottic insufficiency is normal in falsetto phonation)
- stroboscopy limited in cases of aperiodic vibration because frequency detection cannot track rapid, irregular changes effectively, or in cases of diplophonia

Videokymography (VKG)

- camera scans a single line on vocal fold throughout glottal cycle (8000 frames per second)
- provides substantial detail about one point on vocal fold
- no 2-dimensional spatial resolution or coordination between image and auditory signal
- useful in assessing effects of scar and outcomes of surgical treatment of scar, presence of subharmonic vibrations, double or triple VF openings in a single glottal cycle, irregular VF vibrations, and other conditions

High-Speed Video

- provides detailed information about VF function for patients with aperiodic voice, dichotic phonation, vocal fry, scar, and other conditions
- acquires images at 2000 fps; 2-second video capture is played back at 15 frames per second, requires over 4 minutes to view
- can be used to study onset of oscillation, VF tension, stiffness, and mass
- primarily used in research

Electroglottography (EGG)

- uses 2 electrodes on skin of neck over thyroid laminae
- weak, high-frequency current passed through larynx between electrodes
- opening and closing of vocal folds varies the transverse electric voltage in phase with vocal fold vibration
- resulting voltage tracing is the EGG
- can be correlated to stroboscopic images

- allows reproducible, objective determination of the glottal closure pattern
- gives more information about the closed glottis
- more useful than photoelectroglottography and ultrasound glottography
- inverse filtering estimates glottal airflow during an acoustic voice signal, or from airflow related to breathing
- signal filtered to "cancel out" main resonance of the vocal tract
- produces a *flow glottogram*, a representation of voice source as glottal volume velocity waveform
  1. plots transglottal airflow in milliliters per second against time
  2. provides information about open glottis
  3. provides information about the relationship between adductory force and subglottal pressure

OBJECTIVE VOICE ANALYSIS

- performed after physician's evaluation and before evaluations by the SLP and SVS
- very quiet or soundproof room
- equipment for measures of respiratory function, phonatory function, and acoustic signal

Objective Voice Measures

- aerodynamic measures reveal the ability of the lungs and abdomen to provide power to the voice, and the ability of the glottis to release air efficiently
- measures of phonatory function quantify the limits of vocal frequency, intensity, and duration
- acoustic analysis detects and documents numerous subtleties in the voice signal
- laryngeal electromyography may confirm the presence or absence of appropriate neuromuscular function
- perceptual voice evaluation uses validated scales to refine the listener's overall assessment of voice quality

Aerodynamic Measures

- **Pulmonary function testing**: provides readily accessible measures of respiratory function
- **Tidal volume (TV)**: volume of air that enters lungs during inspiration and leaves during expiration in normal breathing

- **Functional residual capacity (FRC):** volume of air remaining in lungs at the end of inspiration during normal breathing, divided into:
  1. **Expiratory reserve volume:** maximal additional volume that can be forcefully exhaled
  2. **Residual volume:** volume of air remaining in lungs after maximal exhalation
- **Inspiratory capacity:** maximal volume of air that can be inhaled starting at the FRC
- **Total lung capacity:** volume of air in lungs following maximal inspiration
- **Vital capacity:** maximal volume of air that can be exhaled following max inspiration
- **Forced vital capacity (FVC):** rate of airflow with rapid, forceful expiration from TLC to residual volume
- **FEV1:** forced expiratory volume in 1 second
- **FEF$_{25-75}$:** maximal midexpiratory flow (also called "midflow")
  1. mean rate of airflow over middle half of the FVC (25%–75%)
  2. deterioration following singing or repeated testing can indicate asthma (*see* Chapter 26, Respiratory Dysfunction)
- **Mean flow rate (MFR):** a measure of glottal efficiency
  1. <u>Normal</u>: Approximately 100 mL/s in males, 92 mL/s in females
  2. calculated by dividing total volume of air during phonation by the duration
  3. subject phonates the vowel /a/ at a comfortable pitch and loudness
  4. simultaneous recordings of frequency and intensity
  5. useful for vocal nodules, laryngeal nerve paresis/paralysis, spasmodic dysphonia
- **Air volume:** measured by use of mask fitted tightly over the face or by phonating into a mouthpiece while wearing a nose clamp
- **Glottal resistance:** calculated from mean flow rate and mean subglottal pressure
- **Subglottal pressure:** measurement requires tracheal puncture or transglottal catheter
  1. can be approximated using esophageal balloon
  2. intratracheal pressure transmitted to balloon through trachea, and is roughly equal to subglottal pressure
  3. can be estimated using plosives (/pa/, /pa/, pa/) through a face mask
- **Phonation quotient:** vital capacity divided by the maximum phonation time
  1. correlates closely with maximum flow rate
  2. provides objective measure of effects of treatment in recurrent laryngeal nerve paralysis and VF masses

Measures of Phonatory Ability

- helpful in treating professional vocalists and useful in assessing results of surgery and other therapies
- values may differ from established norms in trained vocalists
- **Maximum phonation time:** sustain the vowel /a/ for as long as possible following deep inspiration and at comfortable pitch and loudness
- approximately 34 seconds for males, 26 seconds for females
- **S:Z ratio:** divide longest phonation time of /s/ by longest phonation time of /z/
- normally <1.4
- first portion is "voiceless" and second is "voiced," so increased values may indicate increased difficulty with phonation due to vocal fold pathology
- **Frequency range of phonation:** records vocal range from lowest note in modal register to highest falsetto note
- **Physiological frequency range of phonation (PFRP):** disregards quality of voice
- Normal ranges: 36 semitones (males); 35 semitones (females)
- **Musical frequency range of phonation (MFRP):** lowest to highest musically acceptable notes
- 35 semitones for professional singers
- **Vocal registers** (from low to high, may have overlaps of frequency): vocal fry, chest, mid, head, falsetto, whistle; alternative classification: vocal fry, modal, loft, and other classifications
- **Speaking fundamental frequency**
- "normal" value is individualized, varies with age: ~120 Hz (males), 225 Hz (females)
- can be followed objectively over course of voice therapy
- **Frequency-intensity profile:** combines measures into a **phonetogram**
    1. **Glottic efficiency:** ratio of acoustic power at level of glottis to subglottal power
    2. **Subglottic power:** product of subglottal pressure and airflow rate

Acoustic Analysis

- voice disorders may be accompanied by decreased range, intensity, and stability
- acoustic measures can help to recognize and document deviations from normal
- record patient's voice under controlled, repeatable circumstances

- use high-quality microphone at a fixed difference from the mouth
- permits quantitative assessment of vocal progress during and following treatment
- **Fundamental frequency (F0)**: characteristic of individual's speaking voice
- <u>Approximate normal values</u>: 120 Hz (males), 225 Hz (females)
- **Jitter**: the variation in **frequency** of a continuously produced vowel from cycle to cycle
- affected by lack of vibratory control; increased in patients with pathology
- **Shimmer**: the variation in peak-to-peak **amplitude** (in dB) of a continuously produced vowel
- affected by glottal resistance, stiffness, mass lesions of folds
- **Harmonic-to-noise ratio**: ratio between periodic component of vocal fold vibration and glottal noise (in dB) during voiced speech
- represents efficiency of voice production
- decreased in voices with asthenia, breathiness
- some commercial systems use *noise-to-harmonic ratio*
- **Spectrograph**: displays frequency and harmonic spectrum of voice sample
- visual representation of properties of the voice source (vibratory characteristics of the vocal folds) and filter system (resonators or vocal tract)
- time (*x*-axis), frequency (*y*-axis), and intensity (*z*-axis, shading of light versus dark)
- useful clinically for analyzing and tracking changes in characteristics of voice signal over time
- abnormal voice displays greater noise and less energy in the harmonics of the signal
- **Long-time-average-spectrography (LTAS)**: analyzes spectral distribution of speech amplitude over time
- **Cepstral peak prominence**: Fourier transformation of a voice spectrum
- calculated using a voice sentence ("we were away a year ago")
- peak with the highest amplitude
- reliable predictor of dysphonia and breathiness

Classification of Voice Signal Type

- not universally accepted, but useful for considering potential pitfalls in voice analysis
- **Type I**: periodic or nearly periodic signals that display no qualitative changes during the time interval to be analyzed

- if modulating frequencies or subharmonics are present, their energies are an order of magnitude below the energy of the fundamental frequency
- perturbation analysis (jitter, shimmer, and NHR) potentially reliable
- **Type II**: signals with qualitative changes (bifurcations) in the segment to be analyzed or signals with subharmonic frequencies or modulating frequencies whose energies approach the energy of the fundamental frequency
- no obvious, single fundamental frequency throughout the segment
- visual displays such as spectrograms and phase portraits are most useful for understanding the characteristics of the oscillating system
- perturbation analysis is unreliable
- **Type III**: voice signals with no apparent periodic structure
- perceptual ratings are most useful for clinical purposes

Yanagihara Hoarseness Ratings

- **Type I**: regular harmonic components are mixed with the noise component chiefly in the formant region of the vowels
- **Type II**: the noise components in the second formants of /e/ and /i/ predominate over the harmonic components
- slight additional noise components appear in the high-frequency region above 3000 Hz in the vowels of /e/ and /i/
- **Type III**: the second formants of /e/ and /i/ are totally replaced by noise components
- additional noise components above 3 kHz further intensify their energy and expand their range
- **Type IV**: the second formants of /a/, /e/, and /i/ are replaced by noise components
- the first formants of all the vowels often lose their periodic components, which are supplemented by noise components
- more intensive high-frequency components are present

Laryngeal Electromyography (See Chapter 6)

Laryngeal Sensory Testing

- useful in evaluation of both swallowing and voice disorders
- assess sensation with delivery of a pulse of air through an endoscope with known, calibrated duration and pressure
- stimulate internal branches of superior laryngeal nerve and elicit laryngeal adductor reflex
- abnormal findings can prompt further evaluation with swallowing study, therapy for neuropathy, or other interventions

Laryngeal Evoked Brain Stem Response

- **Laryngeal reflex**: internal branch of superior laryngeal nerve, laryngeal loci in brain stem, and recurrent and superior laryngeal nerves
- unilateral stimulation of SLN using a bipolar surface electrode placed between greater cornu of hyoid bone and superior cornu of thyroid cartilage
- <u>Normal</u>: evokes a bilateral adductor response

CHAPTER

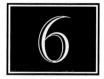

Laryngeal Electromyography

Haig Panossian, Mary J. Hawkshaw, and Robert T. Sataloff

OVERVIEW

- useful in evaluation of various laryngeal disorders
- performed by otolaryngologist, neurologist, and/or physiatrist
- can help establish diagnosis and prognosis in laryngeal paresis/paralysis

Required Equipment

- video monitor for digital display of signal
- surface electrodes
    1. noninvasive
    2. unable to evaluate individual motor units
- needle electrodes
    1. **Monopolar:** active electrode at tip, reference electrode is at remote location on body
    2. **Bipolar:** 2 platinum wires with limited recording range
    3. **Concentric:** electrode at bevel, hollow needle is the reference
    4. **Hooked wire electrode:** introducer needle withdrawn and hook at end of electrode stabilizes position in the muscle
- portable systems for needle guidance for botulinum toxin injections also available

ELECTROMYOGRAM (EMG) EXAMINATION

- evaluates integrity of motor system by recording electrical signals
- examination records motor unit action potentials of muscle fibers

Common Terms

Insertional Activity

- short burst of electrical activity (no more than several hundred milliseconds) produced when needle inserted into muscle
- occurs due to electrical energy of EMG needle, which causes relative change in electrical energy surrounding muscle membrane

Spontaneous Activity

- electrical activity of muscle at rest, which should normally be silent

- presence indicates severe injury with denervation and unstable electrical charges, generally poor prognosis
- occurs 2 to 3 weeks after denervation

Waveform Morphology

- refers to shape, amplitude, and duration of motor unit potential (MUP)
- amplitude correlated with number and strength of muscle fibers innervated by single nerve ending
- duration reflects velocity of neural input (influenced by insulation of nerve)

Recruitment

- increase in number and density of MUPs with increased intensity of voluntary contraction
- reflects degree of innervation (number of active nerve fibers) of a given muscle

Minimal Voluntary Contraction

- 1 or 2 MUPs recorded firing 2 to 5 times/second

Maximum Voluntary Contraction/ Full Interference Pattern

- motor unit recruitment continues until oscilloscope screen is full and single MUPs cannot be distinguished from each other
- decreased recruitment in neuropathy
- in myopathic process, rapid and early recruitment with low amplitude (weak contraction)

Repetitive Stimulation

- stimulate muscle with electrical shocks and record neuromuscular response
- if progressively decreasing response, consider pathology such as neuromuscular junction disorders

Common Abnormal EMG Findings

Polyphasic Waves

- occur when injured nerve regenerates to reinnervate muscle fibers
- early in regeneration process, nerves are small fibers with decreased insulation
- small amplitudes and prolonged duration
- as regeneration progresses, nerves that have regenerated become larger, insulated, and reinnervate more muscle fibers than before
- leads to larger amplitudes and longer duration
- muscle injury (myopathy) with intact nerve demonstrates polyphasic MUP with decreased amplitude and normal-to-decreased duration

Fibrillation Potentials

- spontaneous, single-fiber potentials with amplitudes of several hundred microvolts and less than 2 ms duration, fire at 1 to 50 Hz, typically biphasic/triphasic with initial positive deflection
- commonly seen with denervation, occasionally in myopathic processes

Positive Sharp Waves

- single-fiber contractions of an injured muscle fiber
- large positive deflection of several hundred microvolts lasting <2 ms, followed by negative deflection of 10 to 30 ms, then regular firing at 1 to 50 Hz
- often occur in conjunction with fibrillation potentials 2 to 3 weeks after injury, indicating denervation and axonal loss

Complex Repetitive Discharges

- group of muscle fibers discharge repetitively and nearly synchronously
- abrupt onset and cessation
- discharge rate 5 to 100 Hz with amplitude 100 microvolts to 1 mV
- indicate chronicity in both neuropathy and myopathy

Myotonic Potentials

- repetitive discharges at 20 to 150 Hz and amplitudes of 20 microvolts to 1 mV
- amplitude and frequency wax and wane causing a "dive bomber" sound in EMG speaker
- associated with fibrillation potentials or positive sharp waves

• indicate muscle membrane instability; seen in disorders of clinical myotonia such as myotonic dystrophy

Electrical Silence

• occurs when muscle replaced by fibrotic or lipoid tissue; often old injury

LARYNGEAL EMG

• can help establish diagnosis and guide treatment decisions
• assess both recurrent and superior laryngeal nerves
• concentric or monopolar needle used most often
• test thyroarytenoid (TA), cricothyroid (CT), and posterior cricoarytenoid (PCA) muscles most commonly

Procedure

• patient supine with neck extended, ± shoulder roll
• surface electrode used for grounding electrode (placed on forehead, shoulder, or over clavicle)
• **CT** evaluated by inserting needle lateral to external surface of the junction of the thyroid and cricoid cartilages and approximately 1 cm deep; have patient phonate /i/ starting at low pitch and raising pitch; as vocal folds lengthen, recruitment of muscle should be observed
• **TA** evaluated by inserting needle 5 mm lateral to midline above cricoid cartilage and inserting at 30° to 45° upward angle at approximately 1 to 2 cm depth; have patient phonate /i/ at speaking pitch
• **PCA** evaluated by rotating larynx and passing needle posterior to thyroid lamina at level of cricoid cartilage, taking care not to aim superiorly; have patient sniff sharply and repeatedly
• may also pass needle through thyroid cartilage lamina laterally, or through cricothyroid membrane and cricoid cartilage

Normal Waveform Morphology

• **Biphasic**: upward positive and downward negative spike
• may be polyphasic (1–3 phases) and not necessary pathologic
• <u>Amplitude</u>: 200 to 500 microvolts
• <u>Duration</u>: 5 to 6 ms

Qualitative Analysis

- performed by laryngologist, neurologist, or physiatrist
- listen to amplified signal and view oscilloscope screen
- estimate percentage of normal recruitment response

Quantitative Analysis

- via turns and amplitude analysis
- may be performed with concentric needles
- **Turns**: two successive shifts in amplitude of 100 microvolts or more—measure mean amplitude between turns over time
- smaller muscles demonstrate greater increase in turns and smaller increase in amplitude than large muscles; may limit use in laryngeal muscle evaluation

Lower Motor Neuron and Laryngeal Nerve Disorders

- increased insertional activity, positive wave and fibrillation potentials, complex repetitive discharges
- motor unit potential prolonged with decreased recruitment, incomplete interference pattern, rapid firing of remaining motor units, amplitude variable
- can differentiate VF immobility due to neurologic etiologies from mechanical (ie, arytenoid dislocation or arthrodesis) and assist in confirming side of paresis, which may not be apparent on stroboscopy
- VF immobility etiology can be further differentiated to neuropathy of superior or recurrent laryngeal nerve
- synkinesis may result from aberrant reinnervation of opposing muscles following nerve injury and present clinically with VF immobility despite electrical signal on laryngeal EMG
- evaluate by examining for presence of inappropriate activation on affected side (ie, with needle inserted in TA, electrical signal should not be present with patient sniffing)
- botulinum toxin can be injected to eliminate synkinetic reinnervation; may restore abduction in some patients with bilateral RLN injury and VF immobility

Basal Ganglia Disorders

- insertional activity normal, may have excessive MUPs at rest (incomplete muscle relaxation)
- **Tremor**: rhythmic and periodic MUPs

- **Laryngeal dystonia**: intermittent, sudden increases in muscle activity coinciding with momentary voice arrest; abnormal delay between onset of electrical and acoustic activity; can use EMG-coupled needle to confirm intramuscular injection of botulinum toxin

Muscle Disorders

- insertional activity can be increased or decreased
- myositis and muscular dystrophy may demonstrate positive sharp waves and fibrillation potentials
- MUP short, polyphasic and decreased amplitude, rapid and early recruitment

Neuromuscular Junction Disorders

- insertional activity, recruitment, and interference pattern may be normal initially
- MUPs vary in amplitude and duration with minimal contraction
- **Myasthenia gravis**: autoantibodies block or destroy nicotinic acetylcholine (ACh) receptors at neuromuscular junction
- repetitive stimulation testing may demonstrate progressive decrease in recruitment response
- **Edrophonium (Tensilon/Enlon)**: acetylcholinesterase inhibitor; prolongs presence of ACh in synaptic cleft and therefore increases muscle depolarization
- IV administration causes recruitment to revert to more normal pattern in myasthenia gravis
- Signs of adverse cholinergic reaction: skeletal muscle fasciculations, muscle weakness; give atropine
- Tx: pyridostigmine (Mestinon)—acetylcholinesterase inhibitor (oral)

Upper Motor Neuron Disorders

- insertional activity, amplitude, and duration normal
- decreased recruitment and interference pattern, slow firing of motor unit

SECTION

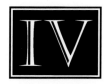

IV

Laryngologic Disorders

CHAPTER

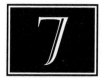

Infectious and Inflammatory Disorders of the Larynx

Justin Ross, Sammy Othman, Mary J. Hawkshaw, and Robert T. Sataloff

PHARYNGITIS

Etiology

- primarily viral (25%–45%); adenovirus is most common
- other common viruses include rhinovirus, enterovirus, influenza A and B, parainfluenza virus, respiratory syncytial virus, and coronavirus
- less common viral causes include Epstein-Barr virus (EBV), herpes simplex virus (HSV), human cytomegalovirus (CMV), and human immunodeficiency virus (HIV)
- group A *Streptococcus* (GAS) causes ~10% to 15% of cases in adults and ~15% to 25% in children
- other known bacterial causes include group C and G Streptococcus, *Fusobacterium necrophorum*, *Arcanobacterium haemolyticum*, *Corynebacterium diphtheriae*, and *Nisseria gonorrhoeae*
- noninfectious causes include allergic, smoking, chemical irritation such as acid reflux, and thermal irritation such as cold weather; mechanical irritation has also been reported

Presentation

- sore throat and fever (most common), dysphagia, headache, neck pain, malaise, exanthem, oral ulcer, cough, conjunctivitis, coryza, cervical lymphadenopathy, abdominal pain
- **GAS presentation**: sudden onset sore throat with difficulty swallowing and patchy, gray-white pharyngeal and tonsillar exudates, fever, anterior cervical lymphadenopathy; occasional "scarlatiniform" (sandpaper) rash that begins in the trunk and spreads to the extremities, but spares palms and soles; may also present with gastrointestinal discomfort, nausea and vomiting, and headache
- **Adenovirus presentation**: sore throat, low-grade fever, conjunctivitis, bilateral cervical lymphadenopathy, rash, myalgia, malaise, and

tonsillar exudates; common in military recruits, day care centers, and other closed-quarter areas

- **EBV presentation**: sore throat, low-grade fever, posterior or generalized lymphadenopathy, hepatosplenomegaly (splenomegaly more common), maculopapular rash on administration of amoxicillin/ampicillin, fatigue, tonsillar exudates; common in children and young adults
- **Pediatric autoimmune neuropsychiatric disorders associated with streptococcal infections (PANDAS)**: acute obsessive-compulsive disorder, tics, and personality changes following GAS infection in children

Diagnosis

- history and physical (H&P), CENTOR criteria (*see* Table 7–1) differentiates between viral and bacterial infection
- heterophile antibody testing may be used if Epstein-Barr virus (EBV) suspected

Treatment

- antibiotics for bacterial origin, symptomatic management if viral
- **GAS**: penicillins (PCN) to prevent acute rheumatic fever and glomerulonephritis; cephalosporins or macrolides if PCN allergic
- Arcanobacterium haemolyticum **and** Corynebacterium diphtheriae: macrolide or a PCN with β-lactamase inhibitor

TABLE 7–1. CENTOR Criteria

Criteria	Points
Absence of cough	+1
Tonsillar exudates	+1
Fever	+1
Tender anterior cervical lymphadenopathy	+1
Age—under 15	+1
Age—above 44	–1

<1: treat as viral infection	
=1: treat as viral or obtain cultures (optional)	Total Points
2–3: obtain throat cultures or rapid strep test	
4–5: consider empiric antibiotics	

- Fusobacterium necrophorum: PCN/β-lactamase inhibitor and metronidazole
- prophylactic antibiotics are generally not recommended except under special circumstances

Complications of Untreated Group A Streptococcus

- **Rheumatic fever**: cardiac sequelae (mitral valve regurgitation), involuntary muscle movements (Sydenham chorea), joint pain, diffuse rash that spares the face (erythema marginatum)
- **Peritonsillar abscess**: present with drooling, uvula deviation, and muffled voice ("hot potato voice"); rarely causes life-threatening respiratory obstruction
- **Retropharyngeal abscess**: drooling with neck pain/stiffness and cervical lymphadenopathy; may cause life-threatening respiratory obstruction, sepsis, and infection of the mediastinum
- **Sinusitis and otitis media**
- **Acute glomerulonephritis:** rare with GAS pharyngitis (much more common in GAS cellulitis)
- **Toxic shock syndrome and necrotizing fasciitis**
- **Lemierre's syndrome**: a septic thrombophlebitis of the jugular vein, is a rare complication, most often attributed to pharyngitis caused by *F necrophorum*

ACUTE SUPRAGLOTTITIS (EPIGLOTTITIS)

Etiology

- generally bacterial with few reported viral cases
- most common cause is *H influenzae*—was type B historically, but now more commonly untyped due to vaccination
- less commonly group A and β-hemolytic streptococci, *S aureus*, *K pneumoniae*, *H parainfluenzae*
- <u>noninfectious causes</u>: thermal, acidic, caustic, mechanical, irritative

Presentation

- progressive dysphagia, odynophagia, and fever over 1 to 2 days
- symptoms will progress to **muffled voice**, **drooling**, stridor, tachypnea, toxic appearance, and **tripoding** in sniffing position, palpable tenderness of the laryngotracheal complex

- adults less likely to present with dyspnea, drooling, stridor, or fever, and more likely to report sore throat, odynophagia, and hoarseness
- severe sore throat and odynophagia present in 90% of adults with epiglottitis

Diagnosis

- H&P including flexible laryngoscopy (gold standard of diagnosis), blood cultures, imaging (lateral neck x-ray), direct laryngoscopy to obtain cultures once airway is secured
- Flexible nasopharyngolaryngoscopy (NPL) may be attempted in adults at bedside if not in significant respiratory distress
- pediatric patients should have NPL in OR due to possibility of noncompliance and subsequent rapid progression of edema
- **Lateral neck x-ray**: thumb print sign (absent in 14%–27%); vallecula sign (loss of normal vallecular aeration)
- computed tomography (CT)/magnetic resonance imaging (MRI) not indicated unless abscess suspected

Treatment

- **intubation over flexible bronchoscope if required for airway protection** (no combination of variables predictive of need for intubation)
- intensive care unit (ICU) admission with continuous pulse oximetry
- **IV antibiotics**: second- or third-generation cephalosporin (gold standard), ampicillin + chloramphenicol (if cephalosporins unavailable or allergic)
- no evidence proving the benefit of racemic epinephrine, steroids, antireflux medication, or humidified air, but often used anecdotally
- extubation and/or discharge from intensive care setting determined by resolution of supraglottic cellulitis confirmed by laryngoscopy

CROUP (LARYNGOTRACHEOBRONCHITIS)

- viral-mediated subglottic edema and glandular hypersecretion
- <u>Etiology</u>: parainfluenza types I, II, III, and IV (most commonly), *M pneumoniae*, adenovirus, respiratory syncytial virus, influenza viruses A and B, *H influenzae*
- most commonly occurs between 6 months and 3 years
- subglottis is the narrowest area of the pediatric airway; 1 mm of subglottic edema decreases airway diameter by 50%

- <u>Presentation</u>: viral prodrome for 1 to 2 days followed by barking cough
- severity determines stridor, suprasternal retractions, and accessory muscle use
- generally nontoxic appearing
- agitation and increased pulse if hypercarbic
- <u>Dx</u>: H&P, imaging (A-P neck x-ray—steeple sign); CT/MRI not indicated
- <u>Tx</u>: determined by severity
  1. **Mild**: managed in primary care or emergency department setting with single oral or IV dose of dexamethasone; helium-oxygen mixtures used to decrease airway turbulence and promote laminar flow—no high-quality evidence promoting use; nebulized cool mist and racemic epinephrine
  2. **Moderate to severe**: hospitalization with symptomatic management required as previously discussed, but therapy is continued during inpatient stay
  3. **Recurrent croup**: indication for direct laryngoscopy and bronchoscopy (DLB); done to rule out subglottic stenosis, cyst, laryngeal cleft, or hemangioma

OTHER INFECTIOUS DISORDERS

Acute Viral Laryngitis

- <u>Etiology</u>: generally viral—rhinovirus (most common), parainfluenza, influenza, adenovirus, respiratory syncytial virus, pertussis
- <u>Presentation</u>: hoarseness, dysphonia, dysphagia, throat pain, cough, globus sensation, low-grade fever, lymphadenopathy
- <u>Dx</u>: H&P
- <u>Tx</u>: complete voice rest or soft, breathy phonation (avoid whispering which causes laryngeal hyperfunction and muscle tension dysphonia), hydration, humidified air, and smoking cessation; avoid antibiotics

Laryngeal Diphtheria

- <u>Etiology</u>: *Corynebacterium diphtheriae* infection; occurs in immunocompromised or unvaccinated patients
- <u>Presentation</u>: silver-gray membranous exudates in pharynx/larynx; progressive hoarseness/pain leading to complete airway obstruction, dysphagia, cardiomyopathy
- <u>Dx</u>: direct visualization and culture—removal of membrane causes bleeding

- Tx: antitoxin and a penicillin, may require intubation and nasogastric tube

Tuberculous Laryngitis

- Etiology: usually contiguous spread from pulmonary *Mycobacterium tuberculosis*
- Presentation: slow and insidious onset (hoarseness, pain, dysphagia, and laryngeal stenosis occur late), granulomatous lesion on the interarytenoid fold (most common in the past), true vocal fold (TVF), or supraglottis
- Dx: direct visualization and deep submucosal biopsy, skin testing (sensitivity lowered by BCG injection), chest x-ray, quantitative interferon gamma assay
- Tx: treat with rifampin, isoniazid, and ethambutol (at least 2 agents) for 6 months; surgical tx of stenosis

Laryngeal Perichondritis

- Etiology: decreased vascular supply due to trauma (usually iatrogenic) and/or radiation, followed by bacterial colonization (gram-negative rod [GNR]); **thyroid cartilage most common site**
- Presentation: tenderness, edema/erythema, hoarseness, dysphagia/odynophagia, fetor, CA joint fixation
- Dx: direct visualization and culture if possible
- Tx: secure airway, fluoroquinolones, incision and drainage, humidified air, corticosteroids, antireflux medications, voice rest

Leprosy (Hansen's Disease)

- **Etiology**: *Mycobacterium leprae*, aerosolized nasal secretions and skin-to-skin transmission; highly contagious but clinical symptoms require long-term contact
- **Presentation**: husky voice, dry cough, globus, hemoptysis, TVF paralysis, cutaneous disease; no odynophagia or dysphonia
- most common site is **epiglottic tip** due to lower temperature, then TVF
- Dx: tissue biopsy/culture; foamy histiocytes with nonstaining bacilli
- Tx: dapsone + rifampin ± clofazimine for 6 months; may require lifelong tx

Syphilis

- Etiology: *Treponema pallidum*, laryngeal involvement in primary or secondary stage

- <u>Presentation</u>: hoarseness, impaired vocal fold mobility, respiratory compromise, granulomatous laryngeal masses, perichondritis, chondritis, obstructive cicatricial fibrosis
- <u>Dx</u>: VDRL/RPR, FTA-Abs, direct visualization and biopsy, CT/MRI
- <u>Tx</u>: penicillin G

Rhinoscleroma

- <u>Etiology</u>: *Klebsiella rhinoscleromatis*, endemic to Central America and Eastern Europe
- <u>Presentation</u>: hoarseness, cough, respiratory compromise; keratotic lesions of nose, pharynx, tongue, and lower airway; **subglottis is most common laryngeal subsite**
- <u>Dx</u>: biopsy and culture—Mikulicz cells (vacuolated bacteria within histiocytes)
- <u>Tx</u>: tetracycline or ciprofloxacin; corticosteroids

Actinomycosis

- <u>Etiology</u>: *Actinomyces* sp., anaerobic saprophyte, normal oral flora
- <u>Presentation</u>: hoarseness, cough, dysphagia in an immunocompromised individual
- <u>Dx</u>: biopsy and culture—granulomas and **sulfur granules**
- <u>Tx</u>: penicillin × 6 months; debridement of scarring and/or necrosis if necessary

FUNGAL INFECTIONS

Blastomycosis

- <u>Etiology</u>: *Blastomyces dermatidis*; round, thick-walled fungus endemic to southeast United States and Mississippi River Valley
- <u>Presentation</u>: laryngeal pyogenic granuloma and fibrosis with multiple microabscesses miliary spread, laryngeal stenosis, arytenoid fixation
- <u>Dx</u>: direct visualization and biopsy, silver stain, CT/MRI
- <u>Tx</u>: amphotericin B, ketoconazole, or itraconazole

Coccidiomycosis

- <u>Etiology</u>: *Coccidiodes immitis*; spherical, thick-walled, endospore-filled fungus endemic to southwest United States and South America

- <u>Presentation</u>: cough, chest pain, fevers, malaise, chills, arthralgias, laryngeal stenosis
- <u>Dx</u>: silver stain with presence of spherules in affected tissue, direct visualization and biopsy, CT/MRI
- <u>Tx</u>: amphotericin B, ketoconazole, or itraconazole

Histoplasmosis

- <u>Etiology</u>: *Histoplasma capsulatum*; found in bat and bird droppings
- AIDS-defining illness (CD4+ <50)
- <u>Presentation</u>: cough, fever, chills, malaise, mediastinitis, laryngeal granulomas
- <u>Dx</u>: silver stain with invasive fungal hyphae in affected tissue, CT/MRI
- <u>Tx</u>: amphotericin B, ketoconazole, or itraconazole

Candidiasis

- <u>Etiology</u>: *Candida albicans*; oval-budding yeast-like fungus; laryngeal manifestations occur in immunocompromised host
- <u>Presentation</u>: upper airway thrush in the immunocompromised host
- <u>Dx</u>: mucosal scrapings—budding yeast cells on microscopy; HIV testing
- <u>Tx</u>: fluconazole

ANGIOEDEMA

Etiology

- edema of skin, respiratory, and/or gastrointestinal mucosal and submucosal tissue secondary to increased vascular permeability
- Allergic subtype: histamine/IgE-mediated, urticarial
- Nonallergic subtype: usually bradykinin-mediated, nonurticarial, hereditary and nonhereditary

Hereditary Angioedema

- usually **autosomal dominant** (Chromosome 11)
- three types identified:
    1. Type 1: low C1 esterase inhibitor (C1 INH) concentration
    2. Type 2: decreased C1 INH function
    3. Type 3: estrogen-dependent (generally related to oral contraceptive use)

Nonhereditary Angioedema

- Idiopathic
- Acquired: development of neutralizing antibodies to C1 INH; onset generally 40 to 50 years of age; recurrent episodes 2 to 5 days in duration
  1. **ACE inhibitor-induced**: bradykinin-mediated; 0.2% of the U.S. population
  2. **Pseudoallergic (drug-induced)**: angiotensin-receptor blockers (1.66 per 1000 person-years); NSAID/ASA (0.1%–0.3%, multiple pathways—histamine, bradykinin, COX inhibition); DPP-IV inhibitors; statins
  3. **Thrombolytics**: plasmin-mediated release of bradykinin; patients given tPA for nonhemorrhagic stroke have an increased risk of angioedema, especially while taking ACE inhibitors (~17%)

Presentation and Diagnosis

- <u>Presentation</u>: differs based on primary mediator (histamine versus bradykinin), upper airway edema common to both
  1. **Histamine-mediated**: rapid onset of sx following exposure; epinephrine responsive anaphylaxis; wheals (urticaria)
  2. **Bradykinin-mediated**: abdominal (50%) and genitourinary discomfort
- <u>Dx</u>: H&P, flexible laryngoscopy, direct laryngoscopy in some cases, imaging not required

Treatment

- <u>Secure airway</u>: if required, intubation via orotracheal versus nasopharyngeal (gold standard) route
- <u>Standard medical therapy</u>: corticosteroids, H1 blocker, H2 blocker, ± epinephrine (if anaphylaxis)
- <u>Discontinue offending agent</u>: ACE inhibitor induced angioedema will usually resolve in <48 hours following discontinuation of medication

C1-INH Protein Replacement Drugs

- **Berinert** (plasma derived): acute tx of adult/pediatric HAE; one study showed no increased efficacy over steroid and antihistamine alone
- **Cinryze** (plasma derived): prophylactic tx of HAE in pts >10yo

- **Ruconest** (recombinant): acute tx of HAE attacks, but not those with laryngeal symptoms

Ecallantide

- <u>Mechanism</u>: kallikrein inhibitor
- indicated for acute tx HAE attacks in pts >11yo
- has shown no increased efficacy versus placebo when both groups received corticosteroid, antihistamine, H2 blocker, and epinephrine
- anaphylaxis (~3%)

Icatibant

- bradykinin-2 receptor antagonist
- indicated for acute tx of HAE attacks in adults
- shown to reduce time to symptom resolution when compared to administration of corticosteroids and antihistamines

Fresh Frozen Plasma (FFP)

- <u>Mechanism</u>: likely due to intravascular volume replacement and supplementation of C1 INH and other degradative enzymes
- shown to decrease intubation frequency (60% versus 35%) and ICU stay (3.5 versus 1.5 days)
    1. use supported by multiple case reports but no randomized controlled trials
    2. small chance of worsening symptoms—likely due to presence of high molecular weight kininogen and kallikrein in FFP
    3. suggested dose of 2 to 4 units

Antifibrinolytics

- <u>Drugs</u>: **tranexamic acid, aminocaproic acid**
- used as prophylaxis against HAE
- reduced attacks by 75% in 50% of tx cohort in one study

CHAPTER

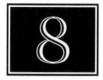

Nonneoplastic Structural Abnormalities of the Larynx

Justin Ross, Mary J. Hawkshaw, and Robert T. Sataloff

VOCAL NODULES

- **bilateral,** fairly symmetric, fibrotic, whitish masses found in the striking zone of the true vocal fold (TVF)
- generally occur at the point of maximum contact on the medial surface
- increase stiffness and bulk of vocal fold surface causing alterations in vibratory characteristics
- Etiology: **voice misuse/abuse**
- Pathophysiology: mechanical stress causes epithelial **basement membrane duplication** and **increased collagen deposition** in the superficial lamina propria (LP)
- Presentation: hoarseness, breathiness, vocal fatigue, loss of range, pressed speech, strap muscle tension and tenderness; uncommonly asymptomatic
- Dx: history and physical (H&P), flexible laryngoscopy, **strobovideolaryngoscopy**
- strobovideolaryngoscopy is essential for differentiation of nodules from cysts
- examination of asymptomatic patients generally reveals nodules on the superior surface rather than in the striking zone—most commonly seen after voice therapy
- stroboscopy can be performed easily in patients >6 years old, and as young as 6 months
- Tx: **voice therapy**, rarely surgery
- voice therapy for at least 6 to 12 weeks results in cure of symptoms and/or lesions ~90% of the time
- **never attempt surgery without a trial of expert voice therapy**
- surgery may result in submucosal scarring and resultant adynamic segment
- behavioral modification during voice therapy should include family members, especially in children who are likely exhibiting learned behaviors
- controversy surrounds operative intervention prior to puberty—if child has complied with voice therapy without resolution of nodules, and if dysphonia causes substantial psychosocial disturbance, it is reasonable to operate prior to voice maturation
- heavy voice use may result in asymptomatic, symmetric or asymmetric, bilateral physiologic swellings that are commonly confused with nodules, **known as pseudocysts**, and generally resolve after 24 to 48 hours of voice rest

LARYNGEAL CYSTS

Introduction

- may occur anywhere within the larynx
- approximately 5% to 10% of all nonmalignant laryngeal lesions
- higher incidence in men, but more symptomatic in women
- epiglottis is the most common site, but largely asymptomatic
- excluding vocal fold cyst, all laryngeal cysts should be evaluated with computed tomography (CT) and magnetic resonance imaging (MRI)
- consideration should be given to endoscopic ultrasound and optical coherence tomography

Vocal Fold Cyst

- **unilateral** or bilateral epithelial-lined sacs within the superficial LP which may protrude onto the vibratory margin
- typically unilateral with contralateral reactive depression or swelling
- increases bulk and sometimes stiffness of overlying epithelium
- occasionally attached to vocal ligament
- more common in females and professional voice users
- Etiology: acquired (voice misuse/abuse, trauma, upper respiratory infection) or congenital (epidermoid cyst)
- Pathophysiology:
    1. *Mucus retention cysts*: arise from obstructed mucus gland and are lined with glandular, ciliary, or oncocytic ductal epithelium
    2. *Epidermoid cysts*: arise from congenital cell rests or invaginated epithelium during mucosal healing; lined with squamous or pseudostratified columnar epithelium; contents are generally caseous
- Presentation: hoarseness, breathiness, vocal fatigue, loss of range, pressed speech, compensatory muscular hyperfunction, diplophonia (common with epidermoid cyst)
- extent of **dysphonia may be less than expected based on size of the lesion, especially if the cyst is compressible**
- voice quality may worsen in the premenstrual or menstrual period
- Dx: H&P, flexible laryngoscopy, **strobovideolaryngoscopy**
- Stroboscopic findings: fluid-filled swelling that deforms on contact with contralateral vocal fold, loss of mucosal wave overlying cyst due to displacement of superficial LP, hourglass glottic insufficiency
- possibly reduced incidence of contralateral reactive lesions relative to vocal fold polyps
- Tx: voice therapy, endoscopic **surgical excision** with microflap or mini-microflap technique

- surgery often necessary, but should be preceded by a trial of expert voice therapy
- ruptured cysts and intracordal tethering increase risk of scar and sulcus formation
- oncocytic retention cysts have thin-walled capsules composed of cuboidal epithelium, and are difficult to dissect without rupturing
- Pseudocysts: compensatory, unencapsulated fluid-filled lesions that form on vocal fold contralateral to a pathologic lesion; resection generally worsens voice

Laryngocele

- symptomatic or clinically apparent dilation of the saccule of Hilton which **communicates** with the laryngeal lumen
- may be filled with air (laryngocele), mucus (laryngomucocele), or pus (laryngopyocele)
- more prevalent in adults, males, glass blowers, those who have chronic obstructive pulmonary disease, and performers (wind and higher brass instrument players, singers)
- highest incidence in the sixth decade
- Etiology: congenital saccular enlargement or laryngeal tissue weakness, obstruction of the laryngeal ventricle (benign or malignant mass)
- commonly occurs secondary to increased pressure in the laryngeal lumen
- Subtypes:
  1. *Internal*: confined to the false vocal fold, medial to the thyrohyoid membrane
  2. *External*: begins in the false vocal fold, extending through the thyrohyoid membrane into the neck
  3. *Combined*: extends both medial to and though the thyrohyoid membrane
- Presentation: **lateral neck mass** that increases in size with intraluminal pressure (external), **laryngeal mass** that inflates with phonation (internal), hoarseness, dyspnea, dysphagia
- laryngopyoceles present with fever, chills, pain, and leukocytosis
- Dx: H&P, flexible laryngoscopy, strobovideolaryngoscopy, **CT/MRI** with contrast
- imaging helpful to differentiate from saccular cyst, abscess, and neoplasia
- Tx: surgical excision via external or endoscopic approach
- endoscopic approach with CO_2 laser effective for small internal laryngoceles

- larger internal and external laryngoceles may benefit from open approach via thyrotomy and/or thyrohyoid membrane

Saccular Cyst

- fluid-filled cyst or pseudocyst of the saccule of Hilton that may protrude into but **does not communicate** with the laryngeal lumen
- represent 25% of all laryngeal cysts
- saccular ductal cysts are epithelial lined, while saccular mucoceles and pyoceles are not
- Etiology: congenital atresia of the laryngeal saccule or obstruction of the ventricular/saccular orifice by mucus retention cyst(s) or neoplasm (benign or malignant)
- Subtypes:
    1. *Anterior cysts*: project medially and posteriorly between the true and false vocal folds into the laryngeal lumen
    2. *Lateral cysts*: project superiorly and posteriorly, elevating and displacing the false vocal fold and aryepiglottic fold; may extend through the thyrohyoid membrane and present as a neck mass
- Presentation: dysphonia, stridor, dyspnea, lateral neck mass, fever, and chills (if pyocele), or no symptoms
- most are asymptomatic (~50%), and the mass is found on autopsy or incidentally during laryngoscopy
- Dx: H&P, flexible laryngoscopy, strobovideolaryngoscopy, **CT/MRI** with contrast, B-mode ultrasonography (especially in children)
- Tx: observation if asymptomatic; surgical excision via external or endoscopic approach, determined by size
- needle aspiration for temporary relief of severe or life-threatening symptoms
- cyst roof excision (marsupialization) and needle aspiration have a high rate of recurrence
- usually excised with endoscopic laser microsurgery, followed sometimes by closure of the defect via microsuture technique

VOCAL FOLD POLYPS

- generally unilateral, gelatinous masses of varying size
- described as gelatinous, fibrinoid, hyaline, angiomatous, mucoid, or myxomatous
- Etiology: cough usually traumatic (vocal abuse/misuse); may have increased risk in the setting of chronic irritation/inflammation (eg, tobacco use, laryngopharyngeal reflux [LPR], etc)

- <u>Pathophysiology</u>: traumatic shearing forces cause damage to the vocal fold microvasculature, increased leukocyte infiltration and mucopolysaccharide deposition in the superficial lamina propria
- <u>Presentation</u>: progressive hoarseness, breathiness, vocal fatigue, loss of range and pitch control, cough, stridor, shortness of breath, globus sensation, dysphagia, muscle tension dysphonia (MTD)
- functional deficits depend on laterality and symmetry of the lesion(s), position relative to the vibratory margin, extent of involved mucosa (eg, pedunculated versus sessile), and pathology
- cover layer mass is functionally decreased in edematous polyps, and increased in the presence of hemorrhage or fibrosis
- <u>Dx</u>: H&P, flexible laryngoscopy, strobovideolaryngoscopy
- <u>Stroboscopic findings</u>: translucent, fleshy, or erythematous mass with preservation of mucosal wave in most cases (~80%), although it may be decreased
- may be preceded by vocal fold hemorrhage
- frequently comorbid with contralateral reactive vocal fold lesion
- large polyps tend to extend into the subglottis
- <u>Tx</u>: relative voice rest, vocal hygiene, voice therapy, corticosteroids, surgery
- occasionally resolve with voice rest, improved vocal hygiene and several weeks low-dose oral corticosteroids
- improved chance of nonoperative resolution in nonsmokers with small polyps
- usually require surgical excision and postoperative voice therapy
- pathologic analysis required for all lesions that do not respond to nonsurgical management or in presence of concerning risk factors (eg, weight loss, TVF paresis, smoker, etc)

Hemorrhagic Polyps

- phonatory trauma causes increased shearing forces resulting in capillary rupture and local extravasation of blood
- increased incidence in coagulopathic patients
- unaddressed hematoma will cause hyaline degeneration, thrombosis, infiltration of inflammatory cells, and collagen proliferation with subsequent scar formation
- if the hematoma remains enlarged rather than flattened with epithelium against muscle and lamina propria 48 to 72 hours after onset, incision and drainage are considered

CONTACT GRANULOMA AND
VOCAL PROCESS ULCER

- unilateral or bilateral lesions usually found on the medial mucosal surface of the vocal process, but may occur anywhere
- <u>Etiology</u>: LPR, intubation, MTD, voice abuse/misuse, iatrogenic Teflon injection, glottic insufficiency with secondary MTD/LCA dominance
- suspect LPR in all cases
- in the absence of reflux or intubation, etiology is almost always phonatory trauma
- forceful adduction with lateral cricoarytenoid (LCA) dominance seen in treatment-refractory granulomas
- <u>Pathophysiology</u>: inflammatory lesions characterized by leukocyte infiltration, collagen deposition, and proliferation of fibroblasts and capillaries
- <u>Presentation</u>: often asymptomatic; occasionally cause laryngeal pain, otalgia, globus sensation, hoarseness, painful phonation, hemoptysis; may scar years after injection
- may mimic more serious lesions like carcinoma, tuberculosis, and granular cell tumor
- <u>Dx</u>: H&P, flexible laryngoscopy, strobovideolaryngoscopy, 24-hour pH monitor
- <u>Stroboscopy findings</u>: pearl-colored or erythematous polypoid lesion, severely decreased mucosal wave (Teflon granuloma)
- video barium swallow if complaints of swallowing disorder
- esophagogastroduodenoscopy (EGD) if long-standing reflux
- decision to biopsy should be guided by history
- recurrent granuloma despite adequate treatment an indication to rule out granulomatous disease (eg, sarcoidosis, tuberculosis, etc)
- <u>Tx</u>: **gastric acid reduction** (PPI ± H2 blocker, antacids, alkaline water), **voice therapy**, **low-dose oral corticosteroids**, corticosteroid injection into lesion base, surgery if refractory
- avoid inhaled corticosteroids that may cause vocal fold atrophy, laryngitis, and *Candida* infection
- re-examine in 1 to 2 months and consider biopsy/resection if unchanged or worsened
- surgical excision performed with cold instruments or laser, followed by corticosteroid injection into wound base; endoscopic or external approach
- refractory granuloma with 24-hour pH monitor proven reflux may be candidates for Nissen fundoplication

- injection of botulinum toxin (Botox) into the LCA has been used in refractory and recurrent cases by decreasing the force of vocal process contact in patients with LCA-dominant closure pattern

Teflon Granuloma

- foreign-body reaction elicited by Teflon when used for injection medialization laryngoplasty
- significant impairment of mucosal wave observed on stroboscopy
- trial of corticosteroids may be attempted, but usually are not helpful
- high rate of recurrence following surgical excision
- abandoned in clinical practice, but many previously injected patients still are seen

REACTIVE LESIONS

- usually result from vocal fold cyst or polyp, but may be caused by any lesion exerting mass effect on the contralateral vocal fold
- Pathophysiology: epithelial hyperplasia and/or development of unencapsulated pseudocysts that develop due to trauma from repeated contact by a primary lesion during phonation; may develop into fibrous nodules or true cysts
- classified based on consistency (fibrous or polypoid) and relationship to the vocal fold edge
- Risk factors: polypoid primary lesion, primary lesion less than one-quarter vocal fold length, never smoker with hoarseness ≥6 months
- smoking may be protective due to reduced shearing forces from vascular congestion and resultant vocal fold edema—not recommended as a therapeutic or preventative strategy
- Presentation: hoarseness, breathiness (relative to size of primary), alteration in range and pitch control, MTD
- Dx: H&P, flexible laryngoscopy, strobovideolaryngoscopy
- Stroboscopic findings: red or white lesion at junction of anterior third and posterior two-thirds of the vocal fold, which may be indented, flat or raised; occasionally hypo- or adynamic
- masses may be polypoid, soft, fibrous, or present as subepithelial pseudocyst, cyst, or fibrotic nodule
- may have sufficient bulk to cause glottic insufficiency
- Tx: voice therapy, corticosteroid injection, endoscopic resection
- usually responds to **voice therapy** following excision of primary lesion
- corticosteroid injection may be a useful adjunct to nonsurgical management or following surgical excision

- surgical excision may be indicated depending on extent and firmness of lesion, subjacent scar, or progression
- fibrous lesions more likely to persist following removal of primary
- recurrence more common in polypoid lesions
- lesions further from vibratory margin more likely to resolve

VOCAL FOLD HEMORRHAGE

- submucosal hemorrhage involving part or the entire length of the TVF
- appropriate management essential to avoid career-threatening chronic changes
- Etiology: precipitated by vocal fold trauma, occasionally associated with mucosal tear
- **Performers**: singing, public speaking, or same as nonperformers
- **Nonperformers**: external laryngeal trauma, phonotrauma (eg, screaming), cough, sneeze
- iatrogenic causes include intubation, oro-/nasogastric tube placement, and endoscopy
- increased incidence in premenstrual or pregnant females and with anticoagulant medication use, especially when combined
- Pathophysiology: increased intravascular pressure (eg, Valsalva), shearing forces, or trauma to the laryngeal complex results in capillary rupture and edema
- unresolved hemorrhage results in secondary fibroblast infiltration and collagen deposition, with resultant stiffness and dysphasia
- Presentation: **sudden hoarseness** (typically), progressive hoarseness, reduced upper range, vocal fatigue, dysphagia (posterior hemorrhage), rarely asymptomatic
- hemorrhage in asymptomatic patients generally isolated to superior surface
- Dx: H&P, flexible laryngoscopy, strobovideolaryngoscopy
- Stroboscopic findings: red blush involving the musculomembranous submucosa, reduction of mucosal wave and amplitude, occasionally incomplete glottic closure, associated hemorrhagic mass, and varicosities and/or ectasias
- hemosiderin staining seen in subacute events
- association with hemorrhagic mass confers a negative prognosis for voice outcomes and for nonsurgical resolution
- Tx: **strict voice rest (1 week)**, address underlying disease, hold antiplatelet and anticoagulant medications, voice therapy, surgical excision of persistent raised hematoma or associated hemorrhagic mass

- singing and public speaking contraindicated for at least 1 week and sometimes as long as 6 weeks
- relative voice rest and serial strobovideolaryngoscopy until normal mucosal wave is restored
- small hemorrhage isolated to the superior vocal fold resolves with observation and no functional impairment in nearly all cases
- consider surgical evacuation if hematoma results in a bulging vocal fold and resorption has not occurred within 2 to 3 days
- excision or laser cautery of causative varicosities/ectasias indicated for recurrent hemorrhage—should be considered after hematoma has resolved

REINKE'S EDEMA

- bilateral accumulation of mucoid, gelatinous material within the **superficial LP** (Reinke's space) along the entire musculomembranous fold
- also known as polypoid degeneration, polypoid corditis, and edematous hypertrophy
- <u>Etiology</u>: smoking, LPR, hypothyroidism, vocal abuse, vocal fold atrophy or paresis
- more common in adults and women
- unilateral Reinke's edema is usually reactive (contralateral lesions or adynamic segments; **ipsilateral or contralateral paresis/paralysis**), but may be malignant
- <u>Pathophysiology</u>: chronic mucosal irritation and increased shearing force result in increased mucopolysaccharide deposition in the superficial LP
- increased expression of fibronectin, laminin, and collagen type IV in associated vascular endothelium
- increased cover mass, but reduced stiffness
- <u>Presentation</u>: hoarseness (low, gruff, husky voice), cough, stridor, vocal fatigue, MTD, but rarely increased vocal effort
- <u>Dx</u>: H&P, flexible laryngoscopy, strobovideolaryngoscopy, laboratory work (TSH, free T4)
- <u>Stroboscopic findings</u>: hyperdynamic amplitude and mucosal wave that is often asymmetric, excessive superficial LP along the vibratory margin that appears translucent
- contact endoscopy demonstrates longitudinal mucosal "blue lines" separating subepithelial pockets within the superficial LP
- unilateral Reinke's edema should always be evaluated for an underlying cause due to potential for malignancy

- <u>Tx</u>: **address underlying cause** (smoking cessation, antireflux medications/fundoplication, diet alteration, thyroid hormone replacement, etc), voice therapy, surgical evacuation if conservative measures fail and patient is unhappy with voice
- do not treat if the patient values a low, masculine voice quality that may confer professional benefits (eg, female trial attorneys, businesswomen)
- senior author (RTS) favors strongly unilateral surgery, with staged surgery on the contralateral vocal fold if there is good mucosal wave preservation on the first side

PROLONGED ULCERATIVE LARYNGITIS

- prolonged, self-limiting inflammatory laryngeal disorder characterized by vocal fold ulcerations and associated mucosal hyperemia and edema
- <u>Etiology</u>: unknown but may have infectious, irritative, metabolic, autoimmune, or idiopathic origins
- may be worsened by irritants (eg, smoking, LPR, inhaled pollutants)
- generally affects healthy individuals who are nonsmokers and nondrinkers
- possibly associated with bacterial biofilms
- <u>Presentation</u>: progressive hoarseness, throat pain, excessive throat clearing, cough, vocal fatigue, loss of high pitches
- <u>Dx</u>: H&P, flexible laryngoscopy, strobovideolaryngoscopy, culture, *Helicobacter pylori* testing (when indicated), rarely biopsy
- <u>Stroboscopic findings</u>: whitish-pink, often raised ulcerations, vocal fold erythema, edema, exudates, stiffness, and reduced mucosal wave and amplitude
- ulcerations always occur on the musculomembranous portion of the vocal fold
- <u>Tx</u>: **antireflux medications**, voice therapy for prevention of compensatory hyperfunction
- serial strobovideolaryngoscopy until resolution of ulcerations
- consider low-dose oral corticosteroids, antibiotics, and antifungals in select cases, but efficacy unproven
- avoid biopsy unless strong suspicion of malignancy
- **ulcerations heal spontaneously** without long-term functional deficits in nearly all cases, but healing may take several months

SULCUS VOCALIS

- longitudinal invagination of vocal fold epithelium due to decreased or absent superficial LP, with associated collagen deposition and deficient capillaries in some types
- <u>Etiology</u>: unknown, but theories include congenital and/or acquired causes
    1. *Congenital*: developmental defect; ruptured epidermoid cyst
    2. *Acquired*: phonotrauma; vascular lesion; postoperative scar
- increased incidence in patients with chronic laryngeal inflammation, cancer, and >40 years of age
- <u>Types</u>:
    1. *Physiologic sulcus (type 1)*: shallow groove with preserved physiologic mucosal wave
    2. *Sulcus vergeture (type 2)*: variable loss of superficial LP and atrophic depression of vocal fold mucosa that is nonadherent to the vocal ligament
    3. *True sulcus vocalis (type 3)*: complete absence of superficial LP and invagination of vocal fold mucosa with variable thickness and hyperkeratosis that is adherent to the vocal ligament
- **Pseudosulcus vocalis**: longitudinal groove inferior to the TVF with similar appearance to type 3 sulci, but extends posteriorly beyond the musculomembranous vocal fold; typically associated with LPR
- <u>Presentation</u>: dysphonia (strained, harsh, reedy quality), breathiness, loss of vocal range, decreased maximum phonation time (particularly type 3), odynophonia, vocal fatigue, fixed pitch elevation, may be asymptomatic
- <u>Dx</u>: H&P, flexible laryngoscopy, strobovideolaryngoscopy
- <u>Stroboscopic findings</u>: longitudinal groove along the vibratory margin, vocal fold stiffness with reduced mucosal wave and amplitude, vocal fold bowing with anterior glottic gap (spindle-shaped glottis), vocal fold varicosities, lateral supraglottic hyperfunction, and may have associated chronic laryngitis and/or benign lesions (eg, polyp, cyst, etc)
- true sulcus vocalis demonstrates significantly reduced amplitude and mucosal wave due to epithelial tethering to vocal ligament
- may be misdiagnosed as transient paresis following upper respiratory infection, presbylaryngis, and postoperative scarring
- <u>Tx</u>: address concurrent laryngeal pathology (LPR, allergic laryngitis, muscle tension dysphonia), voice therapy, surgery
- surgical management must address stiffness and glottic gap—excision of scar-like sulcus and reconstitution of deficient superficial LP (usually fat implantation), buccal graft, false vocal fold flap, releasing incisions, medialization, or other techniques

MUCOSAL BRIDGE

- longitudinal separation of musculomembranous mucosa from underlying vocal fold
- <u>Etiology</u>: generally congenital, but may be related to trauma or sulcus vocalis
- <u>Presentation</u>: ranges from severe dysphonia to completely asymptomatic
- <u>Dx</u>: suspension microdirect laryngoscopy required in most cases
- <u>Tx</u>: surgical excision only when absolutely necessary—may worsen dysphonia

LARYNGEAL WEBS (*See* Chapters 12, 31)

- layer of mucosa connecting vocal folds across the glottic inlet
- may form anteriorly or posteriorly, and in rare cases there is complete laryngeal atresia
- <u>Etiology</u>: congenital (velocardiofacial syndrome—anterior glottic webs), acquired (iatrogenic, intubation, acidic/caustic ingestion, other trauma)
- <u>Pathophysiology</u>:
  1. *Congenital*: failure of the laryngotracheal tube to completely recanalize during the third month of fetal development
  2. *Acquired*: damage to both vocal folds leads to healing that connects the mucosa of opposing segments
- <u>Presentation</u>: dysphonia, stridor, dyspnea with accessory muscle use, often high-pitched voice
- <u>Dx</u>: H&P, flexible laryngoscopy, genetic testing if congenital (**chromosome 22q11.2 deletion**), lateral neck XR (**sail sign**), microdirect laryngoscopy and bronchoscopy
- <u>Tx</u>: observation if asymptomatic, cold knife or CO_2 laser lysis with or without keel placement (may reduce recurrence), laryngofissure may be required for more extensive webs
- keel placement and application of mitomycin C may reduce recurrence
- new, two stage web prosthesis procedure produces sharp anterior commissure

BOWED VOCAL FOLDS

- concave vocal folds (unilateral or bilateral) with variable glottic insufficiency

- <u>Etiology</u>: sulcus vergeture, vocal fold scar, presbylarynx, superior laryngeal nerve paresis/paralysis
- <u>Pathophysiology</u>: varies depending on etiology (structural versus neurological)
- <u>Presentation</u>: **breathiness**, reduced volume, occasionally mild hoarseness, voice fatigue
- <u>Dx</u>: H&P, flexible laryngoscopy, **strobovideolaryngoscopy**
- <u>Tx</u>: voice therapy (sufficient for many patients), injection medialization laryngoplasty, thyroplasty

ARYTENOID DISLOCATION AND SUBLUXATION

- <u>Etiology</u>: upper airway instrumentation (ie, **intubation**, direct laryngoscopy, bronchoscopy, esophagoscopy), external laryngeal trauma, whiplash, idiopathic
- no established risk factors, but may be associated with diabetes, renal failure, autoimmune disease, acromegaly or laryngeal anomalies
- use of stylet during intubation may decrease risk
- **Anterior displacement**: typically from anterior force exerted on arytenoid by laryngoscope blade during intubation; usually prevented by posterior cricoarytenoid ligament; vocal process usually low and medial
- **Posterior displacement**: possibly from posterior pressure generated by tube during intubation; commonly an extubation injury especially if cuff is inflated; vocal process typically high and lateral
- **Anterior complex displacement**: cricoid portion of superior cricoarytenoid joint usually fractured; arytenoid is anteriorly displaced with vocal process high and variable; usually caused by laryngoscope blade during intubation
- anterior blunt neck trauma may cause anterior or posterior dislocation and is usually associated with thyroid cartilage fracture
- trauma-related cricoarytenoid hemarthrosis may result in joint fixation
- <u>Presentation</u>: hoarseness, breathiness, voice fatigue, loss of projection, dysphagia/odynophagia, laryngeal tenderness
- <u>Dx</u>: H&P, external laryngeal palpation, flexible and rigid laryngoscopy, strobovideolaryngoscopy, CT/MRI, laryngeal electromyogram, arytenoid palpation
- imaging may show displacement of arytenoid, widening of cricoarytenoid joint space and/or glottic gap but is less useful in pediatric patients (unossified cartilage)

- <u>Laryngoscopic findings</u>: reduced or absent arytenoid cartilage, true vocal fold mobility, vocal process height asymmetry (low—anterior, high—posterior), posterior glottic chink, glottic gap
- absent jostle sign if joint fixation present
- <u>Tx</u>: direct laryngoscopy and closed reduction (ideal) → open reduction if unsuccessful; voice therapy
- late treatment may lead to joint fixation, necessitating permanent medialization (injection or type 1 thyroplasty) after reduction to align vocal process height
- mobility may be restored if reduction performed within 10 weeks of injury
- restored motion is rarely normal

CHAPTER

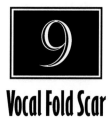

Vocal Fold Scar

Arthur Uyesugi and Jaime E. Moore

INTRODUCTION

- vocal scar results from injury to the vibrating layers of the vocal fold impairing mucosal wave and usually causing dysphonia
- etiologies of vocal fold scar include laryngeal procedures, phonotrauma, congenital causes, radiation therapy, intubation injury, external trauma, and other
- surgery for vocal fold scar produces variable results, and realistic expectations are essential before surgery is performed

ANATOMY OF THE VOCAL FOLDS

- <u>vocal fold (superficial to deep)</u>: squamous epithelium, superficial layer of the lamina propria, vocal ligament (intermediate and deep layers of the lamina propria), and thyroarytenoid muscle
- squamous epithelium and superficial lamina propria (the cover) form the mucosal wave and are chief oscillators during phonation
- symptomatic vocal fold scarring alters phonation by interfering with the mucosal wave and impairing glottic closure
- restoring vocal fold architecture and function is difficult, and impossible in some cases

CLINICAL EVALUATION

History

- onset of dysphonia (time, sudden or gradual, constant or intermittent, improving or worsening, etc)
- symptoms (hoarseness, breathiness, fatigue, effortful phonation, etc)
- vocal habits/hygiene
- vocal requirements
  1. professional voice user
  2. employment
- prior surgery (laryngeal surgery and intubation history)
- <u>comorbid conditions</u>: laryngopharyngeal reflux (LPR)/ gastroesophageal reflux disease (GERD), allergic rhinitis, autoimmune disease, head and neck radiation therapy
- patient expectations

Physical Exam

Strobovideolaryngoscopy

- essential component of examination, reliable interpretation of vocal fold motion with relatively periodic voices
- impaired mucosal wave, diminished amplitude, and glottic insufficiency may be seen
- scar typically is not an isolated laryngeal finding
    1. Associated diagnoses: muscle tension dysphonia, varix and glottic insufficiency
    2. Coexisting diagnoses: laryngeal papilloma, laryngeal cancer, leukoplakia, LPR, and phonotraumatic lesions (ie, nodules, cyst, and polyps)

Additional Testing

- high-speed digital imaging, videokymography, optical coherence tomography, narrow-band imaging, and electroglottography may help in diagnosis
- high-speed imaging able to visualize mucosal wave in highly aperiodic phonation associated with severe vocal fold scarring
- potential imaging modalities include electroglottography, ultrasound, computed tomography (CT), and magnetic resonance imaging (MRI), but their indications are not standardized
- operative evaluation with 0 and 70° telescopes and palpation may be necessary to confirm suspected findings
- **Objective voice assessment**
    1. includes aerodynamic and acoustic assessment and quality of life measures
    2. valuable for diagnosis and evaluation of treatment efficacy
    3. cepstral peak prominence may be particularly useful for vocal fold scars, as it does not rely on a periodic waveform

MANAGEMENT

Nonsurgical Management

- Voice hygiene: essential for voice optimization; includes hydration, avoidance of tobacco smoke, and encouraging safe vocal behaviors
- Voice therapy: typically improves outcomes, and hyperfunctional and compensatory behaviors occur commonly regardless of prior vocal training

- <u>Voice therapy techniques</u>:
  1. *Effective use of the support and resonator systems*: improved vocal intensity, diminished fatigue
  2. *Reduction of compensatory muscle tension dysphonia*: decreased fatigue and effort, improves accuracy of baseline vocal quality assessment
  3. *Resonant voice therapy*: improved mucosal wave and ease of phonatory tasks
  4. *Vocal function exercises and phonation resistance training exercises (PhoRTE)*: improved glottic insufficiency in select cases, especially with mild unilateral scar
- vocal fold scar usually needs to be mature (6 to 12 months) and vocal techniques need to be optimized before conclusions can be made about final voice results
- for vocal scar following head and neck cancer treatment, cancer surveillance needs to be considered before performing extensive reconstructive procedures
- quality of life scales (eg, Voice Handicap Index) can be used to gauge treatment progression

Surgical Management

- consider surgery if voice function is not satisfactory after optimal therapy
- essential for the surgeon and patient to have reasonable expectations
  1. can decrease hoarseness, phonatory effort, and breathiness
  2. can make the voice permanently worse
- surgical options vary depending on the size, location, and severity of scar

Laser and Steroids

- pulsed-dye laser (PDL) has been studied and shown to be effective in select cases, specifically less severe cases of scar
- potassium titanyl phosphate (KTP) has been shown to work in animal models and has been effective in humans
- both lasers usually require multiple treatments to be effective long term
- laser can be combined with injectable steroids
  1. steroid injections alone may be a viable option for select lesions
  2. injecting prior to use of laser can allow the steroid to act as a heat sink to prevent further tissue damage → may inactivate the steroid so reinjection after laser should be considered

3. injectable steroids should be considered as a preventative mechanism during phonosurgery
4. injection of 5-fluorouracil (5-FU) mixed with triamcinolone is highly effective for scar elsewhere and has been used successfully by the author (RTS) for vocal fold scar since 2015

Vocal Fold Medialization

- <u>Options</u>: injection medialization, type I thyroplasty
- treatment of glottic insufficiency is sometimes sufficient, and mucosal surgery can be avoided
- overcorrection can lead to strain, especially in patients with bilateral, extensive scar
   1. thyroid compression can be utilized in the office to help with evaluation
   2. injection medialization can be used as a trial if it is unclear what the voice quality might be after medialization
- procedures to restore mucosal wave should be considered before a thyroplasty

Epithelium Freeing Techniques

- <u>Microscopic direct laryngoscopy with elevation of microflaps</u>: used to release adhesions and excise scarred areas (Z-plasty-like incisions can be used to break up scar)
   1. microflap procedures done with or without implantation of various material to reconstitute the lamina propria
   2. autologous fat superficial implantation: variation of traditional microflap procedure where a mucosal pocket is created with a small access tunnel and is filled with nonmorcellized fat
- <u>External approaches</u>:
   1. Gray's minithyrotomy accesses the superficial lamina propria through a small cartilage window allowing implantation of various materials
   2. microendoscopy of Reinke's space (MERS) is a modification of Gray's minithyrotomy that uses a microendoscope to visualize the dissection space
- once the space is identified and dissected, various materials can be placed to restore the defective superficial lamina propria
- materials used in implantation include bovine collagen, allogenic collagen and fascia, autologous fat and fascia, etc
- autologous fat and fascia produce good results without the risk of foreign-body reactions

Laryngeal Resurfacing

- appropriate for cases of severe vocal fold scar
- vocal folds that are lateralized and extensively scarred
- access can be accomplished via endoscopic approach or transcervical approaches such as laryngofissure
  1. external approaches may be warranted if extensive bulk is needed
  2. bulk can be gained by rotating a pedicled strap muscle flap to fill the defect
- mucosa reconstruction can be accomplished using a buccal mucosa graft and false vocal fold flap using either an endoscopic or external approach

Sulcus Vocalis

- the majority of techniques discussed previously can be used to treat sulcus vocalis, but there are techniques specifically designed for this condition whether congenital or acquired
- Pontes and Behlau suggested a mucosal sling technique that essentially involves multiple releasing incisions
- fat implantation and autologous transplantation of fascia into the vocal fold have been used; implantation of homograft fascia has recently been trialed by the author (RTS)

Research

- absence of the vocal ligament in models can make extrapolation difficult
- the porcine model appears to be most similar to the human vocal fold
- research is progressing to establish potential growth factors, implantable cells (cell therapy), and scaffolding material that can be combined to successfully and reliably genetically reengineer the superficial layer of the lamina propria

CHAPTER

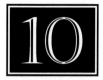

10

Vocal Fold Injury and Repair

Susan L. Thibeault

INTRODUCTION

- Hirano was one of the first to recognize the importance of the microstructure of the vocal fold
- vocal fold has five histological layers of increasing density broken down into two biomechanical layers (the body and the cover)
- body is composed primarily of muscle
- cover has been described as being composed primarily of collagen and elastin
- shape and tension of the cover determine the vibratory characteristics and subsequent vocal source quality
- shape and tension may be modified by lesions arising from the cover, which can alter vocal fold surface configuration and subsequently change vibratory biomechanics
- Gray demonstrated that the normal molecular structure of the lamina propria is constructed of a great deal more than collagen and elastin
- molecular and cell techniques and tools in voice research will likely provide new vistas for diagnosis and treatment of tissue repair in the vocal folds via wound healing

WOUND HEALING

- scar tissue represents poor reconstitution of epidermal and dermal structures at the site of the healed wound
- wound healing begins immediately following injury and is considered to occur in three phases, the inflammatory, proliferative, and remodeling phases
- sequence of repair can be broken down further to hemostasis, inflammation, mesenchymal cell migration and proliferation, angiogenesis, epithelialization, protein and proteoglycan synthesis, wound contraction, and remodeling (Table 10–1)

Hemostasis/Coagulation

- blood vessels hemorrhage in all wounds that either damage the epidermal barrier or damage the underlying structures
- hemorrhage must be truncated by hemostasis
- coagulation cascade consists of intrinsic and extrinsic pathways
- intrinsic pathway is activated when blood is exposed to a negatively charged foreign surface and factor XII is triggered
- extrinsic pathway is initiated when factor VII interacts with tissue factor, an intracellular protein that is expressed in white cells

TABLE 10–1. Summary of Normal Wound-Healing Mechanisms

Stage of Wound Healing	Time Course (Approximate)	Principal Molecular and Cellular Events
Hemostasis/coagulation	Immediately to 1 day postinjury	Formation of fibrin clot at site of injury.
Inflammation	Immediately to 3 days postinjury	Vasoconstriction and vasodilatation at site of injury.
		Presence of neutrophils followed by macrophages, whose function is to phagocytose bacteria and dead tissue and secrete enzymes for tissue breakdown.
Mesenchymal cell migration and proliferation	2 to 4 days postinjury	Fibroblasts migrate into wound site and become predominant cell type.
		Some fibroblasts phenotypically change into myofibroblasts for tissue repair.
Angiogenesis	2 to 4 days postinjury	Formation of fewer larger blood vessels at site of injury.
Epithelization	Hours to 5 days postinjury	Epithelial cell migration to form epithelium and BMZ.
Protein and proteoglycan synthesis	3 to 5 days to 6 weeks postinjury	Formation of ECM through production of proteins, proteoglycans, glycoaminoglycans by fibroblasts.
Wound contraction and remodeling	3 days to 12 months postinjury	Myofibroblasts and collagen mediate contraction.
		Scar remodeling consists of turnover of ECM proteins, proteoglycans, and glycoaminoglycans.
		Apoptosis of myofibroblasts and epithelial cells.

- extrinsic pathway enters the common pathway directly through activation of factor X resulting in the production of thrombin, which catalyzes the conversion of fibrinogen to fibrin, and factor XIII, which stabilizes the fibrin polymer in platelet aggregates
- fibrin becomes the main component of the provisional matrix that provides a scaffold that allows for future migration of inflammatory and mesenchymal cells

- platelets are the first cells to arrive at the wound site, and they adhere to fibrin and release adenosine diphosphate (ADP), which in the presence of calcium stimulates further platelet aggregation
- platelet aggregation directs release of multiple cytokines—platelet-derived growth factor (PDGF), TGF-β, TGF-α, bFGF, platelet-derived epidermal growth factor (PDEFG), and platelet-derived endothelial cell growth factor (PDECGF), which contribute to repair at various times of healing

Inflammation

- inflammation begins shortly after the wound is created and is initiated with intense local vasoconstriction that is replaced by vasodilatation after approximately 10 to 15 minutes
- vasoconstriction contributes to hemostasis and is mediated by circulating catecholamines and the sympathetic nervous system
- vasodilatation generates heat and erythema at the site of injury
- capillaries develop gaps between the endothelial cells, creating edema
- inflammatory factor signaling is a complex process initiated by platelet degranulation and factor secretion, subsequently, recruiting various immune cells to the injury
- signaling for inflammatory factor proteins cyclooxygenase 2 (COX-2), interleukin 1 beta (IL-1β), and tumor necrosis factor alpha (TNF-α) has been documented to occur as early as 1-hour postinjury in the rat vocal fold model
- significant upregulation for nuclear factor kappa beta (NF-κβ), COX-2, transforming growth factor beta (TGF-β1), and IL-1β is observed as early as 4 hours postinjury
   1. IL-1β, NF-κβ, and TNF-α expression peaks at 4 to 8 hours
   2. TGF-β1 expression peaks at 72 hours
- neutrophils arrive shortly following acute inflammation, which serve to engulf foreign material and absorb it using hydrolytic enzymes and oxygen radicals
- neutrophils, albumin, and globulin then penetrate the matrix
- 48 to 84 hours after injury, neutrophils are phagocytosed and destroyed by macrophages
- release of the destructive proteolytic enzymes and free oxygen radicals can damage tissue and be held responsible for persistent inflammation and chronic infection in wounds
- circulating monocytes originating from the bone marrow and blood migrate from the capillaries into the extravascular space
- *Macrophages*: peak at 48 hours and are a primary source of cytokines that stimulate proliferation of fibroblasts and the production of

collagen, TGF-β, PDGF, EGF, and fibroblast growth factor, which promotes tissue formation

1. function to phagocytose bacteria and dead tissue and secrete collagenases, elastases, and tissue inhibitors of metalloproteinases (TIMPs)
2. outnumber neutrophils as the primary cell type from 48 to 72 hours after injury and are replaced by fibroblasts

- 72 hours postinjury, expression levels peak for procollagen 1 and 3 conferring increased fibroblast infiltration and suggesting transition into the proliferative wound-healing phase
- chronic inflammation can occur if there is foreign material or bacteria at the site of injury, and can cause tissue damage and infection, because the neutrophils release destructive proteolytic enzymes and free oxygen radicals that cause damage

Mesenchymal Cell Migration and Proliferation

- mesenchymal stromal cells (MSCs) are multipotent cells with the ability for differentiation to diverse mesenchymal lineages
- circulatory MSCs migrate to the vocal fold injury site and remain at the site for a prolonged period producing growth factors such as vascular endothelial growth factor and hepatocyte growth factor
- mesenchymal cell migration and proliferation occur 2 to 4 days after injury
- cellular recruitment to the wound site consists primarily of fibrocyte recruitment as a precursor to fibroblast differentiation and occurs following the inflammatory phase in the vocal folds
- fibrocytes are a type of inactive mesenchymal cell categorized as a leukocyte subpopulation in peripheral blood that originate from the bone marrow and enter the circulatory system to migrate to the injury site by way of cytokine signaling
- fibroblasts from surrounding undamaged tissue migrate into the wounded matrix in response to chemotactic signals
- specific, reactive fibrocyte population largely unique to vocal fold lamina propria has been found and characterized by intracellular prolyl-4-hydroxylase-ß expression and CD11b expression on the cell surface
- fibroblasts undergo a phenotypic change into myofibroblasts that allows them to repair injured tissue
- presence of myofibroblasts is an indication of tissue injury

Angiogenesis

- angiogenesis restructures new vasculature in the area of injury
- mediated by high lactate levels, acidic pH, and decreased oxygen tensions in the tissue
- basic fibroblast growth factor stimulates angiogenesis, improving vascularization and increasing the number of fibroblasts at the site of injury
- small capillary sprouts forms on venules at the periphery of the devascularized area
- capillary sprouts grow and proliferate into capillaries, which mature through aggregation of many capillaries into fewer larger vessels

Epithelialization

- renewal of the epithelial barrier is essential for repair and begins within hours of injury
- earliest sign of epithelialization is thickening of the basal cell layer at the wound edge
- basal cells elongate, detach from the underlying basement membrane, and migrate into the wound
- migration occurs along collagen fibers in a leapfrog fashion until they reach other cells (contact guidance)
- once contact inhibition is achieved, cells undergo a phenotypic transformation resembling basal-like cells
- compared to normal epithelium newly differentiated basal cells are fewer in number, and the basement membrane zone (BMZ) is atypical
- preserving epithelium and the BMZ improves wound healing
- in the vocal fold there is rapid epithelial regeneration following vocal fold injury with a multilayered confluent epithelium and intercellular junctional complexes returning 3 days postinjury in a rat model and 5 days postinjury in a rabbit model
- recovery of intercellular junction protein E-cadherin and transglutaminase-1 is present 3 to 7 days postinjury
- epithelial barrier remains functionally impaired up to 5 weeks postinjury

Protein and Proteoglycan Synthesis

- fibroblasts that are in the wound begin to produce proteins 3 to 5 days after injury through 14 days postinjury
- major protein synthesized is collagen, which constitutes 50% of the protein found in scar
- collagen types III and I appearing at 1 and 3 days postinjury, respectively

- collagen synthesis is maximum 2 to 4 weeks after injury
- synthesis can be altered by several factors (eg, age, stress, and pressure) and various growth factors (eg, FGF, EGF, and TGF-β)
- collagen type III matrix replaces the fibrin scaffold
- collagen type I offering additional strength to this scaffold
- fibroblasts are responsible for production of the proteoglycans and glycoaminoglycans (HA) at the injured site
- HA production is stimulated by PDGF28 and plays an important role in early wound healing
- HA peaks at 5 days postinjury
- there are no differences in overall density of HA between injured and uninjured vocal folds in different animal models at 2 to 6 months postinjury
- hyaluronic acid synthase 1 (*HAS-1*) gene is upregulated 1 hour postinjury, with peak expression occurring 4 hours after injury
- hyaluronic acid synthase 2 (HAS-2) peaks 16 hours and 72 hours postinjury
- FN is produced throughout all stages of wound healing with particularly strong expression observed 3 to 14 days postinjury
- FN promotes reepithlialization and matrix deposition
- elastin is not synthesized in response to injury
- scar tissue lacks the normal amount of elastin, decreasing the elastic properties of the repaired tissue

Wound Contraction and Remodeling

- **Wound contraction**: centripetal movement of the wound edge toward the center of the wound
- **Myofibroblasts**: likely contribute wound contraction; present on the third day after injury and remain until 21 days postinjury at the periphery of the wound
- **Scar remodeling**: stable collagen accumulation beginning ~21 days postinjury; final stage of wound healing
- apoptosis of epithelial cells and myofibroblasts occurs during remodeling
- **Early immature scar**: present during the first 1 to 3 months following injury; stiff and thick, with elevated procollagen I levels and collagen bundles that are notably less dense but disorganized with less dense elastin
- **Mature scar**: generally thinner and more pliable
- collagen densities and elastin disorganization remain higher than in intact vocal fold tissue despite a return to normal levels of procollagen and elastin at 6 months
- scar remodeling can continue up to 12 months with turnover of collagen in a denser, more organized fashion along lines of stress

- 80% breaking strength is achieved in the new scar tissue via an increase in the number of intra- and intermolecular cross-links between collagen fibers

VOCAL FOLD MANIFESTATIONS OF INJURY AND REPAIR

- <u>Etiology of vocal fold injury</u>: excessive vocal use or phonotrauma, intubation, intentional or incidental resection of laryngeal tissue, inflammation (infection or physical irritants), external laryngeal injury (blunt or penetrating)
- injured tissue causes alterations in normal vocal fold lamina propria viscosity and oscillatory motion

Wound Healing Paradigms in Benign Vocal Fold Lesions

- vocal fold scarring alters the body-cover relationship and inhibits propagation of normal mucosal wave
- relationship between the ultrastructural changes of the ECM and their effect on the viscoelastic properties of the tissue (stiffness and viscosity) presents potential treatment avenues
- rheologically, when compared to the normal lamina propria, scarred vocal fold lamina propria was found to have significantly increased levels of viscosity and stiffness
- **Scarred lamina propria**: new, unorganized collagen, and less elastin distributed in scattered networks, decreased decorin, increases procollagen I, less fibromodulin and elevated FN
- **Vocal fold polyp**: superficial lamina propria edema, decreased FN, less adhesion loss in the BMZ, and increased vascular injury characterize polyps
- **Reinke's edema**: superficial lamina propria edema, increased fibrin, hemorrhage and thickening of the BMZ, and decreased FN transcript levels

Protein's Role in Modulating Vocal Fold Tissue Viscosity (Table 10–2)

- there is a direct relationship between the biomechanical properties of the vocal fold and the constituents of the lamina propria
- relationship between increased tissue stiffness, viscosity, and changes in the fibrous and interstitial proteins not fully understood

TABLE 10–2. Characteristics of ECM Players in Normal and Injured Lamina Propia

ECM Player	Function	Localization in Normal Lamina Propria	Localization in Injured Lamina Propria
Collagen	Provide strength to lamina propria	Density increases across superficial layer of lamina propria to deep layer of lamina propria	Disorganized and decreased in scarred lamina propria Decreased in vocal fold polyps with stiffer mucosal waves
Elastin	Provide stretch and recoil of the lamina propria	Highest density in middle layer of lamina propria	Decreased in scar tissue
Procollagen type I	Precursor to collagen	Unknown in normal lamina propria	Increased in scarred lamina propria
Decorin	Promote lateral association of collagen fibrils to form fibers and fiber bundles in the ECM Binds to fibronectin and TGF-β	Found throughout lamina propria. Highest density is in superficial layer of the lamina propria	Decreased in scarred lamina propria
Fibronectin	Induces cell migration and ECM synthesis. May be involved in the development of fibrosis	Found throughout the lamina propria including the BMZ (specialized lamina propria)	Increased in scarred lamina propria Increased in vocal fold polyps. Higher levels of fibronectin associated with stiffer mucosal waves in vocal fold polyps mRNA levels decreased in Reinke's edema Increased levels in BMZ of nodules
Fibromodulin	Inhibits TGF-β, which upregulates collagen synthesis Plays role in collagen fibrillogenesis	Found in the intermediate and deep layers of the lamina propria	Decreased in scar lamina propria mRNA levels decreased in vocal fold polyps and increased in Reinke's edema

continues

TABLE 10–2. *continued*

TGF-β	Upregulated fibronectin and collagen synthesis	Has not been measured in normal lamina propria	Has not been measured in injured lamina propria
	Downregulates synthesis of decorin		
	Inhibited by fibromodulin		

- increased stiffness, increased viscosity, or decreased mucosal wave characterized by decreased collagen, increased FN, decreased fibromodulin, and decreased decorin
- interstitial proteins play an important role in the organization and regulation of the fibrous proteins
- levels of the interstitial proteins that are directly related to the viscoelastic properties of vocal fold tissue, resultant to their interface with fibrous proteins
- contributing role of interstitial proteins in the fibrous protein architecture may be related to TGF-β
- **TGF-β**: upregulates FN and new collagen synthesis; downregulates the synthesis of decorin in vitro, and is inhibited by fibromodulin; levels unmeasured in vocal fold lamina propria

MICROARRAY ANALYSIS OF VOCAL FOLD WOUND HEALING AND BENIGN VOCAL FOLD LESIONS

- global patterns of gene expression in benign laryngeal disease and healing have been measured with DNA microarray (MA), a high-throughput genomic technology
- following vocal fold injury transcriptional activity appears highest at the 3-day time point and subsides gradually over time
- gene activity in vocal fold injury is associated with cellular remodeling and repair along with muscle differentiation, notably corresponding with the respective temporal stages in the wound healing paradigm
- for polyps and Reinke's edema, transcription profiling has revealed differences in expression of 65 genes allowing for pathologic discrimination

1. <u>Polyps</u>: three overexpressed genes (*SPARC*, *SPARCL1*, and *Col6A3*) are responsible for ECM remodeling, cell growth, and tissue development and repair
2. <u>Reinke's edema</u>: *MAP2K3*, *SOD1*, *GPX2*, *GTSA2*, and *CASP9* genes were overexpressed suggesting that Reinke's edema is associated with changes secondary to oxidative stress

- vocal fold granuloma and vocal fold polyp have two different levels of cellular activity as measured by MA
- upregulated wound healing, inflammation, and matrix remodeling genes differentiate vocal fold granuloma with speculation that a continuous repair response is present for vocal granulomas with an emphasis on the inflammation stage
- downregulated membrane receptor genes for vocal polyps imply anomalies in normal cellular activity, indicating a system inhibition rather than overexpression of ECM
- cluster of epithelial regulated genes highly expressed in vocal fold polyp specifies greater activity in the epithelium compared to normal true vocal fold
- differing reports regarding alterations in the epithelium of vocal fold polyp have been described
- repetitive vocal trauma can be reflected by changes in the BMZ, demonstrating a separation of the epithelium from the underlying dermis

FUTURE DIRECTIONS AND THERAPEUTIC APPLICATIONS

- improved understanding of the alterations in tissue viscosity and elasticity is needed to appreciate fully the biological manifestations of the complexity of wound healing in the vocal fold lamina propria
- research in vocal fold biology has demonstrated that the interactions between the ECM components in vocal fold disease states are complicated
- viscoelastic properties of vocal fold tissue appear to be related to relationships between the fibrous and interstitial proteins
- all vocal fold lesions do not appear to follow a typical wound-healing paradigm
- potential therapeutic applications targeting facets of each of the stages of wound healing have been recent research focus

CHAPTER

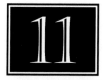

11

Laryngotracheal Trauma

Yolanda D. Heman-Ackah

continues

INTRODUCTION

- incidence of laryngotracheal trauma is estimated to be 1 in 14,000 to 30,000 emergency department visits in the United States
- strangulation injuries are primary cause of death, incidence of 1.17% of all deaths
- <u>Classification</u>: blunt, penetrating, caustic, thermal iatrogenic
- <u>Morbidity from laryngotracheal trauma</u>: voice compromise, dyspnea, dysphagia, chronic airway obstruction
- mortality rate from laryngotracheal trauma ranges from 2% to 17.9%

SCHAEFER CLASSIFICATION SYSTEM FOR SEVERITY OF LARYNGEAL INJURIES

- <u>Grade I</u>: minor endolaryngeal hematoma without detectable fracture
- <u>Grade II</u>: edema, hematoma, minor mucosal disruption without exposed cartilage, nondisplaced fractures
- <u>Grade III</u>: massive edema, mucosal disruption, exposed cartilage, vocal fold immobility, displaced fracture
- <u>Grade IV</u>: grade III with 2 fracture lines or massive trauma to laryngeal mucosa
- <u>Grade V</u>: complete laryngotracheal separation

ADULT FRAMEWORK INJURY

Etiology

- most common mechanisms of fatal laryngotracheal injury
  1. hanging (41%)
  2. strangulation (15.4%)
  3. motor vehicle accidents (15.4%)

4. falls (7.7%)
5. assault from blunt trauma other than strangulation (5.1%)
6. incised wounds (3.8%)
7. gunshot wounds (2.6%)
8. explosions (1.3%)
9. other/unexplained (7.8%)
- most common mechanisms of nonfatal laryngotracheal injury
  1. sport-related physical contact (39%)
  2. physical assault (33%)
  3. penetrating (16.7%-20%)
  4. motor vehicle (11.3%)

Anatomical Considerations

- inferior border of the cricoid cartilage sits at the level of the sixth and seventh cervical vertebrae
- structural barriers to laryngeal injury (in upright position):
  1. overhang of the mandible superiorly
  2. bony prominence of the clavicles and sternal manubrium inferiorly
  3. mass of the sternocleidomastoid muscles laterally
- laryngeal injuries are relatively rare except with a direct blow to the neck

Mechanism of Injury

Anterior Forces

- cause the thyroid cartilage to bend against the cervical vertebrae on impact
- younger larynges (<40 years) are more pliable due to limited ossification
- thyroid cartilage has a point of maximal flexibility, beyond which a fracture occurs as:
  1. single median fracture
  2. single paramedian fracture
  3. comminuted anterior thyroid cartilage fracture
- following fracture of the thyroid cartilage:
  1. cricoid ring is no longer shielded by the thyroid cartilage
  2. vector of force is then distributed onto the cricoid cartilage due to low position in neck
  3. cricoid cartilage has a thin anterior arch that curves laterally into rigidly buttressed tubercle, which increases resistance to lower impact forces in both men and women

   4. cricoid is the only complete cartilaginous ring of the airway, and
      its presence helps to maintain the patency of the airway
- lower-level impact may result in:
   1. single median cricoid cartilage fracture
   2. multiple paramedian cricoid cartilage fractures
   3. the airway is maintained by the remaining structure of the lateral
      buttresses of the cricoid cartilage
- higher-level impact forces result in secondary lateral arch of cricoid
   fracture:
   1. loss of the lateral buttress then can lend to airway collapse
   2. recurrent laryngeal nerve injury from impingement of the nerve
      near the cricothyroid joint

Circumferential Forces

- most frequent cause is strangulation
- can cause fractures of thyroid and cricoid cartilage and hyoid bone

Hanging Injuries

- typically have a vector of force at the level of the thyroid cartilage and
   the hyoid bone
- the cricoid cartilage is rarely fractured
- fracture of the cricoid cartilage should raise the suspicion for
   strangulation and physical assault
- descent is typically several feet, resulting in:
   1. fracture of the thyroid cartilage and hyoid bone
   2. thyrohyoid transection
   3. C1–C2 dislocation, which causes spinal cord injury
- death is usually imminent

Laryngotracheal Separation

- can be caused by severe forces and forces low in the neck
- was relatively common during motor vehicle accidents in adults prior
   to development of airbags and mandatory use of shoulder straps
- usually occurs between the cricoid cartilage and the first tracheal ring
   1. causes displacement of the trachea inferiorly and soft tissue
      collapse into the airway/airway obstruction
   2. strap muscles and surrounding cervical fascia often serve as a
      temporary conduit for air until edema and hematoma cause
      obstruction of this temporary airway
- often concurrent bilateral recurrent laryngeal nerve injury

PEDIATRIC FRAMEWORK INJURY

Anatomic Considerations

- larynx sits higher in the neck in children than it does in adults, and can lie between the second and seventh cervical vertebrae depending on age
- mandible serves as more of a protective shield in the child than it does in the adult
- pediatric larynx is more cartilaginous than the adult larynx (which ossifies)
  1. greater elasticity than the adult larynx
  2. more resilient to external stresses
  3. more mobile than the adult
- children are more likely to sustain soft tissue injuries (ie, edema, hematoma) than fractures of the larynx
- greater risk of airway compromise from small amounts of edema and hemorrhage
- mortality rate in children from laryngeal trauma is 8.7%

Mechanisms of Injury

Telescoping Injury

- typically caused by a fall onto the handlebar of a bicycle
- cricoid cartilage is dislocated superiorly underneath the thyroid lamina

Transection Injuries

- typically caused by more forceful anterior injuries
- snowmobile or all-terrain vehicle causing collision with a cable or wire—often called a "clothesline" injury
- horizontal, linear force low in the neck causes:
  1. compression of the cricotracheal complex against the anterior cervical vertebrae
  2. possible cricotracheal separation
  3. substernal retraction of the trachea due to elasticity of the intercartilaginous ligaments
- commonly fatal, although fascial stenting can at times maintain an adequate airway long enough for an artificial airway to be established
- often associated with injuries to the esophagus, bony cervical spine, spinal cord, and recurrent laryngeal nerves

Hanging Injuries

- young children may accidentally hang themselves while playing
- adolescents may intentionally hang themselves (ie, suicide attempts, internet "challenges")
- fall to hanging usually less than 1 to 2 feet
- rope tightens in the region of the thyrohyoid membrane usually, causing avulsion but not transection
- airway obstruction occurs as the epiglottis is closed over the glottis
- death usually is not imminent (as it is in intentional hanging)

SOFT TISSUE INJURIES FROM BLUNT TRAUMA

Horizontal or Vertical Fractures of the Thyroid Ala

Rupture of the Thyroepiglottic Ligament

- narrowing of the laryngeal lumen
- herniation of pre-epiglottic tissue
- posterior displacement of the epiglottic petiole

Vocal Fold Injuries

- tear of the thyroarytenoid muscle or ligament
- mucosal laceration of the vocal fold
- hemorrhage of the vocal fold
- malposition of the vocal fold from a displaced or overlapping thyroid cartilage fracture

Arytenoid Injuries

- arytenoid mucosal degloving
- arytenoid cartilage or vocal process avulsion
- cricoarytenoid cartilage dislocation

Esophageal/Pyriform Sinus Mucosal Injuries

- laceration
- perforation

Nerve Injury

- <u>Recurrent laryngeal nerve</u>: due to impingement from blunt trauma or transection from separation injuries
- <u>Phrenic nerve</u>: occurs in cases of cricotracheal separation

Other

- pneumothorax/pneumomediastinum: should raise suspicion for associated laryngeal fracture
- mucosal lacerations anywhere along the laryngotracheal complex

Strangulation and Hanging Injuries

- carotid intimal tear in 9.1%
- jugular vein injury in 2.2%
- carotid adventitia rupture in 21.7%

CLINICAL EVALUATION OF BLUNT TRAUMA

- similar for adults and children
- an understanding of the mechanism of injury (vector and degree of force) is extremely important

Initial Assessment
(See Chapter 31 for Pediatric Focus)

- begins with assessment of the airway and signs of airway compromise
- if no airway compromise, start with a complete examination:
  1. palpate the neck
  2. assess voice quality
  3. flexible laryngoscopy: evaluate mobility of vocal folds, patency of upper airway, and integrity of laryngeal mucosa
- serial examination of the airway over 24 to 48 hours if intubation or tracheotomy is not necessary
- **Signs of laryngeal injury**: dysphonia, stridor, vocal fold hemorrhage, endolaryngeal, hemorrhage/hematoma, endolaryngeal laceration, dysphagia/odynophagia, hemoptysis, ecchymosis or abrasions of anterior neck, dyspnea, endolaryngeal edema, subcutaneous emphysema, neck pain, laryngeal point tenderness, loss of laryngeal

landmarks, impaired vocal fold mobility, arytenoid dislocation, exposed endolaryngeal cartilage

Presence of Laryngeal Injury

- if airway stable → computed tomography (CT) of neck/larynx
    1. are there signs of fracture instability? (Table 11–1)
    2. are there indications for surgical exploration? (Table 11–2)
    3. if signs of fracture instability or indications for surgical exploration → proceed to the operating room for surgical exploration and repair (Figure 11–1)
- if airway unstable → secure the airway and then proceed to the operating room for surgical exploration and repair
    1. stabilize the neck to prevent worsening of possible cervical spine injuries
    2. perform tracheotomy at least 2 tracheal rings below the injured segment or through the distal transected segment under local anesthesia

TABLE 11–1. CT Findings That Suggest Fracture Stability

Fracture Type	Displacement	Likely Stable	Management
Single vertical, unilateral	Nondisplaced	Yes	Observe, fixate if symptoms or exam worsen
	Minimally displaced (<1 cartilage width)	Yes	Fixate if immediate or delayed voice change, otherwise observe
	Displaced (>1 cartilage width)	No	Reduce and fixate
Single horizontal, unilateral	Nondisplaced	Yes	Observe, fixate if symptoms or exam worse
	Minimally displaced	Yes	Observe, fixate if symptoms or exam worsen
	Displaced	No	Reduce and fixate
Multiple unilateral	Nondisplaced	No	Reduce and fixate
	Displaced	No	Reduce and fixate
Multiple bilateral	Nondisplaced	No	Reduce and fixate
	Displaced	No	Reduce and fixate

TABLE 11–2. Indications for Operative Evaluation After Blunt Laryngeal Trauma

Laceration of vibrating edge of true vocal fold

Laceration of anterior commissure

Deep laceration of thyroarytenoid muscle

Exposed cartilage

Impaired vocal fold mobility

Arytenoid dislocation

Epiglottis displacement

Herniation of preepiglottic contents

Unstable/displaced laryngeal fractures

Airway compromise

Extensive endolaryngeal edema

3. in cases of severe laryngotracheal trauma, avoid orotracheal and/ or nasopharyngeal intubation (can precipitate complete tracheal separation)
4. if tracheotomy is impossible or inappropriate, consider transglottic jet ventilation

Pediatric Airway Distress (*See* Chapter 31)

SURGICAL EXPLORATION AND REPAIR

Intraoperative Evaluation

- tracheotomy if needed for surgical access to the larynx or for postoperative airway management
- direct laryngoscopy to evaluate endolaryngeal integrity and palpate arytenoids for signs of dislocation (reduce if needed)
- bronchoscopy
- esophagoscopy

Open Exploration and Order of Repair

Repair Mucosal and Thyroarytenoid Muscle Lacerations

- perform within 24 hours of injury

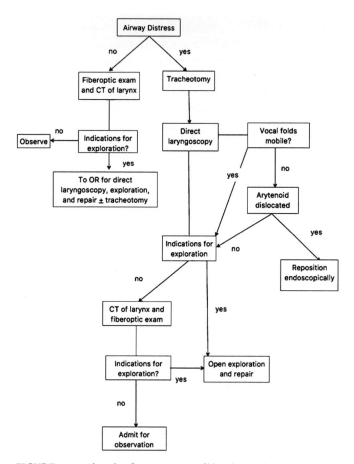

FIGURE 11–1. Algorithm for management of blunt laryngeal trauma.

- repair mucosa at the anterior commissure and vibratory margin of the vocal folds
- promotes healing by primary intention and minimizes granulation tissue formation

Restore Mucosal Cover Over Exposed Cartilage

- local mucosal flaps if necessary
- fine absorbable suture on an atraumatic needle

Reposition the Vocal Ligament at the Anterior Commissure

- preferably access endolarynx via median fractures or paramedian fractures less than 0.5 cm from the midline
- may create a midline thyrotomy if no midline/paramedian access is available
- once vocal ligament addressed, displaced epiglottis or herniated pre-epiglottic contents can be appropriately repositioned

Endolaryngeal Stent Placement

- <u>Indications</u>:
    1. severely comminuted fractures that are not amenable to external fixation
    2. extensive lacerations of opposing mucosa that are not amenable to primary repair of at least 1 side
    3. mucosal injury in the region of the anterior commissure
- stent should be soft and pliable so that it does not cause pressure necrosis
- should be secured to prevent mobilization
- remove in 7–14 days
- place stent prior to fixation of framework injuries

Reduce and Fixate Displaced/Unstable Fractures

- open reduction and fixation with miniplates (ideal)
- figure-of-eight stitch with permanent suture if unable to fixate miniplates
- **Miniplates**: titanium or absorbable 3-dimensional miniplates (low-profile plates ~1.2–1.4 mm) drill bit should be 2 sizes smaller than the screw
- reduce cricothyroid joint dislocations
- laryngotracheal reanastomosis if required

Repair Injuries to the Recurrent Laryngeal Nerve

- freshen the edges of a severed nerve
- reanastomose the epineurium in a tension-free closure
- if a tension-free closure cannot be performed → ansa cervicalis to recurrent laryngeal nerve transfer or hypoglossal to recurrent laryngeal nerve transfer
- if nerve transfer cannot be performed → cable graft using a greater auricular, sural, or homograft nerve

Postoperative Management

- strict voice rest if mucosal repair of the vibratory margin
- place small nasogastric feeding tube at time of surgical exploration for feeding in the immediate postoperative period
- aggressive antireflux protocol
- perioperative antibiotics
- systemic corticosteroids
- routine tracheotomy care to minimize coughing including cool humidified air
- head of bed elevation may help resolve edema

PENETRATING INJURIES

- second most common cause of laryngotracheal injuries in the adult and the most common cause in the pediatric population
- Causes: stab wounds, gunshot wounds, dog bites, explosion injuries

Mechanism of Injury

- direction of the force
- object used to create the force
- injury crosses midline → increases likelihood of upper aerodigestive tract injury

Gunshot Injuries

- note the entrance and exit wounds
- small-caliber, high-velocity bullets produce greater tissue damage than do larger-caliber low-velocity bullets
- handgun bullets: shorter and fly with a straight trajectory, resulting in tissue damage at the site of impact
- shotgun slugs: longer and unstable in their trajectory; tumbling of the slug causes "shock wave" damage to surrounding tissue that may extend several centimeters from the site of impact

Explosion Injuries

- produce diffuse injury to multiple structures in the neck
- require a full neck exploration to identify the full extent of the injury
- structures commonly injured include larynx, trachea, carotid artery, jugular vein, supporting soft tissues of the neck

- laryngeal fractures are typically comminuted → often requires rigid fixation and endolaryngeal stenting

Stab Wounds/Dog Bites

- important to note the location and direction of the entrance wound
    1. injury can occur at a significant distance from site of entry
- patients can appear deceptively comfortable despite impending airway compromise, vascular injuries, and/or esophageal perforations
- high index of suspicion for injuries is necessary
- mortality rates as high as 19%

Assessment of Penetrating Injuries

- assess airway patency: observation versus orotracheal intubation versus tracheotomy dependent on individual situation
- evaluate and control vascular and cervical spine injuries
- assess remaining neck structures
- flexible laryngoscopy if injury crossed midline
- CT scan of the soft tissues of the neck
- esophagram: use water-soluble contrast rather than barium (increased risk of mediastinitis); high false-negative rate of 21%
- esophagoscopy: perform if signs of esophageal perforation (ie, odynophagia, fever, back pain, chest pain, pneumomediastinum)
- Tx: surgical repair if signs of upper aerodigestive tract injury are present (Table 11–3)
- muscle interposition flap between penetrating injury of posterior tracheal wall and anterior esophageal wall

Table 11–3. Indications for Operative Evaluation of Penetrating Laryngeal Injury

- Endolaryngeal lacerations
- Expanding neck hematoma
- Subcutaneous emphysema
- Audible air leak from neck wound
- Hemoptysis
- Laryngeal framework disruption
- Impaired vocal fold mobility
- Endolaryngeal edema
- Dysphagia/odynophagia
- Stridor/dyspnea

CAUSTIC INJURIES (*See* Chapter 31)

- occur in adults and children
- children less than 5 years—ingestions tend to be accidental
- caustic ingestion in adolescents and adults tends to be suicide attempt—produce the most severe injuries
- **Bases**: liquefaction necrosis of muscle, collagen, and lipids; results in progressively worsening injury over time
- **Acids**: coagulation necrosis; damage occurs rapidly and often is superficial
- **Bleaches**: pH close to neutral, endolaryngeal damage is minimal
- **Low-phosphate/nonphosphate detergents**: small amounts can cause severe upper airway edema and airway compromise within 1 to 5 hours after ingestion
- affect the following areas from direct contact: oral cavity, pharynx, esophagus, larynx (epiglottis and supraglottis)
- Tx: admit for airway observation; if edema is present, stabilize airway with tracheotomy—avoid nasotracheal and orotracheal intubation
- irrigate the mouth, pharynx, and laryngeal inlet with water or saline to remove any remnants of the offending agent
- evaluate the esophagus for injury

THERMAL INJURIES

- burn injuries from external fire or inhaled hot air, steam, ember, and other
- thermal insult may extend throughout the supraglottic and glottic larynx, tracheobronchial tree, and lung parenchyma
- evaluate with flexible laryngoscopy and bronchoscopy
  1. presence of carbonized material in the larynx
  2. inflammation in the larynx
  3. edema in the larynx
  4. necrosis in the larynx
  5. may have significant burn injury without signs of edema initially
  6. edema usually comes following resuscitation from hypovolemic shock
- airway protection is primary concern: endotracheal intubation (preferred) or tracheotomy if cannot be intubated
- Complications: laryngeal stenosis, web or nonobstructing scar; may occur several months following injury
- repair is delayed until scar formation has stabilized

IATROGENIC INJURIES

Radionecrosis

- radiation therapy typically causes mucosal drying/xerostomia and laryngeal edema (especially if acute)
- **radionecrosis** occurs in 1% of patients receiving doses 6000 to 7000 cGy
- increased incidence with larger daily fractions
- aggravated by laryngopharyngeal reflux
- difficult to distinguish from tumor recurrence
- often require direct laryngoscopy and biopsy
- T̲x̲: hyperbaric oxygen, consider laryngectomy (partial or total) if conservative management fails

Intubation/Laryngoscopy/Upper Endoscopy (See Chapters 12 and 13)

- often caused by prolonged intubation
- occurs in adults, children, and neonates

Neonates (*See* Chapter 31)

- circumferential granulation tissue, scarring and stenosis of the subglottis results
- cricoid is the narrowest part of the neonatal airway and the most traumatized by the endotracheal tube
- T̲x̲:
    1. <50% stenosis: observation (if asymptomatic), dilation, and/or excision
    2. 50% to 70% stenosis: dilation and/or excision, endoscopic or open excision
    3. >70% stenosis: endoscopic or open (cricoid split ± cartilage grafting, cricotracheal resection); increased likelihood of open procedure with greater degree of stenosis

Adults (*See* Chapters 12 and 13)

- glottis is the narrowest portion of the airway
- posterior glottis supports the endotracheal tube, which can cause ischemic necrosis of the mucosa overlying the vocal process, resulting in:
    1. ulceration

   2. chondritis
   3. granulation (*see* Chapter 8)
   4. scarring
- must remove the endotracheal tube and treat for laryngopharyngeal reflux
- management of resulting laryngotracheal stenosis varies (*see* Chapters 12 through14)

Arytenoid Dislocation (See Chapter 8)

CHAPTER

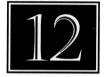

Acquired Glottic Stenosis

Jared M. Goldfarb, Justin Ross, and Joseph R. Spiegel

ANATOMY

Anterior Glottic Stenosis (AGS)

- musculomembranous vocal folds
- anterior commissure
- anterior cricoid lamina

Posterior Glottic Stenosis (PGS)

- posterior two-fifths of the true vocal folds (cartilaginous portion)
- interarytenoid region (posterior commissure): interarytenoid muscle, overlying mucosa
- cricoarytenoid joints (CAJs)
- posterior cricoid lamina

ETIOLOGY

- may be congenital, iatrogenic, trauma (ie, caustic ingestion, thermal injury, blunt/penetrating), related to infection (eg, tuberculosis, diphtheria), autoimmune disease (ie, granulomatosis with polyangiitis, sarcoidosis, amyloidosis), or radiation
- AGS more often congenital than PGS, but rare overall
- surgical intervention to opposing vocal fold mucosal surfaces commonly causes AGS
- AGS and especially PGS are commonly caused by endotracheal intubation
    1. traumatic intubations
    2. prolonged intubation
    3. repeated intubations
    4. large endotracheal tube

EVALUATION

- diagnosis often made after failure of attempted extubation
- some present with persistent dyspnea and or dysphonia after extubation
- increased f0 and persistent falsetto may be seen in anterior stenosis
- anterior or posterior stenosis may present with respiratory distress, biphasic stridor, aphonia (severe stenosis)
- Cohen classification for anterior stenosis originally described in pediatric population (see following text)

Laryngoscopy

- stroboscopy can be useful to determine relative vocal fold tension and height
- video recording especially useful when patients can produce only short "bursts" of voice
- if tracheotomy is present, flexible laryngoscopy from below can be the best visualization of the posterior laryngeal airway

Other Testing

- laryngeal electromyogram can differentiate paralysis from CAJ fixation
- CT neck and chest: contrast not necessary unless a laryngeal neoplasm or abscess or an extralaryngeal lesion is suspected
  1. fine-cut study (1-mm slices) of larynx can demonstrate arytenoid position
  2. other potential sites of airway stenosis assessed
- pulmonary function testing
- objective voice analysis can help determine effects of airflow on voice
- endoscopic and microscopic examination under general anesthesia with palpation of arytenoid complex and interarytenoid region

Anterior Stenosis: Cohen Classification

- Type I: <35% obstruction
- Type II: 35% to 50% obstruction
- Type III: 50% to 75% obstruction
- Type IV: 75% to 90% obstruction

Posterior Stenosis: Bogdasarian Classification

- Type I: interarytenoid scar band separate from interarytenoid mucosa/muscle
- Type II: interarytenoid scarring involving mucosa and muscle
- Type III: interarytenoid scarring with unilateral CAJ fixation
- Type IV: interarytenoid scarring with bilateral CAJ fixation

TREATMENT

- management of underlying gastroesophageal reflux disease/LPR and autoimmune conditions essential

- treat causative infections if indicated
- smoking cessation
- voice therapy can improve postoperative outcomes and avoid secondary laryngeal pathologies (ie, muscle tension dysphonia, polyp, cyst, nodule, scar)
- <u>Surgical indications</u>: dyspnea, bothersome dysphonia
- botulinum toxin injection into thyroarytenoid, lateral cricoarytenoid and interarytenoid muscle following operative intervention may decrease restenosis by restricting adduction
- topical mitomycin C may delay restenosis—no optimized protocol to guide use
- steroid injections may help soften immature scar
- mature scar does not typically respond well to simple scar division and dilation with steroid injection or mitomycin C
- management of multisite stenosis may require a combination of endoscopic and open procedures
- preliminary experience suggests that injection of 5-FU/triamcinolone may be helpful

Anterior Glottic Stenosis

- vertical height of anterior stenosis and involvement of subglottis are more predictive than diameter of treatment success
- surgical intervention of bilateral, opposing vocal fold mucosa increases risk of web
- managed via endoscopic or open approach, often requires keel placement

Endolaryngeal Procedures

- excision typically via cold knife or CO_2 laser
- dilation occasionally performed adjunctively
- mucosal bridges rarely recur with endoscopic excision and steroid injections
- consider 5-FU/triamcinolone injection
- <u>Two-stage excision</u>: thin webs may be managed in two steps to avoid keel placement:
  1. one side is cut along the edge of the vocal fold, and the remaining flap is left attached
  2. 2 weeks are allowed for healing of denuded mucosa
  3. the contralateral side is then divided along the medial edge, and the tissue is removed
- <u>One-stage excision</u>:
  1. division and partial or complete excision of web

   2. often placement of keel or sutured mucosal flap (buccal or **false** vocal fold advancement flap) to cover denuded tissue
   3. removal of keel or endolaryngeal suture (if mucosal flap) in office or operating room based on patient tolerance
- Conversion of web to mucosal bridge: may reduce recurrence
   1. incision made in web at ideal location for anterior commissure
   2. prosthesis/keel is placed for 2 to 3 weeks
   3. remaining mucosal bridge is divided

Keels

- fin-shaped stent fashioned from minimally reactive materials (ie, Silastic, Teflon, metal)
- some evidence that vertical web thickness is more predictive of keel/stent effectiveness
- indicated when adequate amount of mucosa unavailable for flap reconstruction
- **Keel placement**: facilitated by groove carved in thyroid cartilage at anterior commissure (3–4 mm superior, 4–5 mm inferior) usually with CO_2 laser
   1. Internal approach: suture passed through 16-gauge needles or Lichtenberger needle driver inserted into cricothyroid membrane and above thyroid notch → suture attaches to keel which is pulled into place within anterior commissure and is then tied externally → removed in 1 to 3 weeks
   2. External approach: can be achieved via cricothyrotomy incision or following laryngofissure and excision of web → remains in place 1 to 3 weeks
- placement of reinforced Silastic mesh with endoscopic sutures obviates the need for external suturing, but is technically challenging

Open Procedures

- endolarynx accessed via minithyrotomy or laryngofissure
- Indications: Cohen III and IV, if thickness >1 cm, subglottic involvement, or concurrent PGS
- One-stage excision: as previously discussed, but approached via thyroid cartilage
- Anterior cricoid split with cartilage graft: may be successful in concurrent SGS

Complications

- recurrence of web

- vocal fold scar/adynamic segments may form at web excision site
- vocal fold erosion related to keel placement
- vocal fold height and tension asymmetry
- respiratory distress related to keel dislodgement
- granulation at suture/keel site
- subcutaneous emphysema due to violation of endolaryngeal mucosa or thyroid cartilage

Posterior Glottic Stenosis

Tracheotomy

- type I and some type II stenoses can be treated without tracheotomy
- severe type II and almost all type III and IV stenoses require tracheotomy

Endolaryngeal Procedures

- type I simple scar bands can be divided by laser or cold instruments; recurrence is rare
- treatment of type II stenosis involving both mucosa and underlying muscle is controversial because of the need to provide mucosal coverage during healing
- **Microtrapdoor flap:** inferiorly based flap allows submucosal excision of scar followed by redraping of residual mucosa
- **Transverse cordotomy:** perpendicular transection of vocal fold anterior to vocal process extending to cricoid
- **Medial arytenoidectomy:** curvilinear excision of medial arytenoid; option if scar does not extend to vocal process
- **Total arytenoidectomy:** combines arytenoidectomy and transverse cordotomy
- cordotomy and arytenoidectomy procedures typically used for severe type III and type IV stenosis, and can be used to widen the airway sufficiently to allow removal of the tracheotomy

Open Laryngeal Procedures

- generally reserved for severe type II, and type III and IV stenoses, but usually managed endoscopically
- especially useful in high SGS involving posterior glottis
- typically approached via midline thyrotomy below the level of the vocal folds or laryngofissure
- **Excision with mucosal advancement flap or graft:** as described previously, buccal mucosal graft most common

- **Posterior cricoid split with cartilage grafting (*see* Chapter 31):** single- or double-stage repair requiring stent to remain in place for a variable length of time; costal cartilage graft typically used
    1. <u>Single-stage repair</u>: endotracheal tube acts as stent; remains in place 5 to 14 days, decannulated at time of procedure
    2. <u>Double-stage repair</u>: typically 2 to 6 weeks with second-stage endoscopic removal and subsequent decannulation
    3. also may be performed endoscopically; high rates of successful decannulation in pediatric population (>90% reported)

Complications

- granulation tissue
- graft failure
- recurrent stenosis

Outcomes

- in type I and II stenoses outcomes are measured by remaining breathing restriction and voice quality
- in patients with tracheotomy, the goal is decannulation without substantial breathing restriction
- <u>Complicating factors</u>:
    1. obesity
    2. diabetes
    3. underlying pulmonary disease

CHAPTER

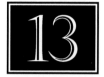

Acquired Subglottic Stenosis

Bhavishya S. Clark, Justin Ross, and Michael M. Johns

INTRODUCTION

- the most common cause of acquired laryngotracheal stenosis (LTS) or subglottic stenosis (SGS) is endotracheal intubation
- patients are commonly misdiagnosed with asthma but fail to improve on inhaled β-agonists
- there is no agreed upon treatment algorithm, both endoscopic and open approaches are utilized
- 95% of cases of SGS are acquired

ANATOMY AND PHYSIOLOGY OF THE SUBGLOTTIS

- inferior arcuate line of true vocal fold (TVF) to lower margin of cricoid cartilage
- extends ~10 mm inferior to anterior commissure and ~5 mm inferior to posterior commissure
- bound ventrally by thyroid and cricoid cartilages and cricothyroid ligament
- bounded laterally by cricothyroid muscle and thyroid cartilage
- larger in males than females
- most narrow region of the pediatric airway is at the cricoid cartilage until age 5
- Poiseuille's equation: airway lumen resistance is inversely proportional to the radius to the fourth power
  1. small changes in subglottic diameter exponentially increase lumen resistance to airflow
  2. 1 mm of circumferential edema in the pediatric subglottis reduces cross-sectional area by 60%
- the subglottis is particularly susceptible to stenosis:
  1. junction between two embryological growth centers
  2. presence of complete cartilage ring
  3. respiratory epithelium vulnerable to injury

CAUSES

Congenital (*See* Chapter 31)

Acquired

- Endotracheal intubation: 90% of cases, injury occurs in the posterior glottis and subglottis where the tube and cuff rest

- Postoperative
    1. high tracheotomy (above second tracheal ring)
    2. cricothyroidotomy
    3. prior surgery of the subglottis (ie, recurrent respiratory papillomatosis, hemangiomas)
- Trauma
    1. blunt force
    2. penetrating laryngeal injury
    3. fume or smoke inhalation
    4. caustic ingestion
    5. foreign body
- Granulomatosis disease
    1. tuberculosis
    2. sarcoidosis: more often found in supraglottis
    3. granulomatosis with polyangiitis (Wegener's granulomatosis): 16% to 23% develop SGS; airway distress due to isolated SGS can be presenting symptom; biopsy of subglottis may be negative, serologic testing is recommended (ie, C-ANCA, ESR)
- Infectious
    1. syphilis
    2. leprosy
    3. typhoid fever
    4. rhinoscleroma caused by *Klebsiella*
    5. blastomycosis
    6. coccidiomycosis
    7. histoplasmosis
- Inflammation
    1. connective tissue disorders
    2. radiation
    3. laryngopharyngeal reflux: higher incidence in patients with SGS
- Laryngeal neoplasm
    1. chondroma
    2. fibroma
    3. papilloma
    4. malignancy

Idiopathic

- typically females (98%) who are perimenopausal (mean age 50.4 years) and Caucasian (95%)
- scar development may be related to *Mycobacterium* sp. bacterial colonization
- diagnosis of exclusion

HISTOLOGY AND PATHOPHYSIOLOGY

- <u>Mucosal lining from lumen inward</u>: columnar ciliated respiratory epithelium, subepithelial connective tissue with a capillary plexus, laryngeal fibroelastic membrane with seromucous glands, loose connective tissue with larger vessels
- <u>Mechanism of stenosis</u>: disruption of the subglottic mucosa or cartilaginous framework, or hematoma formation and then resorption
- <u>Phases of healing</u>: (1) inflammation, (2) proliferation, (3) remodeling
- compression by an endotracheal tube (ETT) or cuff causes pressure necrosis and edema of the mucosa
- disturbance of the mucociliary flow results in bacterial infection with resultant ulceration, perichondritis, and chondritis
- acute stenosis can occur during the inflammation stage
- proliferative stage is characterized by neovascularization, collagen deposition, and reepithelialization with formation of granulation tissue
- remodeling by myofibroblasts creates submucosal fibrosis and scar contraction leading to chronic stenosis
- if cartilage is involved, it may weaken and collapse as it heals leading to tracheomalacia further compounding SGS

CLINICAL EVALUATION

History

- history of prior intubation, duration of intubation, size of the endotracheal tube, number of intubations, traumatic intubations, self-extubations
- trauma: blunt versus penetrating, caustic versus thermal
- prior head and neck surgery or radiation
- medical comorbidities (ie, cardiopulmonary status, diabetes, steroid usage, GERD)
- aero-digestive complaints usually start 2 to 4 weeks after initial trauma or injury
  1. dysphonia
  2. chronic cough
  3. dysphagia
  4. progressive shortness of breath
  5. noisy breathing
- patients commonly misdiagnosed as having asthma → failure of symptomatic improvement after inhaled steroid use should heighten suspicion for LTS

Physical Examination

- Observe for signs of airway distress: inspiratory or biphasic stridor, dyspnea, air hunger, retractions
- Assess voice: quality, loudness, pitch, breathiness, vocal effort
- Comprehensive head and neck exam: focus on nasal cavity, oral cavity, oropharynx, neck, flexible laryngoscopy, rigid strobolaryngoscopy, if possible
- Examine and palpate the neck for signs of trauma
- Flexible laryngoscopy: vocal fold mobility, signs of reflux laryngitis, granulomas, immediate subglottic changes, tracheomalacia, and other abnormalities
- Pulmonary function testing: Simple, sensitive, noninvasive, can assess presence of intrinsic lung disease and flow volume loop
- pH impedance testing and esophagoscopy with biopsy: important to identify LPR and eosinophilic esophagitis as untreated disease worsens surgical outcomes
- Culture: culture of nasal cavity, axilla and rectum (methicillin-resistant *Staphylococcus aureus* [MRSA]), and sputum (*Pseudomonas aeruginosa*)

Direct Laryngoscopy with Tracheobronchoscopy

- exam under general or local anesthesia is gold standard for diagnosis
- discuss potential need for tracheotomy prior to endoscopy (tracheotomy set should be available and ready in room)
- Airway management options (discuss with anesthesia preoperatively):
  1. jet ventilation
  2. intermittent intubation with small (usually 4.0 to 6.0) microlaryngeal/tracheal tube and apnea—may be required for higher-grade stenosis if jet ventilation provides insufficient oxygenation
  3. spontaneous ventilation
  4. local anesthesia with sedation
- Airway examination extends to and includes main-stem bronchi:
  1. assess the diameter of the largest ETT or endoscope that can be passed through the stenosis
  2. examination for other airway abnormalities
  3. after removal of the sizing ETT or endoscope, the stenotic segment may become edematous prompting need for an awake tracheotomy (decrease edema with preoperative steroids)
- documentation includes location (distance from vocal folds and tracheostoma), subsite, length, and presence of secondary stenoses using a sizing ETT or 0° Hopkins' endoscope

Imaging

- <u>Plain film</u>: quick, cost effective; lateral and anterior-posterior views to assess for lumen narrowing; does not provide dynamic evaluation of the airway; not sensitive for identifying milder stenosis
- <u>Airway fluoroscopy</u>: dynamic evaluation of airway, assess vocal fold motion and airway collapse during expiration in children; sensitivity for SGS and bronchial obstruction is 80%
- <u>Computed tomography (CT)</u>: thin cuts through larynx are sensitive and specific; can identify location and length of involvement; aids surgical planning
- <u>Magnetic resonance imaging (MRI)</u>: does not image the cartilaginous framework validly

GRADING SYSTEMS FOR SGS

Cotton-Myer (Figure 13–1)

- created for pediatric population
- based on relative reductions of subglottis cross-sectional area
  1. <u>Stage I</u>: <50% obstruction
  2. <u>Stage II</u>: 51% to 70% obstruction
  3. <u>Stage III</u>: 71% to 99% obstruction
  4. <u>Stage IV</u>: complete obstruction
- suitable for mature, firm, circumferential lesions
- does not reflect length of stenosis or extensions into other subsites

Lano

- does not reflect length of stenosis or lumen diameter
- based solely on involved subsites (glottis, subglottis, trachea)
  1. <u>Stage I</u>: 1 subsite involved
  2. <u>Stage II</u>: 2-subsite involvement
  3. <u>Stage III</u>: 3-subsite involvement

McCaffrey (Figure 13–2)

- does not include lumen diameter
- based on involved subsites, length of stenosis, and mobility of the vocal folds
  1. <u>Stage 1</u>: subglottis or trachea, <1-cm long
  2. <u>Stage 2</u>: subglottis, >1-cm long
  3. <u>Stage 3</u>: subglottis and trachea, >1-cm long
  4. <u>Stage 4</u>: any lesion involving glottis

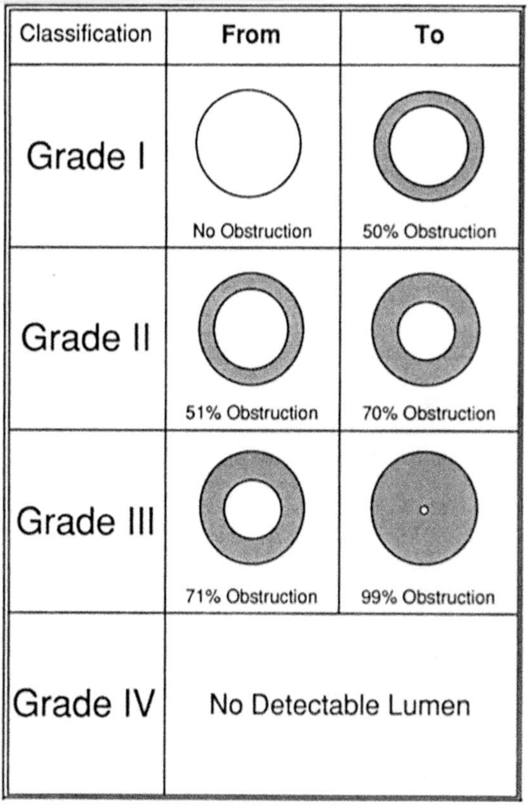

Classification	From	To
Grade I	No Obstruction	50% Obstruction
Grade II	51% Obstruction	70% Obstruction
Grade III	71% Obstruction	99% Obstruction
Grade IV	No Detectable Lumen	

FIGURE 13-1. Cotton-Myer Grading System.

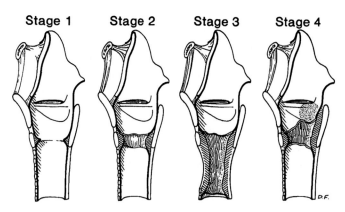

FIGURE 13-2. McCaffrey Grading System.

MANAGEMENT INTRODUCTION

- stenosis may involve one or more airway segments
- etiology of isolated SGS is more likely idiopathic than traumatic
- <u>Risk factors</u>: endotracheal intubation, obesity, LPR
- frequently misdiagnosed as asthma and recurrent upper respiratory infection
- airway patency is primary goal, preservation of swallowing and voice is secondary
- unless originating from autoimmunity or malignancy, surgery is treatment of choice
- may be managed endoscopically or open
- intraoperative ventilation typically done with jet ventilation or alternating intubation and apnea to optimize visualization
- multilevel stenosis >1 cm in vertical height is inherently more difficult to treat
- open procedures are typically more effective for higher-grade and multilevel stenosis

MEDICAL MANAGEMENT

- mild-grade SGS causing minimal functional impairment can be monitored closely with serial endoscopic exams
- inhaled corticosteroids may have a beneficial effect
- <u>Antireflux agents</u>: proton pump inhibitors ± H2 receptor antagonists
- <u>Antibiotic prophylaxis</u>: treatment of MRSA and *Pseudomonas* colonization improves rates of postoperative infection following open airway surgery
- <u>Intralesional steroid injection</u>: may be used as an adjunct to excision and dilation; alternatively, serial office injections may improve pulmonary function testing and dyspnea in idiopathic SGS
- <u>Mitomycin C application</u>: antimetabolite produced by *S caespitosus*; inhibits fibroblast proliferation; efficacy varies, but may increase interval between excision/dilation procedures
- <u>Experimental treatments</u>:
    1. intralesional lipid-encapsulated 5-fluorouracil: increased airway diameter has been shown in an animal model
    2. *Rapamycin*: low-dose administration prevented progression of laryngotracheal stenosis in an animal model
    3. *Methotrexate*: increased duration between procedures in an animal model

ENDOSCOPIC REPAIR

- associated with few complications, low morbidity, short operative time, and short length of hospitalization
- <u>Indications</u>: grades I to III stenosis ± ongoing inflammation; lack of cartilage involvement, including tracheomalacia; no external compression; identifiable airway lumen
- <u>Techniques</u>: dilation (rigid or balloon), laser resection, microsurgical debridement
- <u>Adjunct treatment</u>: mitomycin C application or steroid injection can increase interval between endoscopic treatments
- recurrence rate after endoscopic dilation remains high → higher-grade stenosis is associated with increased probability of restenosis
- unlikely to require repeat intervention if progression-free after ~2.5 years

Dilation

- rigid or radial-expansion balloon dilators have roughly equivalent outcomes
- radial incisions or wedge resection typically performed prior to dilation
- equivalent interval to reoperation comparing excision + dilation versus dilation alone
- average 10 to 13 months until repeat excision/dilation required
- application of mitomycin C may increase symptom-free interval between interventions
- improves subjective voice outcomes, with worse results expected in multilevel stenosis and when stenosis involves area within 2 cm of the true vocal folds
- safely performed as an outpatient
- ~70% will require repeat excision/dilation procedures

Endoscopic Laser Excision

- CO_2 or Nd:YAG
- radial cuts or wedge excision of fibrosis with laser avoids circumferential inflammation and tracheal edema
- may be performed in concert with micro-trapdoor flap in adults with stenosis <1 cm in length; some advocate tracheotomy if flap >4 mm to prevent airway occlusion secondary to large flap
- <u>Benefits</u>: laser use delays collagen maturation, minimizes deep tissue injury, enables precise control, allows hemostasis

- <u>Risks</u>: bleeding, tracheal perforation, tissue edema, reformation of stenosis (success rates 66%–80%)

Microsurgical Debridement

- 4 mm subglottic blade
- <u>Benefits</u>: rapid, no risk of airway fire or laser plume
- <u>Relative contraindication</u>: high vascular lesions
- <u>Risks</u>: potential for tracheal perforation leading to tracheoesophageal fistula

OPEN REPAIR

- <u>Relative indications</u>: grade III or IV stenosis, failure of endoscopic repair, cicatricial stenosis, combined stenosis >1 cm in vertical length, tracheomalacia, loss of cartilage, previous history of bacterial infection associated with tracheotomy, posterior glottic stenosis with arytenoid fixation
- <u>Relative contraindications</u>: severe associated systemic or cardiac diseases, stenosis not yet stabilized with severe ongoing inflammation
- patient is intubated prior to surgery regardless of presence of tracheotomy

Expansion Procedures

- <u>Indications</u>: ≥2 failures to extubate, weight >1.5 kg, spontaneous breathing for at least 10 days, FiO_2 <30%, no requirement for antihypertensives for >10 days, no active respiratory infection, no congestive heart failure in prior 30 days
- performed in adults or children
- typically performed with cartilage graft sutured, anchored, and/or held in place by internal stenting
- <u>Complications</u>: wound infection, suture line granulomas, re-intubation, injury to recurrent laryngeal nerves, anastomotic dehiscence with restenosis, dislodgement of stent, voice alteration, graft failure, pneumothorax or pneumomediastinum

Internal Laryngeal Stenting

- <u>Indications</u>: support for bone or cartilage grafts, splint for mucosa/epidermal grafts or laryngeal fractures, prevent approximation of

denuded mucosal surfaces while healing, preserve lumen following reconstruction where malacia would result in loss of airway
- <u>Stent options</u>: endotracheal tube, Montgomery T-tube (single lumen, Silastic), Aboulker stent (double cannula, Teflon), Silastic stent, ETS Poirot, or laryngeal stent (may be custom made by surgeon)
- duration of stenting and ideal type of stent are controversial
- <u>Soft stents</u>: indicated for interposition between denuded mucosal surfaces and splinting mucosal/epidermal grafts; less likely to cause granulation
- <u>Rigid stents</u>: indicated for splinting some fractures and cartilage grafts or providing support for weak cartilaginous framework
- mucosal healing or epidermal/mucosal graft integration typically requires only 1 to 3 weeks of stenting
- posterior cricoid cartilage grafts typically require between 2 weeks to 3 months of stenting (more secure grafts require the least amount of time)
- if development of mature scar is required to secure structural framework in cases of deficient cartilage, stenting may be required for months to >1 year

Graft Materials and Practice

- free grafts are used more commonly for luminal augmentation than pedicled grafts
- <u>Free grafts</u>: costal cartilage (most common), auricular cartilage, thyroid alar cartilage, nasal septal cartilage, hyoid; autograft or homograft
- <u>Pedicled grafts</u>: hyoid-sternohyoid graft, thyroid-cartilage-sternothyroid graft
- <u>Costal cartilage</u>: typically harvested from fifth rib; ideal graft material due to thickness and abundance
- <u>Thyroid alar cartilage</u>: elliptical graft is harvested from superior thyroid ala lateral to midline; done during expansion procedure; provides limited material—typically useful only in small children
- graft should be inset with intact perichondrium facing endoluminally
- length and width are highly customized
- anterior grafts are typically longer and wider than posterior grafts
- endoluminal surface of anterior cricoid grafts should be carved into a modified boat shape (typically elongated hexagon or ellipse), and externally facing surface acts as a flange and should remain flat
- posterior cricoid grafts typically carved into a boat shape with anterior and posterior flanges; can be secured in place by insetting posterior flanges in subperichondrial pocket

Anterior Cricoid Split (ACS) With or Without Cartilage Graft

- <u>Indications</u>: anteriorly based grades II to III subglottic stenosis, especially if extending to anterior commissure; ACS without graft is a viable option for grade I stenosis in infants
- vertical midline incision through lower thyroid cartilage, cricoid, and first two tracheal rings
- if used, graft is sutured or wired in place
- ETT left in place for 7 to 14 days to act as a stent in ACS without graft, and 2 to 4 days in ACS with graft
- ACS without graft less likely to be effective in higher-grade stenosis but has roughly equivalent outcomes whether performed endoscopic or open
- typically performed in infants with or without tracheotomy, but has been successful in adults
- may obviate need for tracheotomy
- successful extubation in ~70%

Posterior Cricoid Split (PCS) With or Without Cartilage Graft

- <u>Indications</u>: posteriorly based grades II to III SGS with superior extension, especially if involving posterior glottis
- posterior lamina approached endoscopically or via anterior cricotracheal fissure to avoid the anterior commissure; laryngofissure an option if co-occurring grades III to IV posterior glottic stenosis
- equivalent outcomes whether performed endoscopically or open in pediatric patients
- endoscopic approach less common in adults—difficulty with transection due to ossification of cricoid
- scar tissue need not be excised but may be if excessive
- interarytenoid muscle can be divided if fibrosed
- graft material secured via suture or carved flanges that fit into the subperichondrial plane anterior to the tracheoesophageal party-wall
- rigid internal stenting for at least 3 months if no graft is used
- stenting is of variable length following PCS with graft (depends if single- or double-stage procedure)

Laryngotracheal Reconstruction (LTR)

- <u>Indications</u>: effective for grades III to IV and refractory grade II SGS; preferred in children over cricotracheal resection due to ability of continued growth

- division of the anterior and posterior ± lateral walls of the cricoid cartilage with interposition of a cartilaginous graft(s)
- technically, laryngotracheal augmentation with a cartilage graft counts as LTR (eg, ACS and PCS)
- performed as one- or two-stage procedure—determined by timing of decannulation:
  1. Single-stage: ETT acts as the stent (tracheotomy removed at end of surgery if present); direct laryngoscopy and bronchoscopy performed 7 to 10 days post-op to determine candidacy for extubation
  2. Double-stage: tracheotomy is performed (if not present already) and suprastomal stent or Montgomery T-tube is placed; preferred in patients with more advanced disease or comorbidities (ie, cardiac, neuromuscular, etc)
- repair at early age improves speech outcomes and obviates morbidity from tracheotomy
- decannulation outcomes (~90%) similar for single- versus double-stage LTR
- Risk factors for decannulation failure: diabetes, GERD, grade IV stenosis
- multiple postoperative endoscopic dilations and T-tube requirement may predict decannulation failure

Segmental Resection

Cricotracheal Resection (CTR)

- resection of obstructing mucosa, scar, and cartilage with primary thyrotracheal anastomosis
- may require laryngotracheal release maneuvers to maximize resection length
- decannulation rates of ~95%
- may be performed primarily or as salvage
- Indications: grades III to IV and refractory grade II SGS, high tracheal stenosis involving subglottis, adult, at least 3 to 4 mm of normal lumen exists below the vocal fold
- Procedure:
  1. removal of anterior half of cricoid lamina, mucosa overlying posterior cricoid lamina, and first several tracheal rings
  2. neck is kept in flexion (Grillo stitch) for 7 to 10 days postoperatively to minimize tension on the anastomosis
  3. patient may be extubated in the operating room or delayed
- for complicated multilevel stenosis, extended CTR may include expansion procedure, arytenoid lateralization or arytenoidectomy

- <u>Complications</u>: wound infection, suture line granulomas, injury to recurrent laryngeal nerves, anastomotic dehiscence, recurrent stenosis, aspiration, arytenoid prolapse

Laryngotracheal Release Maneuvers

- <u>Options</u>: suprahyoid, infrahyoid, thyrohyoid (associated with dysphagia), right hilar, intrapericardial release
    1. release maneuvers used to maximize resection length (up to 7.5 cm or 5–6 tracheal rings)
- <u>Suprahyoid release</u>: more common in revision cases; average length of tracheal resection 4.4 cm; increased risk of aspiration and vocal fold dysfunction (5%)
- <u>Right hilar release</u>: blunt dissection along lateral borders of trachea, followed by division of inferior pulmonary ligament; provides minimal length, but provides access to pericardium
- <u>Intrapericardial release</u>: U-shaped incision around inferior pulmonary vein

Tracheotomy

- performed while patient is awake
- for patients in acute airway distress, with absolute contraindications to general anesthesia, or to allow time before more definitive surgical treatment
- can be a definitive treatment or be used to secure the airway for subsequent endoscopic or open procedures
- tracheotomy dependence more likely in iatrogenic and autoimmune than idiopathic or traumatic etiologies
- tracheotomy dependence greater in grade III or IV stenosis and BMI >30
- decannulation rates higher for open versus endoscopic management
- successful decannulation is associated with lower stenosis grade in LTR, but not CTR

PREVENTION

- <u>Choose appropriate ETT</u>:
    1. low-pressure, high-volume cuff minimizes mucosal injury
    2. recommend size 7.0 or smaller in adults
- <u>Avoid accidental extubation</u>:
    1. secure tube to minimize movement
    2. minimize patient movement

- monitor cuff pressure routinely $\rightarrow$ should allow for air leak at less than the capillary perfusion pressure (20–30 cm H_2O, 18–22 mm Hg)
- minimize duration of intubation $\rightarrow$ consider early tracheotomy if prolonged intubation is anticipated
- minimize need for multiple intubations
- use antireflux medications in patients who are intubated or have signs and symptoms of GERD/LPR
- early endoscopic treatment of acute inflammatory airway lesions with intralesional steroids, laser reduction, balloon dilatation has been shown to minimize stenosis formation
- identify patients with long-term intubation, extubation difficulties, or those who develop dyspnea weeks after extubation

CHAPTER

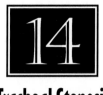

Tracheal Stenosis

Jared M. Goldfarb and Joseph R. Spiegel

INTRODUCTION

- tracheal stenosis is defined as the narrowing of the trachea producing airway obstruction
- can be caused by a variety of congenital or acquired conditions
- may present with complaints ranging from mild dyspnea to life-threatening airway obstruction
- congenital tracheal stenosis (CTS) is almost always eventually fatal without intervention

ANATOMY

- the trachea extends superiorly to the cricoid cartilage and inferiorly to carina
- the adult trachea is typically 11 to 13 cm long with a diameter of approximately 2.2 cm in men and 1.7 cm in women
- diameter correlates with patient height
- bifurcates at the level of T4–T5 (carina)
- thoracic inlet is the border between cervical and thoracic trachea

EMBRYOLOGY

- derives from respiratory diverticulum
- tracheal dilation and bifurcation occurs in weeks 3 to 4 → abnormalities during this period often cause **more severe CTS**
- early tracheal cartilage forms in weeks 8 to 10 → abnormalities during this period often cause **less severe CTS** with fewer associated anomalies

CONGENITAL TRACHEAL STENOSIS (CTS)

Presentation

- **biphasic stridor** immediately after birth, tachypnea, nasal flaring, apnea, wheezing, labored breathing, sternal/rib retractions, shortness of breath, cyanosis
- may see head hyperextension to attempt to open airway
- poor feeding, dysphagia, failure to thrive
- frequent respiratory infections (**most common eventual cause of death**)
- findings most often noted during first several weeks of life

Associated Anomalies

- bronchial stenosis, aplastic lungs
- **pulmonary artery sling (30%–50% of CTS patients)**
- congenital heart defects
- laryngomalacia and bronchomalacia
- subglottic stenosis
- hydrocephalus
- trisomy 21
- imperforate anus
- single kidney
- tracheoesophageal fistula
- diaphragmatic hernia
- lack of gallbladder
- cleft lip or palate

Classification Systems

- Morphologically has been defined by (Cantrell):
  1. generalized hypoplasia
  2. funnel-shaped stenosis
  3. segmental, hourglass shaped stenosis (**most common form, >50% of cases**)
- Classes by associated anomalies (Hoffer):
  1. *Class 1*: short segment stenosis
  2. *Class 2*: extensive stenosis with associated anomalies **except** heart and lung disease
  3. *Class 3*: extensive stenosis with heart or lung disease
- Severity described in terms of (Elliot):
  1. narrowness of trachea
  2. extent of tracheal involvement
  3. involvement of bronchi
  4. presence of complete tracheal rings

ACQUIRED TRACHEAL STENOSIS

Etiology

- Trauma: intubation (most common), tracheotomy, thermal burns, chemical injury
  1. usually related to pressure against mucosa → inflammation, fibrosis, contracture, and necrosis of tracheal cartilage
  2. prolonged intubation: can lead to stenosis within 36 hours, risk increases with duration of intubation, most often occurs at **cuff site**

3. <u>poor tracheostomy tube positioning</u>: excessively superior, most commonly at **site of stoma**
- <u>Infection</u>: tuberculosis (**most common infectious cause**), diphtheria, syphilis, histoplasmosis, blastomycosis
- <u>Systemic inflammatory conditions</u>: granulomatosis with polyangiitis, sarcoidosis, amyloidosis, polychondritis, scleroderma; likely to cause stenosis at **multiple levels** of the trachea
- <u>Neoplasia</u>: direct tumor invasion greater than tracheal metastasis, mass-related external compression (ie, vascular anomaly, lymphadenopathy or thymus, thyroid, lung, esophageal, and mediastinal masses); benign primary masses of the trachea rarely cause tracheal stenosis
- <u>Iatrogenic</u>: tracheal stents (granulation ends of stent), radiation therapy
- <u>Tracheopathia osteochondroplastica</u>: development of submucous osseous and/or chondrus nodules sparing posterior membranous aspect of trachea
- <u>Idiopathic</u>: most common at level of cricoid and in women, progressive disease often requires resection and possibly palliation if recalcitrant

Clinical Presentation

- dependent on etiology, location of stenosis and degree of obstruction
- <u>History</u>: cough, wheezing, shortness of breath, frequent respiratory infections, poor sputum clearance, symptoms persist despite bronchodilators, recent intensive care unit admission or intubation
- dyspnea on exertion (tracheal diameter ~0.8 cm) and stridor (<0.5 cm)
- <u>Physical</u>: often unremarkable, stridor, labored breathing, neck scars or masses, rashes

DIFFERENTIAL DIAGNOSIS

- external compression of trachea
- asthma
- foreign-body aspiration
- gastroesophageal reflux
- pulmonary infection
- neurological causes of apnea
- tracheomalacia

DIAGNOSIS

- lateral and frontal chest radiographs: mediastinal shift, tracheal compression or narrowing, vascular malformations
- Computed tomography or magnetic resonance imaging: nonenhancing studies of the neck and chest are the best **initial imaging studies** for evaluation; virtual bronchoscopy or contrast studies may be necessary
- esophagram
- pulmonary function testing as initial evaluation and follow-up metric
- echocardiogram to evaluate for vascular malformations
- bronchography (rarely used)
- **Bronchoscopy:** definitive but carries risks of further damage; rigid preferred over flexible because it can secure the airway and is both diagnostic and therapeutic
- Serology: inflammatory and autoimmune markers as indicated

MANAGEMENT

Airway Management

- always stabilize airway first
    1. intubation is often difficult and calls for a small endotracheal tube
    2. may also attempt jet ventilation
    3. may need to ventilate with helium carrier
    4. may require continuous positive airway pressure or bilevel positive airway pressure
    5. tracheotomy usually unnecessary as stenosis is often in the distal trachea
    6. extracorporeal membrane oxygenation (ECMO) may be necessary if intubation or tracheotomy are not achievable
- comanagement of associated congenital anomalies
- intensive care level management required for airway and hemodynamic monitoring

Medical Management

- systemic management of inflammatory or autoimmune etiologies with steroids or immunomodulators
- systemic and local antimicrobial management for infectious etiologies
- consider concurrent use of mucolytics, nebulizers, and chest physical therapy

Surgical Management

- balloon or bougie dilation
- tissue destruction with laser therapy (**Nd-Yag most common**), electrocautery, brachytherapy, or cryotherapy
- excision of narrowed area with primary anastomosis
    1. preferred method in short segment stenosis when possible
    2. chin to chest sutures (Grillo stitch) can be used postoperatively to maintain flexion
- tracheal lumen reconstruction with costal cartilage or pericardial grafts
- sliding tracheoplasty
- posterior tracheal division with esophageal integration (repair of cardiovascular malformations at same time is recommended)
- synthetic stent placement
- long-term tracheostomy with T-tube placement

Complications

- granulation and granulomas at surgical site and at location of endotracheal tube
    1. ciprofloxacin with dexamethasone can be used to help prevent granulation tissue while
    2. mitomycin-C is used without substantial evidence to prove its efficacy
- tracheomalacia
- pneumonia
- tracheitis
- mediastinitis
- recurrence

CHAPTER

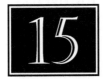

Benign and Premalignant Lesions of the Larynx

Haig Panossian, Justin Ross, Mary J. Hawkshaw, and Robert T. Sataloff

TERMINOLOGY

- **Hyperplasia**: thickening of epithelial surface
- Pseudoepitheliomatous hyperplasia reactive or reparative overgrowth of squamous epithelium with no cytological evidence of malignancy; may be mistaken for malignancy
- **Keratosis**: presence of keratin on epithelial surface
- **Parakeratosis**: presence of nuclei in keratin layer
- **Metaplasia**: change from one histologic tissue type to another
- **Dysplasia**: cellular aberration and abnormal maturation
  1. <u>Mild</u>: changes within inner third of surface epithelium
  2. <u>Moderate</u>: involves one-third to two-thirds
  3. <u>Severe</u>: from two-thirds to full thickness
- **Carcinoma in situ**: full-thickness changes in epithelium with intact basement membrane
- **Koilocytosis**: cytoplasmic vacuolization of squamous cell suggestive of viral infection

LEUKOPLAKIA (*See* Chapter 16)

- any white lesion of a mucus membrane
- may be benign, premalignant, or malignant
- <u>Physical examination</u>: flexible laryngoscopy with or without narrow-band imaging (NBI), stroboscopy
- NBI demonstrates pathologic angiogenesis by selecting wavelengths 415 and 540 nm, which are preferentially absorbed by hemoglobin in superficial neovascular lesions
- thick dark spots within well-demarcated dark area and proliferation of dilated and abnormal intraepithelial capillary loops (IPCLs) have shown histopathologic correlation for high-grade dysplasia or malignancy
- <u>Dx</u>: observation of altered mucosal wave or extent not sufficient to predict risk for malignancy; can consider initial removal of offending agents (smoking, alcohol, reflux, inhalational steroids) followed by repeat examination, but threshold for biopsy and pathology examination must remain low
- molecular markers that may be identified by gene expression microarrays under investigation
- rates of malignant transformation vary in literature, believed to be approximately 8% to 10%
- <u>Tx</u>: based on pathology examination; similar to CIS (following)

ERYTHROPLAKIA

- red lesion of a mucous membrane
- more likely than leukoplakia to have underlying malignancy
- <u>Dx</u>: biopsy and pathology examination necessary
- <u>Tx</u>: based on pathology examination; similar to CIS (following)

CLASSIFICATION SYSTEMS OF DYSPLASIA

Friedman

- <u>Laryngeal intraepithelial neoplasm (LIN)-I</u>: mild or minimal dysplasia
- <u>LIN-II</u>: moderate dysplasia
- <u>LIN-III</u>: severe dysplasia and CIS

Kleinsasser

- <u>Class I</u>: simple squamous cell hyperplasia
- <u>Class II</u>: squamous cell hyperplasia with atypia
- <u>Class III</u>: CIS

CARCINOMA IN SITU (CIS)

- malignant epithelial neoplasm without invasion (distinguishes from true carcinoma)
- may appear as leukoplakia, erythroplakia, or hyperkeratosis
- not a required precursor to SCCa, but commonly coexist
- <u>Dx</u>: biopsy and pathology examination
- <u>Tx</u>: smoking and alcohol cessation; if biopsy positive, requires further examination for invasive SCCa; surgical resection; in-office photodynamic therapy with topically applied 5-aminolevulinic acid (5-ALA); external beam radiation especially if multiple or recurrent lesions, involvement of anterior commissure or patient with limited ability to follow-up
- high likelihood of malignant transformation; rates vary widely in literature but believed to be approximately 30%
- requires frequent surveillance as recurrence or malignant transformation may occur at different site than original lesion

RESPIRATORY PAPILLOMA

- ubiquitous in population with small percentage showing clinical expression
- bimodal age distribution; children under age 5 and adults in third to fourth decade
- adult onset more common in males (64%–90% in recent American studies)
- 1500 to 2500 new cases diagnosed in United States each year
- <u>Etiology</u>: **Human papillomavirus (HPV)**—primarily by low malignant risk strains **6, 11**, and less commonly 16, 18
  1. circular, nonenveloped dsDNA virus encodes proteins that result in dysregulation of proliferation, genetic stability, and apoptosis
  2. infection may cause asymptomatic, benign neoplastic, or oncogenic changes
  3. <u>E6</u>: interferes with p53 tumor suppressor
  4. <u>E7</u>: interferes with pRB tumor suppressor
  5. <u>L1</u>: capsid protein on external surface of virus; used for currently available vaccines
- transmission in children likely due to HPV-positive mothers; delivery via infected birth canal believed to increase rate of transmission but likely multifactorial
- transmission in adults believed to be sexually transmitted, but may be reactivation of latent disease
- cofactors for growth may include concomitant herpes simplex virus type 2 (HSV-2) and laryngopharyngeal reflux (LPR); unknown if local irritants impact disease expression but believed to influence recurrence
- <u>vaccination for HPV</u>: early studies have shown a decrease in incidence and may prevent recurrence
- <u>Presentation</u>: hoarseness, chronic cough, failure to thrive, stridor
- <u>Pathology</u>: papillary fronds with multilayered benign squamous epithelium surrounding fibrovascular core; varying degree of cellular atypia; varying amount of basal layer hyperplasia with presence of koilocytes
- <u>Dx</u>: flexible laryngoscopy, direct laryngoscopy, NBI
- <u>Tx</u>: LPR control; avoid smoking, alcohol; direct laryngoscopy with resection (*see* Chapter 33 for details); combination of cold steel, powered instrumentation, and laser treatment with use of cidofovir and/or Avastin (*see* Chapter 30, Laryngology and Medication, and Chapter 32, Laryngeal Laser Surgery)
- biopsy indicated at initial treatment for viral typing
- HPV-11 has been reported to have higher malignancy rates, while HPV-16 and -18 are higher-risk strains in other sites of the head and neck

- benign biopsy may be misleading, and malignant transformation should be suspected in patients with airway obstruction, reduced vocal fold mobility, dysphagia, subglottic extension, and cervical adenopathy
- rates of malignant transformation vary widely but are most common in patients who have history of receiving XRT
- usually require multiple operations at regular intervals for disease control
- avoid tracheotomy unless in case of severe respiratory distress (rarely acute)

GRANULAR CELL TUMOR

- rare soft tissue schwannoma, primarily occurring in the head and neck (~50%)
- increased incidence in females, black patients, and the third to sixth decades of life
- primary subsite in the head and neck region is the **tongue** (~33%)
- laryngeal lesions are rare (~3%–10%)
- within the larynx >50% occur on the true vocal fold (TVF)
    1. <u>Adults</u>: **posterior TVF** including arytenoid vocal process
    2. <u>Pediatrics (rare)</u>: anterior TVF and subglottic area
- <u>Histopathology</u>: large polymorphic cells with pale-staining and excessively granular, acidophilic cytoplasm; small, vesicular, chromatically dense nuclei; commonly contain myelinated nerve fibers
- Sudan Black B, **PAS, neuron-specific enolase**, and **S-100** positive
- biologically malignant, but histologically benign lesions are typically larger, grow faster, and are rapidly invasive
- <u>Presentation</u>: hoarseness, breathiness, dysphagia, otalgia, stridor, hemoptysis; fleshy, usually solitary, painless mass seen on direct visualization
- multiple lesions (10%) more prevalent in black patients, and associated with underlying genetic condition (eg, LEOPARD syndrome, neurofibromatosis)
- malignancy is rare (<2%) but carries a poor prognosis
- <u>Dx</u>: magnetic resonance imaging (MRI) with and without gadolinium, microdirect laryngoscopy (MDL) with biopsy
- easily mistaken for laryngeal granuloma due to typical presentation on posterior one-third of TVF
- insufficiently deep biopsy may lead to misdiagnosis as squamous cell carcinoma due to secondary pseudoepitheliomatous hyperplasia in surrounding epithelial tissue

- most reliable criterion for malignancy is metastasis to sites that are atypical for multiple benign lesions such as regional lymph nodes, lungs, bones, and viscera
- <u>Tx</u>: surgical excision with negative margins is curative (2%–8% for benign lesions)
- high recurrence rate for malignant lesions (~30%)

LIPOMA

- benign, fatty tumors with a low rate of malignant conversion
- most common benign soft tissue neoplasm
- rarely present in the larynx or hypopharynx
- increased incidence in obese patients and >40 years of age
- <u>Histopathology</u>: encapsulated mass of histologically normal white adipocytes
- <u>Presentation</u>: depends on site affected (false vocal folds most common laryngeal site); commonly breathiness, dysphonia, reduced maximum phonation time, vocal fatigue, dysphagia, stridor
- airway compromise common with laryngeal lipomas
- multiple lipomas are associated with female gender, neurofibromatosis, multiple endocrine neoplasia syndromes, and Bannayan syndrome
- rapid growth may indicate malignant liposarcoma
- <u>Ddx</u>: laryngocele, pharyngocele, saccular cyst, retention cyst, liposarcoma
- <u>Dx</u>: CT (encapsulated area with low attenuation); **MRI (T1: high signal, T2: low signal, T1 w/contrast: no enhancement)**
- <u>Tx</u>: surgical excision of lesion with intact pseudocapsule is curative (recurrence rate 4%–5%)

AMYLOIDOSIS

- local and/or systemic deposition of insoluble, fibrillar proteins
- rarely presents in the larynx, accounting for 1% of laryngeal tumors
- primary immunoglobulin light-chain amyloidosis (AL) is the most common type in larynx, nasopharynx, trachea, and lungs
- **false vocal fold** is the most common laryngeal subsite
- <u>Etiology</u>: laryngeal lesions usually secondary to immunocyte dyscrasias or mucosa-associated lymphoid tissue (MALT) lymphoma
- <u>Histopathology</u>: accumulation of insoluble, extracellular proteins organized in **cross-β-pleated sheets**; commonly perivascular

- **Subtypes**:
  1. <u>Systemic</u> (85%): (a) **primary**: monoclonal plasma cell dyscrasias produce AL; (b) **secondary**: multiple myeloma, chronic infection and inflammatory diseases (amyloid associated protein, AA), hemodialysis (Aβ2M); (c) **hereditary**: familial Mediterranean fever causes production of (AA); (d) **senile**: deposition of amyloid transthyretin (ATTR), usually in cardiac tissue
  2. <u>Localized</u> (15%): any nonsystemic deposition of amyloid (eg, Alzheimer's disease, atrial amyloidosis, type 2 diabetes, medullary islet cell tumor)
- <u>Presentation</u>: dysphonia, dysphagia, breathiness, cough, stridor, respiratory distress, xerostomia, **macroglossia** (19% of all systemic amyloidosis), waxy oral and cutaneous lesions (ecchymosis, petechiae, nodules, papules, plaques), alopecia, neuropathy
- <u>Dx</u>: MDL with biopsy (polypoid or granular appearance); **apple-green birefringence under polarized light with Congo red stain**; urine and serum immunoelectrophoresis; CT/MRI echocardiogram (if cardiac involvement suspected)
- <u>Tx</u>: treat underlying condition, surgery geared toward maximizing phonatory and respiratory outcomes—total excision unnecessary and usually unsuccessful, subglottic and tracheal disease may benefit from an open approach, CO_2 laser excision may be appropriate, open and endoscopic approaches carry risk of postoperative scarring, local and systemic steroids are ineffective in controlling disease

CARTILAGINOUS TUMORS OF THE LARYNX

- rare (<1%) tumors arising from hyaline cartilage
- unknown etiology, but may be related to abnormal ossification later in life
- primarily arise from the **posterior endolaryngeal surface of cricoid cartilage** (~75%)
- other laryngeal sites include **thyroid cartilage** (17%) and **arytenoid cartilage** (5%)
- <u>Histologic subtypes</u>:
  1. **Chondrometaplasia**: multiple benign, mucochondroid, nodular lesions surrounded by soft tissue matrix
  2. **Chondroma**: homogenous, hypocellular lesions without atypia; more common in children; typically <2 cm
  3. **Chondrosarcoma**: increased cellularity relative to chondroma (>40 nuclei/HPF) with atypia, pleomorphism, and mitotic

figures; may present as scattered foci within a chondroma; more
common in adult males; rare locoregional metastasis, distant
spread more common (8%–14%)

4. Cartilaginous constituents of other neoplasms

- chondroma represents 72% to 80% of cartilaginous tumors, though
  some reviews indicate chondrosarcoma is much more prevalent
  (>50%) due to misclassification of low-grade malignant lesions
- vascular invasion common in both chondroma and chondrosarcoma
- Presentation: stridor, hoarseness, breathiness, dyspnea, dysphagia,
  neck mass
- Dx: flexible laryngoscopy, strobovideolaryngoscopy, CT (**matrix
  calcifications**), MRI, bone scan, preoperative biopsy
- bone scan usually can differentiate chondroma from low-grade
  chondrosarcoma
- may present with widely spaced arytenoid cartilages (**arytenoid
  hypertelorism**)
- Surgical options:
    1. **Conservative surgical excision**: endoscopic or open based
       on size; must obtain negative margins; hemicricoidectomy or
       arytenoidectomy may be required
    2. **Total laryngectomy**: indicated for recurrent, high-grade, or
       anaplastic chondrosarcoma, and irreparable damage to laryngeal
       framework
- high rate of local recurrence

LARYNGEAL SCHWANNOMA

- encapsulated benign soft tissue neoplasia consisting of Schwann cells
- very rare benign laryngeal tumor (0.1%–1.5%)
- peak incidence between 20 and 50 years of age
- most commonly arise from false vocal folds and aryepiglottic folds
- majority are nonpedunculated (86.5%)
- most are single, sporadic lesions
- multicentric schwannomas seen in neurofibromatosis type 2 (NF2)
  and schwannomatosis
- Risk factors: radiation exposure, genetic (eg, NF2)
- Histology:
    1. **Antoni A** (hypercellular, spindle cell bundles) and **Antoni B**
       (hypocellular, loose stroma) regions
    2. **Verocay bodies** (palisading nuclei)
    3. fibrous capsule attached to intact nerve
    4. axons not found in tumor
    5. signs of tumor degeneration

- <u>Presentation</u>: hoarseness, dysphonia, dysphagia, globus sensation, stridor, respiratory distress
- pedunculated lesions more likely to cause airway obstruction due to ball-valving
- <u>Dx</u>: flexible and rigid laryngoscopy, MRI w/contrast
- **MRI**: intermediate signal (isodense to muscle) on T1, hyperintense on T2, homogenous enhancement with contrast; no cartilage erosion or surrounding tissue invasion
- incisional biopsy has low diagnostic yield (47%) and increased recurrence
- <u>Tx</u>: observation unless symptomatic or growth, surgery generally curative, possibly radiotherapy
- size will remain stable in majority of schwannomas, and 5% to 10% will shrink
- <u>Surgical options</u>:
  1. **Endoscopic**: cold knife or laser; indicated for small pedunculated lesions; low rate of complications; high rate of recurrence for pedunculated lesions
  2. **Open**: via thyrotomy or pharyngotomy; indicated for nonpedunculated and large lesions; increased risk of vocal fold paresis/paralysis/immobility

CHAPTER

16

Laryngeal Neoplasia

Travis Weinsheim, Luke J. Pasick, and Christopher E. Fundikowski

OVERVIEW

- second most common head and neck cancer
- male:female ratio 7:1
- median age 65
- incidence has decreased in United States, possibly associated with decline in tobacco use
- <u>Risk factors</u>: smoking, alcohol consumption, prior radiation exposure, gastroesophageal reflux, human papillomavirus, wood dust, polycyclic hydrocarbons, asbestos
- smoking and alcohol use together yield a multiplicative risk (odds ratio = 177)
- tobacco, alcohol, or a combination of the two substances are responsible for 72% of head and neck cancer when compared with other risk factors
- ~40% of patients are diagnosed with stage III or IV disease
- overall 5-year survival is 60.9%
- <u>Presentation</u>: hoarseness, ear pain, aspiration, globus sensation, dysphagia, odynophagia, stridor, neck mass, cough, exertional dyspnea
- can affect one or more laryngeal subsites: supraglottic, glottic, and subglottic

SUBSITES AND BOUNDARIES

Supraglottic

- extends from the epiglottis to the ventricular apices
- approximately 32% of laryngeal cancers
- ciliated pseudostratified columnar epithelium
- primary drainage to nodal levels II to IV with bilateral involvement common

Glottic

- extends from the junction of true vocal fold and ventricle to 1 cm below true vocal folds
- most common site of laryngeal cancer, ~51%
- histologically different from supraglottis and subglottis as it is stratified squamous epithelium
- poor lymphatic network with subsequent uncommon nodal metastasis

- bilateral adenopathy uncommon with unilateral lesions
- drainage to nodal levels II to IV

Subglottic

- begins 1 cm below true vocal folds and extends to the inferior limit of the cricoid cartilage
- approximately 2% of laryngeal cancers
- ciliated pseudostratified columnar epithelium
- primary drainage to nodal levels VI (including Delphian node), IV, and upper mediastinum
- poor prognosis

TUMOR BIOLOGY AND PATHOLOGY

- progression from premalignant lesion to laryngeal carcinoma is dependent on genetic alterations of the following genes
  1. Cyclin D1
  2. p53
  3. p16 (not prognostic at this time for laryngeal cancer)
- squamous cell carcinoma is histologically responsible for 95% of laryngeal cancer
- verrucous squamous cell carcinoma is a well-differentiated variant with low probability of metastasis
  1. treatment consists of single-modality therapy
  2. radiation therapy less effective due to slow growth
- adenocarcinoma represents 1% of laryngeal cancers and is distributed in supraglottic and subglottic regions as these are the areas with most of the mucinous glands in the larynx
- rarely, malignant minor salivary gland tumors arise from subepithelial mucous glands and are most commonly located in the subglottis and supraglottis
  1. **Adenoid cystic carcinoma**: most common minor salivary gland tumor of the larynx (32%–69%); characterized by indolent growth pattern, tendency to spread perineurally, and most commonly metastasizes to lung
  2. **Mucoepidermoid carcinoma**: second most common minor salivary gland malignancy of larynx (15%–35%); low, intermediate, or high grade (confused with squamous cell carcinoma on histologic analysis)
- other subtypes include spindle cell carcinoma, fibrosarcoma, chondrosarcoma, neuroendocrine tumors

PREMALIGNANT LESIONS (*See* Table 16–1)

Management

- <u>Hyperplasia</u>: no intervention or routine observation required
- <u>Mild dysplasia</u>: routine observation with laryngoscopy
- <u>High-grade dysplasia</u>: consider local resection or radiation
    1. decision between modalities should factor in morbidity of the procedure and the location of the lesion
    2. prior history of radiation → consider laser resection

Recurrent Laryngeal Papillomatosis
(See Chapter 15)

- human papillomavirus (HPV) 6, 11, 16, 18, 42, 43, and 44
- 1% to 7% transform to squamous cell carcinoma (SCC)
- presence of HPV has not shown to be prognostic in laryngeal cancer
- high rate of co-infection with multiple subtypes

TABLE 16–1. Histopathologic Classifications

Histopathologic Grade	Description	Risk of Malignant Transformation
Hyperplasia (with or without keratosis)	Increased number of epithelial cells without abnormal appearance of cells or architectural atypia	0%
Mild dysplasia	Mild loss in uniformity in epithelial cells in regard to size, shape, and distribution of mitotic figures; also including loss of architectural orientation	5%
Moderate dysplasia	Atypical loss in uniformity in epithelial cells in regard to size, shape, and distribution of mitotic figures; also including loss of architectural orientation	15%
Severe dysplasia (Carcinoma in situ)	Cells that appear atypical, resemble malignancy, and involve the entirety of the epithelial thickness but do not breach basement membrane	40%
Invasive carcinoma	Malignant cells that invade past the basement membrane	NA

STAGING (BASED ON AJCC EIGHTH EDITION)

Important note: the following is clinical TNM staging. There is a separate pathologic staging system for regional lymph nodes (N) (AJCC eighth edition). The pathologic staging may only be performed after the neck dissection specimen is provided to the pathologist. The clinical and pathologic staging differs when there is extranodal extension (ENE) on pathologic examination when a single ipsilateral lymph node is less than 3 cm. The pathologic stage is N2a and clinical stage N3b in the above scenario.

Primary Tumor (T)

Supraglottic

- <u>T1</u>: limited to one subsite; normal vocal fold mobility
- <u>T2</u>: extends to an adjacent subsite of supraglottis, glottis, or region outside of supraglottis (ie, base of tongue, vallecula, medial wall pyriform sinus); no fixation of larynx
- <u>T3</u>: limited to larynx with vocal fold fixation or invasion of the following: pre-epiglottic space, paraglottic space, inner cortex of thyroid cartilage, or postcricoid region
- <u>T4a</u>: extends through outer cortex of thyroid cartilage or to structures outside of the larynx (ie, trachea, soft tissue of neck, strap muscles, thyroid, esophagus, deep extrinsic muscles of tongue)
- <u>T4b</u>: encasement of carotid artery, invasion of prevertebral space or mediastinum

Glottic

- <u>T1a</u>: limited to one vocal fold
- <u>T1b</u>: involves both vocal folds
- <u>T2</u>: tumor extends to supraglottis or subglottis or decreased vocal fold mobility
- <u>T3</u>: limited to larynx with vocal fold fixation or invasion of inner cortex of thyroid cartilage or paraglottic space
- <u>T4a</u>: extends through outer cortex of thyroid cartilage or to structures outside of the larynx (ie, trachea, soft tissue of neck, strap muscles, thyroid, esophagus, deep extrinsic muscles of tongue)
- <u>T4b</u>: encasement of carotid artery, invasion of prevertebral space or mediastinum

Subglottic

- <u>T1</u>: limited to subglottis
- <u>T2</u>: extends to vocal folds
- <u>T3</u>: limited to larynx with vocal fold fixation or invasion of inner cortex of thyroid cartilage or paraglottic space
- <u>T4a</u>: extends through outer cortex of thyroid cartilage or to structures outside of the larynx (ie, trachea, soft tissue of neck, strap muscles, thyroid, esophagus, deep extrinsic muscles of tongue)
- <u>T4b</u>: encasement of carotid artery, invasion of prevertebral space or mediastinum

Clinical Regional Lymph Nodes (cN)

- <u>N0</u>: no regional lymph node metastasis
- <u>N1</u>: metastasis to single ipsilateral lymph node, 3 cm or smaller without extranodal extension (ENE)
- <u>N2a</u>: metastasis to single ipsilateral lymph node, 6 cm or smaller without ENE
- <u>N2b</u>: metastasis to multiple ipsilateral lymph, 6 cm or smaller without ENE
- <u>N2c</u>: metastasis to bilateral or contralateral lymph node; 6 cm or smaller without ENE
- <u>N3a</u>: metastasis to lymph node measuring 6 cm or larger without ENE
- <u>N3b</u>: metastasis to a lymph node, any size, with ENE

Pathologic Regional Lymph Nodes (pN)

- <u>N0</u>: no regional lymph node metastasis
- <u>N1</u>: metastasis to single ipsilateral lymph node, 3 cm or smaller without ENE
- <u>N2a</u>: metastasis to single ipsilateral lymph node, 3 cm or smaller with ENE or metastasis to single ipsilateral lymph node, 3 to 6 cm without ENE
- <u>N2b</u>: metastasis to multiple ipsilateral lymph, 6 cm or smaller without ENE
- <u>N2c</u>: metastasis to bilateral or contralateral lymph node; 6 cm or smaller without ENE
- <u>N3a</u>: metastasis to lymph node measuring 6 cm or larger without ENE
- <u>N3b</u>: metastasis to single ipsilateral lymph node, larger than 3 cm with ENE or metastasis to single contralateral lymph node with ENE or metastasis to multiple ipsilateral, contralateral, or bilateral lymph nodes with ENE

Distant Metastasis (M)

- <u>M0</u>: no distant metastasis
- <u>M1</u>: distant metastasis

TREATMENT (*See* Table 16–2)

Supraglottic

Stages I and II (T1 and T2, N0)

- primary radiation therapy with surgical salvage for failure versus supraglottic laryngectomy
- decision is based on experience of individual surgeon, availability of equipment, location of tumor, and preoperative functionality of the patient
- transoral resection suitable for radiation therapy salvage
- consider ability to obtain clear margins at anterior commissure
- voice outcomes can be similar as radiation therapy in experienced hands

Stages III and IV

- advanced disease typically treated with dual modality
- late-stage disease with a functional larynx may be treated with organ preservation therapy (eg, radiation therapy ± chemotherapy)
- late-stage disease with a dysfunctional larynx (poor swallowing and poor voice) should be considered for primary surgical intervention

T, N, M	Stage
TABLE 16–2. Laryngeal Cancer Staging	
Tis, N0, M0	Stage 0
T1, N0, M0	Stage I
T2, N0, M0	Stage II
T3, N0, M0 or T1-3, N1, M0	Stage III
T4a, N0, M0 or T1-4a, N2, M0	Stage IVa
T4b, Any N, M0 or Any T, N3, M0	Stage IVb
Any T, Any N, M1	Stage IVc

1. radiation therapy ± chemotherapy for primary treatment of a dysfunctional larynx is likely to worsen voice and swallowing function
2. patients who undergo primary surgical therapy may also need risk-adapted adjuvant therapy based on nodal positivity and extranodal extension

- consider total laryngectomy with risk-adapted adjuvant therapy for patients undergoing surgical intervention
- typical selective neck dissection will include levels II through IV

Glottic

Stages I and II (T1 and T2)

- managed with limited radiation and possible surgical salvage or definitive primary surgical intervention
- radiotherapy traditionally believed to have better voice outcomes—controversial and no data definitive on early or late voice outcomes
- survival is equivalent between radiation and surgery
- does not require elective neck dissection due to low probability of nodal metastasis

Stages III and IV (T3 and T4)

- T3 with functional larynx may be treated with organ preservation therapy
- T3 with poor swallowing and poor voice should be considered primary surgical candidates with risk-adapted adjuvant therapy
- T4a cancers are primarily treated with total laryngectomy with risk-adapted adjuvant therapy
- consider paratracheal dissection

Subglottic

- least common site for laryngeal cancer
- no large randomized controlled clinical trials have investigated the optimal treatment of subglottic laryngeal cancer
- treatment may consist of nonoperative management versus total laryngectomy with risk-adaptive management based on stage
- selective neck dissection for nodal disease
- consider paratracheal compartment metastasis when considering surgery or radiation therapy

SURGICAL APPROACHES

- with the goal of preserving maximal patient quality of life, and survival, surgical approaches range from microlaryngeal surgery to total laryngectomy
- "conservation laryngeal surgery" describes procedures that result in partial preservation in order to preserve voice, speech, and swallow functions
    1. patient must have at least one functional cricoarytenoid joint and one laryngeal valve free of disease
    2. laryngeal valve may be any of the following: epiglottis, false vocal fold, true vocal fold
- any laryngeal surgery that is organ preserving or partial in nature requires consent for possible total laryngectomy

Transoral Surgery

Transoral Laser Microsurgery

- mainstay approach utilized since the 1970s with comparable functional and oncologic outcomes in experienced hands
- patient factors such as inability to extend neck, large mandibular tori, and large transverse diameter of mass may preclude this approach
- reduced morbidity and improved functional outcomes compared with open approach
- European Laryngological Society Classification (2008)
    1. I: subepithelial
    2. II: subligamental
    3. III: transmuscular
    4. IV: total cordectomy
    5. V: extended cordectomy
       Va: encompasses contralateral vocal fold and anterior commissure
       Vb: includes arytenoid
       Vc: encompasses subglottis
       Vd: includes ventricle
    6. VI: cordectomy for cancer of anterior commissure, extended to one or both vocal folds, without infiltration of thyroid cartilage

Transoral Robotic Surgery

- amount of surgeon experience correlates with improved patient selection and a decreased rate of conversion to open procedure
- application has been explored for glottic, supraglottic, and total laryngectomy
- higher cost when compared to transoral laryngeal microsurgery

Open Surgery

Vertical Hemilaryngectomy (Partial Laryngectomy)

- resection of vocal fold and portion of thyroid cartilage en bloc
- Variations:
    1. frontolateral for lesions involving anterior commissure
    2. posterolateral for lesions involving unfixed ipsilateral arytenoid

Supraglottic Laryngectomy

- resection of structures superior to thyroid and arytenoid cartilages, and true vocal folds
- baseline pulmonary function and swallow evaluation necessary
    1. FEV1/FVC <50% yields greater risk for aspiration
    2. high postoperative aspiration risk
    3. swallowing rehabilitation necessary

Supracricoid Partial Laryngectomy

- resection includes thyroid cartilage, paraglottic space, and true vocal folds
- spares uninvolved arytenoid cartilages, cricoid cartilage, hyoid
- possible reconstruction of defect
    1. cricohyoidopexy (if epiglottis is removed)
    2. cricohyoidoepiglottopexy (if epiglottis is spared)
- requires tracheotomy
- baseline pulmonary function testing similar to supraglottic laryngectomy
- patients with cricohyoidopexy over 60 years old at increased risk of postoperative pulmonary complications
- salvage surgery after radiation failure

Near Total Laryngectomy

- voice-sparing procedure via a voice shunt through patient's tissues
- resection of hemilarynx and anterior of contralateral vocal fold
- possible resection of ipsilateral cricoid and proximal trachea
- preservation of one arytenoid required to prevent aspiration
- permanent tracheostomy required

Total Laryngectomy

- resection of true and false vocal folds, thyroid, cricoid, and arytenoid cartilages, epiglottis, hyoid, and proximal trachea

- no connection between pharynx and trachea, no aspiration risk
- permanent stoma created
- <u>Indications</u>:
    1. nonfunctional T3, and T4 lesions
    2. hypopharyngeal lesion with postcricoid involvement
    3. chondrosarcomas of cricoid or thyroid cartilages
- recurrent disease after failed organ preservation treatment
- consider ipsilateral hemithyroidectomy in transglottic tumor, or direct extension into thyroid gland
- monitor thyroid function q6mos-1yr following surgery
- *see* Table 16–3

Postoperative Complications

- clean-contaminated procedures pose increased risk of infection
- pharyngocutaneous fistulas between skin and resection site
    1. previous radiation and chemoradiation increase risk
- prophylactic vascularized flaps decrease fistula incidence in salvage total laryngectomy
- aspiration risk after conservation laryngeal surgery, tolerated with good pulmonary function
- perichondritis and chondritis of exposed cartilage
- airway fires may occur in transoral laser microsurgery—laser safe tube is recommended
- stenosis of stoma, pharynx, or esophagus

COMMUNICATION AFTER LARYNGECTOMY

- writing instead of voice is an acceptable alternative that is always available

Esophageal Speech

- all other methods compared to esophageal speech
- air from mouth or pharynx forcefully propelled into esophagus with tongue is expelled → vibration of mucosa of pharyngoesophagus → articulated into speech with tongue, lips, and teeth
- 26% of patients can learn

TABLE 16-3. Surgical Options

Endoscopic and Robotic	Indications	Contraindications
Transoral laser microsurgery	T1, T2, select T3	Inadequate transoral access; bilateral arytenoid cartilage involvement; subglottic extension >1 cm
Transoral robotic surgery	Transoral resection of tumors unresectable by laser microsurgery; based on individual patient and surgeon experience	

Open

Vertical hemilaryngectomy	T1-T3	Subglottic extension >10 mm anteriorly or >5 mm posteriorly; fixed vocal fold; posterior commissure or interarytenoid involvement
Supraglottic laryngectomy	T1, T2 supraglottic; T2, T3 supraglottic extending to base of tongue; T3 supraglottic with preepiglottic space	Vocal fold immobility; involvement of cartilage or pyriform sinus beyond upper medial wall; postcricoid or interarytenoid extension; poor pulmonary or swallowing function
Supracricoid partial laryngectomy	Supraglottic with ventricle, epiglottis, and anterior false vocal fold involvement; supraglottic extending to glottis, paraglottic space, ± vocal fold mobility; transglottic with decreased vocal fold mobility	Subglottic extension; cricoid, thyroid perichondrium, or bilateral arytenoid involvement; poor pulmonary function
Total laryngectomy	Nonfunctional T3, T4 cancer; hypopharyngeal with postcricoid involvement; recurrence after organ-preserving therapy; chondrosarcoma; poor pulmonary function	

Artificial Larynx

- rapidly learned, relatively inexpensive, and does not interfere with other forms of alaryngeal speech
- a device is pressed against the neck → mechanical sound is transmitted to tissues and spaces in neck → oral cavity used to emanate words

Tracheoesophageal Puncture (TEP)

- one-way valve allows air into esophagus → air is expelled into pharyngoesophagus causing vibration of opposing mucosal surfaces → oral cavity is used to articulate speech in a similar fashion as esophageal speech
- can be created primarily or secondarily—at the time of the procedure or 6 to 8 weeks after radiation therapy has ceased
- stomal size of 2 cm or greater is important to allow placement and does not compromise airway
- 20% to 40% of patients have difficulty due to spasm of cricopharyngeus, inferior and middle constrictors
    1. performing generous cricopharyngeal myotomy may decrease risk
    2. injection of Botox has been shown to be effective in postlaryngectomy patients with pharyngoesophageal spasm
- *see* Table 16–4

TABLE 16–4. Alaryngeal Speech

Method	Advantages	Disadvantages
Esophageal speech	Hands free, natural sounding voice	Difficult to learn, quiet, short duration
Electrolarynx	Rapidly learned, loud, inexpensive	Not hands free, battery dependent, mechanical sounding voice
TEP	Well hidden, natural sounding voice	Risk of aspiration or esophageal prolapse, requires maintenance and replacement

SECTION

V

Neurolaryngology

CHAPTER

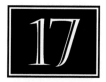

Laryngeal Neurophysiology

Justin Ross, Mary J. Hawkshaw, and Robert T. Sataloff

INTRODUCTION

- laryngologists should be versed in the neurophysiology of laryngeal function
- speech, swallowing, respiration, and airway protection rely on highly complex and integrated system composed of multiple structures within the peripheral (PNS) and central nervous systems (CNS)

MOTOR FUNCTION (*See* Chapter 3)

- vagus nerve (CN X) provides innervation to laryngeal musculature via the recurrent laryngeal nerve (RLN) or the external branch of superior laryngeal nerve (eSLN)
- cell bodies of CN X motor neurons reside in the nucleus ambiguus of the ventral-lateral medulla
- descending corticobulbar tracts decussate above the medulla, containing bilateral input
- upon reaching the nucleus ambiguus, motor innervation is separated into left or right
- **lesions above nucleus ambiguus → bilateral impairment** of laryngeal function, contralateral side is usually most affected
- **lesions at or below nucleus ambiguus → unilateral impairment** of laryngeal function
- cortical input to laryngeal motor nerves is bilateral and arises from multiple brain sites
- under normal circumstances, laryngeal neuromuscular activity is constant but varies with different activities (eg, inspiration, expiration, phonation, cough)
- the number of neuromuscular junctions in laryngeal muscles is greater than other muscles, suggesting improved fine motor control

SENSORY FUNCTION

- **internal branch of SLN (iSLN) →** mucosa of the aryepiglottic folds (AEF), laryngeal surface of epiglottis, vestibule and true vocal folds (TVF)
- **RLN →** subglottis, trachea, spindles of intrinsic muscles, sometimes portions of vocal folds
- **glossopharyngeal nerve (CN IX) →** posterior oropharynx
- laryngeal afferents can detect pressure, touch, taste, pH, and airflow
- posterior pharyngeal afferents detect pressure, touch, taste, and pH

- tracheal afferents detect pressure and food/liquid
- loss of laryngeal sensation can result in dysphagia/aspiration, and can be assessed during flexible laryngoscopy by gently contacting the AEF on each side

LARYNGEAL REFLEXES

- stimulation of sensory afferents (iSLN) may result in laryngeal adductor response (LAR), cough, swallow, and/or respiration
- all laryngeal sensory information travels through the nodose and/or jugular ganglion and the nucleus tractus solitarius (NTS), eventually reaching the medullary central pattern generators that integrate inputs and determine motor activity

Laryngeal Adductor Response (LAR)

- reflexive contraction of bilateral thyroarytenoid muscles (TA) in response to stimulation of laryngeal mucosa
- important for airway protection when liquid or food contacts laryngeal mucosa
- Neural pathway: stimulation of laryngeal mucosal mechanoreceptors → sensory afferents (iSLN) → nodose ganglion (NG) → nucleus tractus solitarius (NTS) → nucleus ambiguus (NA) → motor efferents (RLN) → bilateral vocal fold adduction
- contraction occurs first in the ipsilateral vocal fold (~16 ms), and then the contralateral (~60 ms)
- continuous, intense stimulation of mucosal afferents also can cause sustained vocal fold adduction and exhalation that can be catastrophic
- patients with absent LAR may be at increased risk of aspiration pneumonia
- LAR can be used in sensory testing

Cough

- sequence of activities including rapid inhalation, TVF adduction, increasing subglottic pressure, and finally abrupt airflow through the glottis
- protective mechanism that clears substances that stimulate the laryngeal or tracheal mucosa
- Neural pathway: stimulation of subglottic (primary) or vestibular mucosa → iSLN → nodose or jugular ganglion → NTS → dorsal motor nucleus of CN X (DMV) → ventral respiratory group (VRG)

→ NA or nucleus retroambiguus (NRA) → RLN (NA), phrenic nerve and spinal motor nerves (NRA) → respiratory and laryngeal muscle activation
- also initiated by stimulation of CN X sensory afferents in the external auditory canal (Arnold's nerve), trachea, lungs, heart, and stomach

Central Pattern Generators

- **Central pattern generators (CPGs):** activation patterns of interneurons in medullary integrative regions that determine the excitatory or inhibitory signals that project to motor neurons in the nucleus ambiguus
- responsible for reflexive activation or suppression of LAR, cough, respiration, and/or swallowing
- laryngeal sensory afferents modulate activation of CPGs in a task-specific manner (eg, while swallowing, respiration, and LAR are inhibited and vocal folds adduct)

VOCALIZATION

- larynx is responsible for phonation and pitch modulation
- the voluntary and complex nature of human vocal control relative to other primates is due in large part to complex neural systems rather than anatomic differences alone
- mastication, swallowing, speech (phonation and articulation) and facial expression arise from the ventral sensorimotor cortex (vSMC)
- <u>Mammalian vocalization system</u>: noncortical system that controls spontaneous voicing, present in primates and humans, activated during emotive vocalizations; cingulate cortex → periaqueductal gray → pons → nucleus retroambiguus → NA
- <u>Voluntary vocalization</u>: arises from the ventral prefrontal cortex that projects inputs to the laryngeal motor cortex (LMC) within the vSMC
- voicing is initiated in the dorsal and ventral LMC, while pitch control during speech and singing arises from the dorsal LMC alone
- cortical voice control is thought to arise primarily from the left hemisphere
- feedback loops in the basal ganglia and cerebellum may be involved with learned vocal patterns

CHAPTER

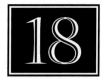

Vocal Fold Paresis and Paralysis

Justin Ross, Mary J. Hawkshaw, and Robert T. Sataloff

INTRODUCTION

- injury to the vagus nerve, superior laryngeal nerve (SLN) or recurrent laryngeal nerve (RLN) resulting in true vocal fold (TVF) denervation
- paresis refers to partial denervation, while paralysis implies complete denervation
- can originate centrally (motor cortex, nucleus ambiguus) or peripherally (vagus, SLN, RLN)
- Seddon classified histologic manifestations of peripheral nerve injury
  1. **Neurapraxia**: injury without damage to axons, resulting in temporary neural dysfunction
  2. **Axonotmesis**: injury to the myelin sheath and axons
  3. **Neurotmesis**: complete discontinuity of nerve (eg, transection)
- degree of peripheral nerve injury most commonly described by Sunderland classification (Table 18–1)
- <u>Etiology</u>: iatrogenic, trauma, infection, neoplasia (compression or infiltration), neurologic disease, collagen vascular disease, idiopathic
- paralysis typically results from complete nerve transection
- arytenoid cartilage subluxation, dislocation, and joint fixation may cause decreased TVF mobility that is misdiagnosed as paresis/paralysis
- absence of jostle sign seen in arytenoid dislocation and fixation, but not severe TVF paresis and paralysis
- neoplasia or neurologic insult can impair motor function through damage to any region of the neural pathway

TABLE 18–1. Sunderland Classification

Degree of Injury	Seddon Classification	Histologic Description	Wallerian Degeneration	Recovery Without Repair
1	Neurapraxia	Edema/compression, ± demyelination	No	Complete
2	Axonotmesis	Axonal injury	Yes	Complete
3	Axonotmesis	Endoneurial disruption	Yes	Partial
4	Axonotmesis	Perineurial disruption	Yes	Minimal
5	Neurotmesis	Transection (epineurium)	Yes	None

Source: Adapted from Sunderland (1990).

- <u>Presentation</u>: dysphonia, hoarseness, breathiness, aphonia, loss of upper range, vocal fatigue, compensatory muscle tension, sometimes with palpable laryngotracheal complex tenderness, choking/aspiration
- associated with benign vocal fold lesions (eg, nodule, cyst, Reinke's edema, polyp), particularly paresis because of compensatory hyperfunction and other causes

Recurrent Laryngeal Nerve (RLN)

Functional Anatomy

- branches from vagus nerve in the root of the neck and usually courses around the subclavian artery (right RLN) or ligamentum arteriosum (left RLN), travels superiorly within the tracheoesophageal groove, and usually penetrates the larynx posteriorly at the cricothyroid joint
- right RLN approaches the larynx at a more oblique angle than the left
- nonrecurrent laryngeal nerve occurs only on the right (0.5%), except in situs inversus
- provides motor innervation to intrinsic laryngeal adductors (thyroarytenoid [TA], interarytenoid [IA], lateral cricoarytenoid [LCA]) and abductors (posterior cricoarytenoid [PCA])
- IA is the only muscle that receives bilateral motor innervation; function is poorly understood, but could provide posterior adduction due to medial compression
- unilateral RLN injury produces breathy, soft voice with possible diplophonia, dysphagia, and aspiration

Adductors

- unilateral TA or LCA denervation results in glottic insufficiency, breathy voice, and increased risk of aspiration
- will occasionally assume a median or paramedian position in the subacute to chronic phase (weeks)
- bilateral denervation is characterized by pronounced TVF bowing and breathy voice or aphonia initially
- over time voice often improves and airway worsens

Abductors

- unilateral PCA paresis/paralysis typically causes anteromedial subluxation of the arytenoid resulting TVF medialization
- bilateral PCA denervation may result in airway obstruction

Etiology

- <u>Iatrogenic</u>: surgery, intubation (cuff or tube contact), mediastinal radiation, I-131 therapy
- <u>Surgical</u>: anterior approach to cervical spine > thyroidectomy > carotid endarterectomy > thoracic surgery (left RLN)
- greater risk during anterior cervical spine surgery (up to 21%) than thyroidectomy (up to 13%)
- thoracic RLN can be damaged during patent ductus arteriosus (PDA) ligation, aortic aneurysm repair, coronary artery bypass grafting (CABG), and other open thoracic procedures
- <u>Mechanism</u>: transection, crush, suture/staple, traction, thermal
- <u>Neoplasia</u>: thyroid mass, lymphoma (neck or mediastinum), lung cancer (upper lobe), central nervous system (CNS) mass
- compression by large thyroid goiters
- <u>Infection</u>: Lyme disease, syphilis, EBV, herpes virus, other
- idiopathic denervation thought by some to have a viral etiology
- <u>Neurologic</u>: multiple sclerosis (MS), amyotrophic lateral sclerosis (ALS), syringomyelia, myasthenia gravis, Guillain-Barré, Parkinson's disease, stroke, other
- <u>Systemic</u>: systemic lupus erythematosus (SLE), amyloidosis, porphyria, polyarteritis nodosa, familial hypokalemic periodic paralysis, Gerhard's syndrome (laryngeal abductors), diabetic neuropathy
- <u>Traumatic</u>: blunt or penetrating

Recovery

- axonal regrowth occurs at a rate of ~1 to 3 mm/day
- injuries greater than Sunderland stage II often result in functional deficit
- reinnervation increases/preserves muscle bulk, but may not provide functional benefit
- nonselective reinnervation by mixed adductor/abductor nerve fibers occurs often → synkinesis
- **Synkinesis**: simultaneous activation of adductor and abductor laryngeal muscles
- evaluation of suspected synkinesis performed with laryngeal electromyography; typically seen as simultaneous activation of thyroarytenoid and posterior cricoarytenoid muscles on affected side
- classification of synkinesis described by Crumley (Table 18–2)
- airway compromise may occur in type III synkinesis due to tonic adduction of TVFs, particularly in bilateral RLN

TABLE 18–2. Crumley Synkinesis Grading		
Synkinesis Grade	**Vocal Fold Movement**	**Voice Quality**
Type I	Little to none	Normal
Type II	Spastic	Poor
Type III	Tonic adduction	Normal
Type IV	Tonic abduction	Breathy voice

Source: Adapted from Rubin and Sataloff (2017).

paralysis—may be treated with botulinum toxin injection of the adductor muscles
- increased risk of aspiration in type IV synkinesis due to tonic abduction of TVFs

Superior Laryngeal Nerve (SLN)

Functional Anatomy

- branches off of the vagus nerve inferior to the nodose ganglion, splits into two branches at the hyoid (internal and external divisions)
- internal SLN (iSLN) pierces the thyrohyoid membrane to provide sensory innervation to endolaryngeal mucosa at and above the level of the TVFs
- external SLN (eSLN) provides motor innervation to the cricothyroid muscle; primarily responsible for pitch change by increasing TVF longitudinal tension
- voice changes noticed by singers due to decrease of vocal range and instability during soft upper midrange singing; noticed by speakers as loss of projection

Etiology

- causes include those affecting the RLN with some exceptions
- most common cause overall likely viral neuritis secondary to herpes simplex or upper respiratory infection
- thyroidectomy is the most common surgical cause; important to ligate superior thyroid artery close to thyroid capsule if unable to identify SLN visually
- isolated injury to eSLN can occur without impairment of iSLN

Presentation

- poor vocal performance with loss of pitch control through midrange and often above, especially during soft singing
- vocal fatigue, hoarseness, breathiness, lower volume, and decreased projection
- compensatory muscle tension dysphonia
- comorbid phonotraumatic lesions (eg, cyst, nodule, polyp, hemorrhage) from compensatory muscle tension
- occasional upper laryngeal anesthesia if iSLN affected; often presents as choking, throat clearing, dysphagia, aspiration, and occasionally as neuropathic pain
- palatal hypoesthesia (ipsilateral reduced gag) seen in iSLN dysfunction

EVALUATION

Introduction

- complete history including neurologic symptoms, recent illness, prior surgery, intubations, trauma, chronicity, tobacco/alcohol/drug use, vocal changes and habits
- complete head and neck exam
- cranial nerve examination including gag reflex and palatal elevation/ deviation
- perceptual and objective assessment of voice
- laryngeal mirror examination followed flexible and rigid laryngoscopy with stroboscopy
- magnetic resonance imaging (MRI) or computed tomography (CT) with contrast covering skull base to aortic arch; include brain or at least brain stem to include the nuclei associated with the SLN and RLN
- laryngeal sensory testing
- swallowing assessment when symptoms are present

Laryngoscopy

- <u>Findings</u>: asymmetrical abduction and/or adduction (RLN), and/or longitudinal tension (eSLN); vocal fold bowing (eSLN); asymmetrical vocal process height and posterior laryngeal tilt (eSLN) classically but inconsistently toward the side of paresis; hypopharyngeal pooling of secretions (iSLN or RLN)
- evaluate motion abnormalities by having the patient perform multiple repeated phonatory tasks

- other options include repeated, alternating /i/ - /hi/; repeated /pa/ - /ta/ - /ka/
- glissandos (slides) alter TVF tension and are helpful in the evaluation of eSLN
- vocal process height discrepancies may become evident at high pitch (abnormal—lower)
- floppy epiglottis is often seen in bilateral eSLN paralysis

Laryngeal Electromyography (See Chapter 6)

TREATMENT

Voice Therapy (See Chapter 37)

- most patients with unilateral RLN paralysis will obtain satisfactory voice and airway with voice therapy alone, but success depends on several factors including the severity of the paresis/paralysis
- essential to establish preoperative baseline, increases patient compliance, and improves psychological readiness for surgery
- corrects compensatory hyperfunction and preemptively optimizes postoperative phonation
- should include pre- and postoperative sessions
- addition of specialized singing training can accelerate therapeutic benefit
- least success in patients with bilateral paralysis

Surgical Management (See Chapter 33)

Indications

- Nerve transection: early reinnervation at time of injury unless excised intentionally or other prohibitive factors
- Nerve injury (crush, stretch, thermal, etc): observation with temporary injection TVF medialization
- Aspiration: early TVF medialization
- Professional voice user: early TVF medialization to meet vocal demands
- Desire for increased voice quality and volume
- Laryngeal electromyogram (LEMG) findings indicating poor prognosis (ie, fibrillations, positive sharp waves)

Injection Laryngoplasty

- medialization technique during which a material is injected lateral to the thyroarytenoid muscle
- many different materials can be used
- goals of therapy include improved glottic closure and vocal quality, reduced aspiration
- can be performed awake or under general anesthesia
- <u>Indications</u>: unilateral vocal fold paresis or paralysis, vocal fold bowing, presbylarynx, glottic insufficiency
- <u>Materials</u>: Teflon, saline, voice gel, Gelfoam, fat, fascia, collagen, AlloDerm, hyaluronic acid, calcium hydroxylapatite

Type I Thyroplasty

- technique in which autologous cartilage or synthetic material (eg, Gore-Tex) is implanted medial to the thyroid cartilage to permanently medialize the vocal fold
- may be performed with arytenoid adduction or arytenoidopexy for persistent, symptomatic posterior glottic gap
- may be performed in combination (staged) with lipoinjection medialization
- arytenoid mobilization or repositioning might be required if long-term RLN paralysis results in cricoarytenoid joint ankylosis

Reinnervation

- goals of therapy are to prevent atrophy and increase/maintain bulk of laryngeal muscles
- reinnervation has been attempted with ansa cervicalis, phrenic nerve, preganglionic sympathetic neurons, hypoglossal nerve, vagus nerve, homograft nerve, and nerve-muscle pedicles
- synkinesis occurs often, even with excellent technique
- improved vocal quality and mucosal wave, as well as decreased aspiration have been reported
- RLN reinnervation can improve long-term (>3 years) vocal quality and adduction over injection medialization alone in patients with total denervation or LEMG
- ansa to RLN reinnervation can reduce spastic synkinesis, improve mucosal wave, and stabilize the arytenoids; limited benefit if injury older than 2 years or patient is >60 years old; branch innervating sternothyroid or sternohyoid used because they have limited activity during phonation and respiration
- ansa to sternothyroid to TA

- innervated TA to denervated TA via nerve interposition graft reported in animal models, and has shown decreased synkinesis and increased adduction
- injection of vincristine into the PCA in an animal model of unilateral RLN injury demonstrated preferential adductor reinnervation, and has a favorable toxicity profile
- phrenic to PCA reinnervation relies on shared activation during inspiration
- nimodipine suggested as a nontemporal treatment option in nontransection injury—may improve chance of successful recovery

Laryngeal Pacing

- induction of muscle contraction via electrical stimulation
- requires afferent (input) and efferent (output) limbs
- source of the afferent limb is based on laterality of paralysis: unilateral (contralateral TA or LCA), bilateral (phrenic nerve)
- efferent limb is connected to the nerve (vagus or RLN), nerve muscle pedicle, or denervated muscle
- optimal stimulation frequency, intensity, and pulse duration is muscle dependent
- few human studies have been performed, but in one study respiratory and voice outcomes were superior in unilateral pacing compared with posterior cordotomy
- another study demonstrated successful decannulation of over half of patients with BVFP

BILATERAL VOCAL FOLD PARALYSIS (BVFP)

- <u>Etiology</u>: surgery, malignancy, intubation, idiopathic, CNS, trauma, radiation
- thyroid surgery most common (~27%) in adults
- esophageal cancer is malignancy most likely to cause BVFP
- <u>Presentation</u>: depends on position of vocal folds; stridor and/or respiratory distress (adducted), aspiration, and/or breathiness (abducted)
- <u>Surgical options</u>:
  1. cordotomy/cordectomy
  2. arytenoidectomy
  3. suture lateralization
  4. phrenic-PCA reinnervation

    5. tracheotomy

    6. laryngeal pacing

- primary goal of therapy is to establish airway patency via lateralization of one or both vocal folds
- tracheotomy may be required in the acute setting
- impairment of postoperative voice quality common
- cordotomy and arytenoidectomy are typically performed with CO_2 laser via endoscopy; complications include granuloma, posterior glottic scar/stenosis, and perichondritis
- suture lateralization is a reversible technique useful in pediatric congenital BVFP as it is often self-limiting, and used in adults in selected cases
- limited success shown with phrenic-PCA reinnervation
- one study demonstrated successful decannulation and improvement of voice quality in the majority of patients who underwent bilateral, combined phrenic to PCA and hypoglossal to TA reinnervation
- injection of botulinum toxin into bilateral TA may provide temporary relief of airway symptoms and avoid or prolong time to tracheotomy

PEDIATRIC VOCAL FOLD PARALYSIS
(*See* Chapter 31)

- second most common congenital laryngeal anomaly (~10%) and cause of neonatal stridor
- Etiology: CNS or cardiac anomaly, birth trauma, iatrogenic, mediastinal mass, neoplasia, blunt trauma
- pediatric BVFP typically is caused by a CNS disorder, most commonly Arnold-Chiari malformation
- Presentation: stridor, aspiration, feeding difficulty, weak/breathy cry, airway obstruction (BVFP)
- BVFP generally presents at birth
- Dx: history and physical, evaluation of cry, attention to neurologic exam, flexible/rigid laryngoscopy, direct laryngoscopy and bronchoscopy, MRI w/contrast (skull base to aortic arch), ± LEMG
- Tx: medialization and/or reinnervation (unilateral); stabilization of airway with intubation or tracheotomy, and lateralization (bilateral)
- up to 65% resolve spontaneously by 12 months
- tracheotomy is the gold standard for BVFP, but patent airway has been achieved with cricoid split and suture lateralization procedures
- temporary suture lateralization is employed in some centers to avoid tracheotomy and may allow a reversible option in cases with spontaneous recovery

CHAPTER

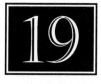

Laryngeal Dystonia

Justin Ross and Aaron J. Jaworek

INTRODUCTION

- involuntary contraction of intrinsic and/or extrinsic skeletal muscles of the larynx
- symptoms generally are aggravated or induced by activation of affected muscle(s)
- primary (genetic, idiopathic) or secondary (acquired)
- may be part of a generalized, segmental, or focal dystonia and classified as spasmodic, tonic, or mixed
- most laryngeal dystonias are primary (idiopathic)
- botulinum toxin type A injection is the most common treatment for laryngeal dystonia
- treatment for generalized or segmental dystonia includes baclofen, benzodiazepines, anticholinergics, and dopamine blocking or depleting agents in recalcitrant disease
- surgical options for laryngeal dystonia include selective denervation, reinnervation, myectomy, and nerve stimulation, and for segmental or generalized dystonia include intrathecal baclofen pump and deep brain stimulation

SPASMODIC DYSPHONIA (SD)

Introduction

- focal dystonia affecting adductor and/or abductor muscles of the larynx
- affects fluency during phonation characterized by strangled and/or breathy breaks
- female predominance (2:1)
- average age of onset is 62 years
- likely related to a primary central nervous system (CNS) disturbance in the laryngeal motor cortex (LMC) and subcortical structures (basal ganglia, thalamus, cerebellum)
- associated with corticobulbar/corticospinal tract demyelination and reduction of axonal density
- primitive phonations (eg, grunts, startles, cries) arising in cingulate cortex are unaffected
- can be associated with torticollis, writer's cramp, and extrapyramidal dystonia
- associated gene mutations include TOR1A (DYT1), TUBB4 (DYT4), and THAP1 (DYT6)

Adductor Spasmodic Dysphonia (ADSD)

- 90% of patients with SD
- irregularly interrupted, strangled, strained, staccato breaks with voiced sounds during connected speech
- affects the thyroarytenoid (TA), lateral cricoarytenoid (LCA), and interarytenoid (IA) muscles

Abductor Spasmodic Dysphonia (ABSD)

- 10% of patients with SD
- breathy breaks with voiceless sounds during connected speech
- affects the posterior cricoarytenoid (PCA) muscles and occasionally cricothyroid (CT) muscles

Mixed Spasmodic Dysphonia (MSD)

- concomitant ADSD and ABSD with staccato and breathy breaks during connected speech

Evaluation

History

- onset frequently associated with preceding viral infection or stressful life event
- nearly equal occurrence of sudden and gradual onset
- sudden onset suggests secondary SD until proven otherwise
- sudden onset and identification of a preceding event are more common in women with SD
- psychiatric disorders are rarely causative
- <u>Risk factors</u>: cervical dystonia; tremor; upper respiratory infection; childhood mumps, measles, or rubella; heavy voice use; stressful life event; recent surgery; pregnancy; trauma
- concomitant vocal tremor in 29% to 54%
- prevalence of tremor 2.8 times higher in patients with SD than general population
- may arise as a manifestation of an underlying neurologic syndrome, drug toxicity, genetic disorder, or autoimmune phenomenon (Table 19–1)
- <u>Family hx</u>: meningitis, cervical dystonia, torticollis, writer's cramp, tremor, neurologic disease, or gene mutation
- Differential diagnosis (*see* Table 19–2)

TABLE 19-1. Diseases Associated With Laryngeal Dystonia and Lab Assessment

Disease	Lab	Abnormal
Wilson disease	Serum ceruloplasmin	Low
Gout	Serum and urine uric acid	High
Polycythemia		
Myeloid metaplasia		
Psoriasis		
Sickle cell		
Alcohol abuse		
Thiazide diuretics		
Lactic acidosis/ketoacidosis		
Renal failure		
Lesch-Nyhan		
Tay-Sachs	Lysosomal enzymes in peripheral WBC	High
Metachromatic leukodystrophy		
Malignancy	α-Fetoprotein (AFP)	High
Ataxia-telangiectasia		
Ataxia-telangiectasia	Serum immunoglobulins (IgA, IgG, IgM)	Low
Multiple myeloma		
Muscular dystrophy	Serum lactate	High
Delirium tremens		
Diseases of cell damage (myocardial and pulmonary infarct)		
Liver disease	Acanthocytosis	High
Abetalipoproteinemia		
Mitochondrial disease		
Mitochondrial disease	Serum LDH	High
Metabolic diseases	Serum CPK	
	Urine amino acids	
	Urine organic acids	
Muscular dystrophy	Creatine kinase (DK)	High
Polymyositis		
Dermatomyositis		
Diseases of cell damage (myocardial and pulmonary infarct)		

TABLE 19–2. Differential Diagnosis for Spasmodic Dysphonia

Condition	Characteristics
Vocal Tremor	• **rhythmic** pitch and intensity modulation • present during sustained vowel phonation • tremor frequency ~5–10 Hz
Dysarthria	• disordered articulation (lingual) • frequently with a slow rate of speech • upper motor neuron symptoms possible (eg, hypertonia, hyperreflexia, spasticity)
Muscle Tension Dysphonia	• pressed, raspy, or strained voice • odynophonia, globus may be present • neck muscles often tight and tender
Psychogenic/Functional Dysphonia	• symptoms can be intermittent • voice may normalize while distracted or sedated • infrequent co-occurrence with tremor

Physical Examination

- comprehensive head and neck evaluation
- observe for presence of an essential tremor (head, neck, hand/wrist)
- palpate neck musculature to assess for concomitant muscle tension dysphonia
- neurologic evaluation with attention to cranial nerves, cerebellar function, and systemic conditions (eg, parkinsonism, ALS, multiple sclerosis, myasthenia gravis, etc)
- musculoskeletal examination if muscle spasm suspected including attention to cervical spine
- referral to speech-language pathologist (SLP) experienced in phonatory disorders for additional voice assessment and voice therapy with attention to reduction of concomitant MTD

Perceptual Evaluation of Voice

- **ADSD predominant**: need connected speech with voiced sounds (eg, /ē/, /ā/, /b/, /d/, /g/), listen for strangled, strained, staccato breaks
  1. ask patient to count in a single breath from 80 to 89
  2. ask patient to repeat "We eat eggs every Easter" or "We mow our lawn all year long"

- **ABSD predominant**: need connected speech with voiceless sounds (eg, /h/, /sh/, /s/, /p/), listen for breathy breaks
    1. ask patient to count in a single breath from 60 to 69
    2. ask patient to repeat "How high is Harry's hat?" or "Harry hit the hammer hard" or "The puppy bit the tape"

Strobovideolaryngoscopy

- flexible and rigid laryngoscopy with continuous and stroboscopic light
- <u>Associated findings</u>: supraglottic hyperfunction (MTD), glottic insufficiency, vocal fold paresis/paralysis, laryngeal tremor, hyperadduction, hyperabduction, paradoxical vocal fold movement, phonotraumatic lesions, dysdiadochokinesia (cerebellar), reflux laryngitis, and other sources of inflammation
- have patient count 60s and 80s, ADSD and ABSD sentences
- have patient perform sustained vowel such as /ē/, for tremor
- have patient sing a song (eg, Happy Birthday)

Laryngeal Electromyography (LEMG)

- can differentiate SD from other neurologic disorders
- delay between signal and audible phonation ~500 ms to 1 s (normal is 0–200 ms)
- may find normal muscle activity with superimposed spasmodic bursts
- localizes spasmodic regions of involved muscles
- TA most commonly involved in ADSD
- equivalent TA and LCA involvement in ADSD with tremor
- IA involvement also seen in ADSD with tremor
- simultaneous spasm of adductor and abductor muscles may occur in ABSD
- often used as a guide for intramuscular placement of botulinum toxin injection

Objective Voice Measures

- establishes pretreatment baseline and evaluates treatment efficacy
- likely to find pretreatment compensatory strategies such as pitch and intensity modulation
- relative average perturbation typically elevated
- perturbation measures can be difficult to interpret due to spasm
- can identify concomitant vocal tremor

Imaging

- obtain magnetic resonance imaging (MRI) with and without gadolinium of brain
    1. imaging may reveal secondary cause of SD (eg, infarct, demyelination, deposition, vascular malformations, neoplasm)
    2. causative basal ganglia and putamen infarcts have been reported
- CNS lesions are less likely to be causative
- consider MRI of the neck extending from skull base to aortic arch if vocal fold paresis/paralysis evident
- functional MRI
    1. limited to research applications
    2. increased activity in sensorimotor cortex and basal ganglia-thalamocortical system during symptomatic speech

Other Testing Considerations

- **Neurolaryngologic panel**: CBC, CMP, TSH, Free T4, TG ab, TPO ab, ACh-R ab panel, FTA ab, Lyme titer with reflex to Western Blot, ANA with subtypes, RF, CCP ab
- **Dystonia panel**: ceruloplasmin, uric acid, lactate, LDH, AFP, CK, IgA, IgM, IgG, urine amino acids, and urine organic acids
- **Genetic testing**: **low yield**, not cost effective

Treatment

Medications

- baclofen, phenytoin, and sodium oxybate occasionally beneficial
- β-blocker (eg, propranolol) for concomitant vocal tremor
- alcohol improved symptoms in >50% of SD patients with or without tremor
- these medications should not be considered as first-line therapy

Speech Therapy

- may improve vocal strain and fatigue by eliminating compensatory hyperfunction (MTD)
- singing therapy useful in patients with reduced symptoms while singing
- rarely curative, but has synergistic benefits with pharmacologic or surgical therapy

Neuromuscular Blockade

- <u>Mechanism</u>: inhibition of acetylcholine release from presynaptic cholinergic neurons at the neuromuscular junction
- most common is botulinum toxin type A (onabotulinum, abobotulinum, incobotulinum)
- botulinum toxin type B (rimabotulinum) used when treatment response diminishes secondary to development of antibodies to botulinum toxin type A (very rare)
- laryngeal Botox total dose range: 0.1 to 30 mouse units (MUs)
- <u>Initial dosing</u>:
    1. ADSD = 0.5 to 1.5 MU to each vocal fold (TA) and can be administered simultaneously
    2. ABSD = 5 to 15 MU to PCA administered to **one side only**
- dose adjustments made based on clinical effect and duration of initial side effects
- onset of action typically occurs in 1 to 3 days, with maximal effect in 1 to 2 weeks
- typical duration of effect is 3 months with longer durations possible at higher doses
- <u>Complications</u>:
    1. <u>ADSD</u>: dysphagia, aspiration, breathy voice
    2. <u>ABSD</u>: dysphagia, dyspnea (high risk with bilateral injection)
- aspiration and breathy voice can last 1 to 2 days up to 2 to 4 weeks following injection
- <u>Contraindications</u>: botulinum allergy, development of antibodies, current aminoglycoside use, pregnancy, lactation, underlying neuromuscular disease such as myasthenia gravis, at risk for aspiration
- <u>Relative contraindication</u>: viral upper respiratory infection at time of injection may result in diminished Botox effect
- higher Botox failure rates with ABSD (~30%–40%) compared to ADSD (~5%)
- some patients with ABSD respond well to injecting the CT muscles (CT muscle predominance suggested when spasms decrease with lower pitched phonation); caution with this approach in singers
- consider surgery when Botox ineffective or if patient wishes to discontinue Botox injections

Botox Injection Procedure

- dilute Botox with sterile preservative-free saline to yield 25 MU/mL to 10 MU/mL
- load hypodermic 1-mL syringe with solution and attach Teflon-coated, 27-gauge × 1.5-inch needle

- position patient in seated upright position or supine with neck extended
- palpate and identify landmarks (thyroid cartilage, cricoid cartilage, and CT membrane)
- wipe skin clean with alcohol pad
- (optional) apply topical anesthetic or subcutaneous injection with lidocaine
- **ADSD**: insert needle through CT membrane midline with trajectory 15° to 30° lateral and 30° cranial into desired TA muscle under continuous EMG guidance
  1. <u>Tips</u>: staying submucosal can reduce risk of cough or laryngospasm during injection; confirm proper placement with phonation (/ē/)
  2. <u>Alternatives</u>: transnasal with sclerotherapy needle via working channel laryngoscope, peroral, trans-thyrohyoid, trans-thyroid cartilage
- **ABSD**: insert needle posterolateral behind thyroid cartilage into PCA muscle under continuous EMG guidance
  1. <u>Tips</u>: manually rotate thyroid cartilage to expose the PCA muscle during injection; the muscle typically lies more inferiorly than expected (at level of cricoid cartilage posteriorly); spreading out the injection over 2 to 3 sites within the PCA can improve outcomes since the muscle has a large surface area; to avoid injection into the pharyngeal musculature listen for EMG signal during swallow (undesired) versus sniffing in through nose (desired)
  2. <u>Alternative</u>: via CT membrane penetrating through cricoid cartilage posteriorly
- inject desired Botox dose after listening for characteristic intramuscular signal activity on EMG

Laryngeal Framework Surgery

- <u>Type 1 thyroplasty</u>: permanent vocal fold medialization technique used in ABSD; concurrent PCA myoplasty has demonstrated effectiveness in selected cases
- <u>Type 2 thyroplasty</u>: permanent lateralization technique used in ADSD; good long-term clinical outcomes and reduction of VHI

Neurectomy, Myectomy, and Neuromodulation Techniques

- <u>TA myectomy</u>: endoscopic or transcervical excision of the TA muscle with ablative technique

1. long-term (>12 months) improvement of symptomatic speech, Voice Handicap Index (VHI), and stroboscopic findings
2. may be more effective than type 2 thyroplasty in cases of severe ADSD

- <u>TA neurectomy</u>: aka selective laryngeal adductor denervation (SLAD); transcervical procedure with posterior thyrotomy, identification and transection of recurrent laryngeal nerve (RLN) branch to TA muscle
    1. unilateral first, with second-stage contralateral surgery based on patient response
    2. concurrent reinnervation with ansa cervicalis (SLAD-R) and/or partial LCA myotomy may be beneficial
    3. better results when compared to botulinum toxin injection in some studies
- <u>PCA neurectomy</u>: transcervical procedure with transection of RLN branch to PCA muscle
- <u>Selective nerve stimulation</u>: promising results with carryover of effect in limited number of studies, applicable to ADSD and ABSD

OTHER LARYNGEAL DYSTONIAS

Vocal Tremor (VT)

- involuntary, rhythmic vocal pitch oscillations with sustained phonation
- resting, postural, and/or kinetic
- may originate from palate, base of tongue, pharyngeal walls, intrinsic and extrinsic muscles of the larynx, and neck musculature
- tremor may be horizontal or vertical dominant
- <u>VT range</u>: 3 to 12 Hz
- <u>VT average rate</u>: 4 to 5 Hz
- <u>Associated conditions</u>: essential tremor, spasmodic dysphonia, Parkinson's disease (PD), inflammatory neuropathy, upper and lower motor neuron disorders, cerebellar disorders, muscle tension dysphonia
    1. <u>Parkinson's disease</u>: 4 to 6 Hz, VT present in ~75%, typically mandibular tremor, primarily at rest
    2. <u>Essential tremor (ET)</u>: 4 to 10 Hz, sporadic or familial, VT present in 15% to 30%, postural or kinetic
    3. <u>Spasmodic dysphonia</u>: <8 Hz, VT present in ~25%, irregular amplitude, kinetic
- <u>Presentation</u>: dysphonia; tremor of oral, velopharyngeal, and/ or respiratory structures; hypertonic or spastic neck musculature;

symptoms corresponding to underlying neurologic condition (eg, Parkinson's disease)

- <u>Dx</u>: Perceptual evaluation for characteristic traits, laryngoscopy, labs (see SD section), LEMG, speech-language pathology evaluation, Vocal Tremor Scoring System (VTSS), consider labs and imaging (MRI)
- VTSS rates vocal tremor based on severity at anatomic subsites
- <u>Tx</u>: voice therapy (SLP), propranolol or primidone trial, dopamine agonists (Parkinson's disease), baclofen and sodium oxybate (SD), botulinum toxin, surgery
- **Botulinum toxin A injection**: useful for idiopathic, essential VT, and SD-related vocal tremor
  1. <u>Horizontal predominant tremor</u>: injection to bilateral TA muscles
  2. <u>Vertical predominant tremor</u>: injection to bilateral strap muscles
- **Deep brain stimulation**: implant placed in bilateral thalamus (cauda zona incerta, ventral intermediate nucleus)

Paradoxical Vocal Fold Movement (PVFM)

- involuntary vocal fold adduction on inspiration
- <u>Etiology</u>: laryngeal dystonia (can be component of larger dystonia—respiratory, cervical) psychogenic (anxiety, panic attack), underlying CNS disorder
- likely multifactorial
- often misdiagnosed as asthma, may see clipping of inspiratory loop on spirometry
- "pseudo-PVFM"—inspiratory stridor related to Bernoulli effect observed in bilateral RLN paralysis, amyotrophic lateral sclerosis, cricoarytenoid joint dysfunction, Reinke's edema, and clavicular breathing
- laryngopharyngeal reflux (LPR) often present (~80%), but causation not definitive
- <u>Presentation</u>: adolescent female athlete with inspiratory stridor during exertion; airway emergency although rarely requires surgical airway (attacks break before becomes true emergency)
- <u>Natural course of disease</u>: may resolve spontaneously as patient ages
- <u>Dx</u>: H&P, strobovideolaryngoscopy—baseline laryngoscopy and repeat while patient reproduces symptoms with exertion, labs, imaging (see SD section), 24-hour pH monitoring (impedance), LEMG, pulmonary function tests (PFTs)
- PFTs and pH monitoring can evaluate for asthma and reflux-induced laryngospasm/PVFM, respectively
- LEMG demonstrates recruitment of adductor muscles on inspiration; can rule out pseudoparadoxical abduction

- <u>Tx</u>: respiratory behavioral retraining, psychotherapy, biofeedback, LPR treatment, Botox injection (bilateral TA) if refractory to therapy, response to Botox can also be diagnostic

Singer's Dystonia

- task-specific dystonia present only during singing
- female preponderance, typically presents in middle age
- affects adductor and/or abductor muscles, adductor type more common
- <u>Presentation</u>: symptoms similar to SD when singing, may only involve certain pitches, conversational speech typically unaffected
- <u>Dx</u>: similar to workup for SD, evaluation by singing voice specialist
- <u>Halstead criteria</u>:
    1. <u>LEMG</u>: increased recruitment of TA or PCA at affected pitch
    2. <u>Spectrography</u>: widely spaced vertical striations (adductor-type), aphonic breaks (abductor-type)
    3. reproducible instability when singing scales without evidence of muscle tension
- <u>Tx</u>: singing voice therapy, Botox injection

CHAPTER

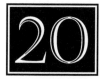

Neurologic Disorders Affecting Airway and Voice

Justin Ross, Mary J. Hawkshaw, and Robert T. Sataloff

DYSARTHRIA

Introduction

- **Dysphonia**: **voice disorder** generally involving to the larynx
- **Dysarthria**: **articulation disorder** caused by impairment of strength, speed, and coordination of nervous systems and musculature responsible for speech production
- Etiologic classification of neurologic voice disorders:
  1. <u>Flaccid paresis/paralysis</u>: lower motor neuron (LMN)
  2. <u>Spastic paresis/paralysis</u>: upper motor neuron (UMN)
  3. <u>Dyskinetic movement disorder</u>: extrapyramidal system
  4. <u>Ataxia</u>: cerebellar
  5. <u>Apraxia</u>: cortical and subcortical
  6. Mixed disorders
- <u>Etiology</u>: vascular, metabolic, iatrogenic, traumatic, infectious, motor, idiopathic
- symptomatic character can point to etiology
- commonly occurs with essential tremor and/or action myoclonus if origin is a brain stem lesion
- injury to the dentate, red, or inferior olivary nucleus may cause palatopharyngeal myoclonus in addition to dysarthria
- <u>Dx</u>: history and physical (H&P), flexible and rigid laryngoscopy, stroboscopy, blood work, **magnetic resonance imaging (MRI) with contrast** (head to aortic arch), laryngeal electromyography (LEMG)
- thorough evaluation of cranial nerves is essential (eg, smile, whistle, gag, tongue movement)
- <u>Tx</u>: treat underlying condition, neurology consultation

Flaccid Dysarthria

- paresis or paralysis of one or more muscles of articulation
- results from diseases affecting brain stem structures, peripheral motor nerves, and/or neuromuscular junction
- <u>Etiology</u>: myasthenia gravis, neoplasia/stroke affecting brain stem, motor nerve injury/infection, Guillain-Barré syndrome (GBS), sarcoidosis, Lyme disease, progressive bulbar palsy (PBP), amyotrophic lateral sclerosis (ALS)
- <u>Presentation</u>: tongue wasting and fasciculations, lip laxity, occasionally dysphagia and drooling
- <u>Speech pattern</u>: slurred, garbled, difficulty with vibratives initially, progressive difficulty with lingual and labial consonants when tongue and lip musculature involved, nasal speech if palate involved

- site of lesion determines presentation: high vagal—breathy, whispered, nasal; low vagal—hoarse, breathy, diplophonic (no effect on palatal resonance)
- lingual consonant (eg, /la/, /ta/) enunciation impaired with injury to hypoglossal nerve, ALS
- labial consonant (eg, /p/, /m/, /b/) enunciation impaired in GBS, Lyme disease
- nasality common in PBP, myasthenia gravis, diphtheria, poliomyelitis

Spastic Dysarthria

- impairment of articulation usually arising from disease of the corticobulbar tracts
- <u>Etiology</u>: ALS, stroke, neoplasia, demyelinating disease
- <u>Presentation</u>: exaggerated facial and palatal reflexes (eg, jaw jerk, gag), impaired emotional control (inappropriate laughter and crying)
- speech may be unaffected by unilateral disease due to cross-innervation by both motor cortices
- secondary insult to the contralateral corticobulbar tract often results in rapid onset of symptoms
- dysarthria more common in left-sided unilateral upper motor neuron disease (hemispheric stroke)
- <u>Speech pattern</u>: thick, strained/strangled, slow, harsh, hypernasal, indistinct consonants like flaccid dysarthria

Hypokinetic Dysarthria

- impairment of articulation commonly arising from disease of the extrapyramidal system
- <u>Etiology</u>: Parkinson's disease (PD), progressive supranuclear palsy
- <u>Presentation</u>: symptoms of PD (rigidity, resting tremor, vocal tremor, bradykinesia, postural instability, shuffling gait, micrographia, dysarthria)
- <u>Speech pattern</u>: decreased volume, monoloudness, monopitch, increased rate of speech, mumbling, slurring, difficulty speaking while walking

Hyperkinetic Dysarthria

- impairment of articulation arising from disease of the extrapyramidal system
- <u>Etiology</u>: Huntington's disease (HD), dystonia musculorum deformans, cerebral palsy (CP), Gilles de la Tourette syndrome

- <u>Presentation</u>: "hiccup speech," choreic or myoclonic movements, may be associated with emotional lability and impaired word finding
- may be spasmodic (eg, Tourette syndrome) or dystonic (eg, HD, CP)
- <u>Speech pattern</u>: increased volume, harsh, highly variable rate, pitch, annunciation, uncoordinated speech and breathing, unexpected breaks

Ataxic Dysarthria

- impairment of articulation arising from acute and chronic cerebellar disease
- <u>Etiology</u>: multiple sclerosis (MS), heat stroke, anoxic encephalopathy, alcohol intoxication, neoplasia, stroke, other cerebellar diseases
- <u>Presentation</u>: dysdiadochokinesis, ataxic gait and arm movement, symptoms of MS (eg, paresthesias, blurred vision, decreases visual contrast and color perception, bladder dysfunction)
- <u>Speech pattern</u>: variable—slurring, monopitch, slow and irregular speech, vocal tremor; resonance generally unaffected in pure ataxic dysarthria
- difficult to diagnose site of lesion based on speech pattern alone

Mixed Dysarthria

- arises from lesions or neurologic conditions affecting multiple subsites
- **Spastic-flaccid**: bilateral corticobulbar lesions with vagal nerve paralysis, common in ALS
- **Spastic-flaccid-ataxic** or **Spastic-ataxic**: seen in MS depending on extent of demyelination
- **Spastic-ataxic-hypokinetic**: alone or in combination seen in Wilson's disease

STUTTERING

- speech motor disorder characterized by (1) speech blocks, (2) repetitive syllables, sounds, and words, and (3) prolongation of sounds
- male predominance
- strong monozygotic twin concordance
- may produce a significant, negative impact on psychosocial well-being
- associated with anxiety disorders, and is exacerbated by stress
- improved fluency while singing
- <u>Etiology</u>: idiopathic, genetic, neurodegenerative disease, brain injury, stroke

- age of onset varies depending on subtype (persistent developmental versus acquired neurogenic)
- posited to arise from abnormal neural activation resulting in inappropriate timing of articulation and speech motor function
- Tx: voice therapy is the gold standard, pharmacotherapy has limited application (inconsistent results in the literature), botulinum toxin is not recommended

Persistent Developmental Stuttering

- polygenetic
- likely arises from bilateral cortical abnormalities in the cerebellum, anterior cingulate cortex, supplementary motor area, and/or right frontal operculum
- onset typically 2 to 4 years old, with relatively high lifetime incidence (~10%)
- persistence into adulthood is ~1%, and is predicted by later onset, extended duration, family history of adult stuttering, and reduced communication skills
- characterized by stutter occurring at the initial syllable or word
- similar quality of stutter found in Parkinson's disease

Acquired Neurogenic Stuttering

- generally arises from subcortical lesions (particularly basal ganglion), but can originate from any affected brain region
- more common in lesions involving the left hemisphere
- characterized by frequent repetition and sound prolongation, but less common broken or blocked syllables and words

NEUROLOGIC DISORDERS

Parkinson's Disease (PD)

- PD is a progressive movement disorder resulting from degeneration of dopaminergic neurons in the substantia nigra
- etiology is unknown but is thought to be a combination of genetic and environmental factors
- genetic mutations identified in up to 10% of patients with PD
- higher risk in patients with an affected first-degree relative, pesticide exposure, and head trauma
- nicotine and caffeine use are slightly protective
- voice and speech affected in >70% of PD patients

- <u>Presentation</u>: bradykinesia, hypokinesia, akinesia, shuffling gait, rigidity, resting tremor, postural instability, flat affect, dementia (late stage), impaired communication (verbal and nonverbal)
- may have comorbid depression and anxiety
- <u>Speech pattern</u>: weak, breathy, aprosodic, monopitch, monoloudness, slow speech, short periods of speech interrupted by silent hesitations, difficulty with labial and lingual consonants, hypokinetic dysarthria
- diminished or irregular airflow due to disordered respiratory muscle activity may limit duration or regulation of prolonged speech
- reduction or alteration of nasal consonant production due to effect on nasal airflow
- <u>Laryngoscopy</u>: disordered abduction and adduction, true vocal fold (TVF) atrophy, phase asymmetry, bilateral TVF paralysis possible in late stages, tremor in some cases, soft voice or incompetent glottic closure
- can have reduced or slowed vertical laryngeal movement and TVF abduction on deglutition
- <u>Medical Tx</u>: carbidopa/levodopa, dopamine receptor agonists (ropinirole, pramipexole), monoamine oxidase inhibitors (MAO-I), anticholinergics, amantadine; voice therapy (eg, Lee Silverman Voice Treatment and others) improves overall speech quality
- <u>Surgical Tx</u>: evidence supports bilateral deep brain stimulation over best medical therapy for management of dyskinesias; management of voice complaints typically begins with a trial of temporary injection medialization (eg, collagen) followed by permanent medialization if there was a good response

Myasthenia Gravis (MG)

- autoimmune disease caused by formation of acetylcholine receptor (Ach-R) autoantibodies that degrade Ach-R at the neuromuscular junction
- can have systemic or local effects
- anti-Ach-R antibodies are found in serum 80% to 90% of patients with systemic MG, 50% to 60% in ocular MG, but in a minority of patients with laryngeal myasthenia (LMG)
- typical age of onset is 50s and 60s in men, and 50s and 60s in women
- <u>Presentation</u>: ptosis, diplopia, generalized weakness, dysphonia, dysphagia, oromandibular/facial muscle weakness, anterior cervical muscle tension, voice fatigue
- 6% of patients will present with dysphonia, and 60% will develop it over their disease course
- <u>Speech pattern</u>: weakness, breathiness, hoarseness, vocal fatigue with intermittent aphonia, hypernasality, stridorous (if abductors affected)

- <u>Dx</u>: strobovideolaryngoscopy, laryngeal electromyography (LEMG) with Tensilon test, anti-Ach-R antibody titer, neck and chest computed tomography with contrast
- LEMG with improvement of voice quality following administration of Tensilon (edrophonium) test is usually confirmatory
- should obtain anti-Ach-R antibodies, anti-striatal antibodies and MUSK antibodies, but typically normal in isolated LMG
- CT or MRI is gold standard to rule out thymoma and differentiate from other mediastinal pathology
- <u>Laryngoscopy</u>: unilateral (SLN-type) or bilateral (fluctuating) TVF paresis, supraglottic hyperfunction (muscle tension dysphonia), glottic insufficiency
- <u>Tx</u>: voice/singing therapy, **pyridostigmine**, referral to neurologist/rheumatologist if refractory to corticosteroids, azathioprine, tacrolimus, mycophenolate, or eculizumab; presence of thymoma warrants thoracic surgery consult and possible excision
- thymectomy is often curative—risk factors for lack of treatment response include well-differentiated carcinoma, >55 years old, thymectomy >1 year following onset of symptoms

Postpoliomyelitis Syndrome

- generalized neuromuscular dysfunction occurring years following acute poliomyelitis, affecting up to 80%
- initial condition marked by infection and damage of anterior horn cell motor neurons causing generalized weakness and rarely complete paralysis (1%–5%)
- <u>Etiology</u>: likely due to continuous innervation-denervation and resultant oversprouting of motor neurons
- <u>Speech pattern</u>: likely breathiness, weakness, and other qualities suggestive of TVF paresis
- <u>Laryngoscopy</u>: TVF paresis/paralysis most commonly, supraglottic hyperfunction, glottic insufficiency
- may see weakness of respiratory musculature and resulting diminished airflow
- <u>Tx</u>: voice therapy, surgical management depends on extent of muscular involvement

Multiple Sclerosis

- CD4+ T-cell-mediated demyelinating disorder affecting the central nervous system (CNS)
- increased risk if affected first-degree relatives and/or twins, Epstein-Barr virus infection, vitamin D deficiency, and tobacco use

- <u>Presentation</u>: syndrome typically heralded by optic neuritis, incomplete myelitis, or brain stem syndrome, and then has a relapsing and remitting course with accumulation of debilitating sensory and motor symptoms; both dysphonia and dysarthria can develop
- <u>Speech pattern</u>: spastic, mixed flaccid, or ataxic dysarthria, scanning speech (long pauses between syllables or words), vocal instability
- <u>Dx</u>: H&P, MRI brain/spine, cerebrospinal fluid sampling (oligoclonal bands)
- <u>Tx</u>: refer to neurologist, medications (ie, corticosteroids, INF-β, glatiramer, natalizumab, etc), speech and swallowing therapy

Diphtheria

- infection of the upper respiratory tract secondary to *Corynebacterium diphtheriae*, which can progress to paralysis of related musculature over time in ~21% of patients
- <u>Onset of paralysis</u>: soft palate (1–4 weeks) → pharynx, larynx, diaphragm (5 weeks) → peripheral neuropathy (8–12 weeks)
- weak phonation similar to postpoliomyelitis syndrome, but always self-remitting
- <u>Tx</u>: horse serum antitoxin and antibiotics (oral macrolides >6 months, IM penicillin <6 months)

Cerebrovascular Accident (CVA)

- interruption of blood flow secondary to ischemic obstruction (thrombus or embolism) or intracranial hemorrhage
- sudden loss of neurologic function can be focal to generalized depending on location and extent of CNS damage
- commonly results in dysphonia, dysarthria, dysphagia, and aspiration
- dysarthria is much more common (up to 30%) than vocal fold paresis/paralysis
- vocal fold paralysis generally only occurs in CVA affecting brain stem structures
- infarct location and deficit:
  1. <u>Cortical/subcortical pathways</u>: uncoordinated TVF movement, decreased laryngeal sensitivity → dysphonia, aspiration
  2. <u>Broca's area</u> (posterior inferior frontal lobe): expressive aphasia
  3. <u>Wernicke's area</u> (posterior superior temporal lobe): receptive aphasia
  4. <u>Internal capsule/corona radiata</u>: pure pseudobulbar palsy
  5. <u>Nucleus ambiguus/nucleus solitarius</u>: TVF paresis/paralysis and diminished laryngeal sensation → dysphonia, aspiration

6. <u>Hypoglossal nucleus</u>: dysarthria with impairment of lingual consonant formation
7. <u>Wallenberg's syndrome</u> (lateral medullary infarct): secondary to obstruction of the posterior inferior cerebellar artery—commonly associated with dysphagia and dysphonia
- early recovery of voice quality improves chance of complete recovery
- multiple systems are generally affected and may have indirect effects on voice (ie, dementia, depression, dysphagia, reflux disease, diminished pulmonary function, obstructive sleep apnea)
- <u>Dx</u>: strobovideolaryngoscopy, LEMG (6 weeks to 3 months after CVA), bedside swallow evaluation, modified barium swallow (MBS), flexible endoscopic swallow evaluation with sensory testing (FEEST), ± manometry and/or esophagoscopy
- patients with paresis/paralysis and early motor unit recovery on LEMG may benefit from temporary medialization which may improve success of voice rehabilitation
- <u>Tx</u>: depends on deficit, voice therapy always indicated
  1. **Glottic insufficiency**: injection laryngoplasty, thyroplasty type I ± arytenoid adduction, arytenopexy, nerve-muscle pedicle graft
  2. **Palatal or laryngeal myoclonus**: botulinum toxin type A
  3. **Dysarthria**: speech therapy to improve tongue mobility and coordination
  4. **Ventilator dependence**: early tracheotomy decreases long-term effects on voice and airway
  5. **Excess oral secretions**: glycopyrrolate, salivary gland botulinum toxin type A injection, submandibular gland excision, ligation of Stensen's duct, tympanic neurectomy

Amyotrophic Lateral Sclerosis (ALS)

- progressive and incurable degenerative disorder of upper and lower motor neurons
- average onset is 56 years old, although it can occur at any age
- death results from respiratory complications within 3 years in the majority of patients
- <u>Presentation</u>: tongue fasciculations, muscle weakness or spasm, drooling, new onset of co-occurring dysphonia and dysphagia in a healthy patient
- early bulbar palsy seen in >25%
- <u>Speech pattern</u>: slow rate, decreased phonation time, breathiness, mixed dysarthria (ie, difficulty with labial consonants, slurred or spastic), hypernasality, harsh voice, tremor, flutter

- objective voice testing may reveal abnormalities prior to onset of perceptible changes
- <u>Dx</u>: H&P, complete neurologic examination, strobovideolaryngoscopy, MRI, LEMG
- <u>Laryngoscopy</u>: aperiodicity, TVF spasm and/or weakness, paradoxical adduction, glottic insufficiency, variable TVF frequency and amplitude
- <u>Tx</u>: incurable; management of secretions and aspiration includes glycopyrrolate, salivary gland chemodenervation, excision, or duct ligation, tracheotomy, and/or laryngeal diversion procedures

Huntington's Chorea

- autosomal dominant (chromosome 4) neurodegenerative disorder affecting the striatum
- average age of onset is 25 to 45 years
- <u>Presentation</u>: depression (most common early symptom), involuntary movements including tics and choreic gait, contorted movements (ie, neck hyperextension) in later stages, dysphagia, dysarthria, emotional lability, aggression, dementia, death
- <u>Speech pattern</u>: increased volume, harsh, highly variable rate, pitch, annunciation, uncoordinated speech and breathing, unexpected breaks

Multiple-System Atrophy (MSA)

- progressive, demyelination neurodegenerative disorder
- previously included 3 subtypes: Shy-Drager syndrome, olivopontocerebellar atrophy, and striatonigral degeneration
- now categorized based on predominant symptoms: parkinsonian (MSA-P) versus cerebellar (MSA-C)
- autonomic symptoms are common to both subtypes
- <u>Presentation</u>: orthostatic hypotension, erectile dysfunction, urinary incontinence, parkinsonian or cerebellar symptoms, dysphonia, dysphagia, occasional laryngeal stridor
- <u>Speech pattern</u>: breathy, strained, monoloudness, decreased loudness, monopitch, rate modulation; MSA-P is similar to PD but with consciously slow speaking rate and excess hoarseness; MSA-C theoretically would cause an ataxic dysarthria
- <u>Laryngoscopy</u>: unilateral or bilateral vocal fold paresis/paralysis (commonly abductor), paradoxical vocal fold movement
- <u>Tx</u>: typically done for stridor, includes cricoarytenopexy, cordotomy, tracheotomy
- poor response to levodopa compared with PD

Tourette Syndrome

- autosomal dominant neuropsychiatric disorder characterized by multiple motor tics and at least one vocal tic
- age of onset is ~7 years old
- tics are voluntary movements that are typically brief, repetitive, and purposeless
- vocal tics occur in up to 50%, and may include sounds, words, coprolalia, echolalia
- coprolalia has an incidence of ~10%
- often comorbid with obsessive compulsive disorder and attention deficit disorder

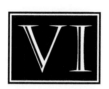

SECTION

VI

Laryngologic Manifestations of Systemic Diseases

CHAPTER

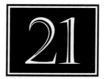

Voice Disorders in the Elderly

Karen M. Kost and Justin Ross

INTRODUCTION

Overview

- incidence of vocal complaints in the elderly is ~12% to 35%
- one-third of individuals >65 years have occupational voice requirements
- undesirable characteristics of an older voice are not a necessarily due to aging
- severity of dysphonia are related to laryngeal changes, the functional status of the patient, coexisting morbidities, pulmonary reserve, medications, and cognitive function
- dysphonia and hearing loss frequently coprevalent—negatively impacts psychosocial quality of life (QOL)

Presbyphonia

- physiological process of vocal aging including morphological changes in the mucosa, muscle, and cartilage
- diagnosis of exclusion
- <u>Coprevalent diagnoses</u>: laryngeal muscle atrophy, vocal fold paresis/paralysis, benign vocal fold lesions (polyps, nodules, cysts, papillomas), chronic inflammatory laryngitis (reflux-related conditions, autoimmune disorders, medication-induced conditions), acute inflammatory laryngitis (viral, fungal, and bacterial), muscle tension disorders, neurologic disorders (essential tremor, Parkinson's, poststroke, spasmodic dysphonia, amyotrophic lateral sclerosis), vocal malignancies, vocal fold immobility/hypomobility (mechanical)
- <u>Presentation</u>: breathiness hoarseness, reduced projection, excessive throat clearing and phlegm, vocal fatigue, cough, raspiness, pitch breaks, loss of range, globus sensation, tremor, and dysphagia
- <u>Dx</u>: history and physical (H&P), flexible and rigid laryngoscopy, stroboscopy
- <u>Stroboscopic findings</u>: vocal fold **bowing** and **atrophy**, **glottic insufficiency**, prominent vocal processes, spindle-shaped glottic chink, soft vocal fold closure, reduced amplitude and mucosal wave, supraglottic hyperfunction
- related findings include laryngopharyngeal reflux (LPR), muscle tension dysphonia (MTD), true vocal fold (TVF) paresis, vocal fold mass, varicosities and ectasias, mild Reinke's edema
- <u>Other related conditions</u>: coronary artery disease, cerebrovascular disease, pulmonary disease, obesity, stroke, diabetes, cancer, diet, hearing loss, vision loss, swallowing dysfunction, arthritis, neurological dysfunction (ie, tremor), gastrointestinal disorders, cognitive dysfunction

AGE-RELATED LARYNGEAL CHANGES

Introduction

Histologic Changes

- larynx undergoes extensive anatomic and physiologic change during adulthood and with advancing age
- Cellular changes: decreased cellularity, reduced number of organelles responsible for protein synthesis, reduced production of extracellular matrix
- Superficial lamina propria (SLP): thickening or edema of the superficial layer, degeneration or atrophy of elastic fibers, decreased number of myofibrils
- Cricoarytenoid joint (CAJ): surface irregularities and disorganization of collagen fibers
- Laryngeal cartilages: progressive calcification and/or ossification

Thyroarytenoid (TA) Histology

- TA differs from other skeletal muscle in fiber size, contractile protein profiles, mitochondrial content, aging patterns
- similar differences have been found in other laryngeal muscles
- rapidly contracting and fatigue resistant, suited for respiration, cough, and phonation
- contains type I (slow twitch), IIx and IIa (fast twitch), and hybrid fibers
    1. Medial aspect: slow twitch fibers
    2. Lateral aspect: fast twitch
- increased levels of mitochondria found in the posterior cricoarytenoid, cricothyroid, and TA muscles relative to limb skeletal muscle
- small motor units, each motor neuron innervates a few fibers
- sensory information via mechanoreceptors, chemoreceptors, taste buds, and free nerve endings

General Age-Related Changes of the Larynx

- **Sarcopenia**: loss of muscle mass, strength, and quality
- loss in muscle mass generally not noticed until deficits extend beyond threshold levels
- likely the result of metabolic, neurologic, hormonal, and environmental factors
- loss of TA muscle mass occurs with aging, but patterns of fiber loss not defined

- <u>Mechanical changes</u>: reduced contractile force, speed, and endurance
- <u>Neurologic changes</u>: no net loss of TA nerve fibers, but increased number of myelin-abnormal and myelin-thinning fibers, suggesting an active process of degeneration and regeneration; decrease in the size and number of SLN myelinated fibers → decreased laryngeal sensation
- <u>Metabolic changes</u>: mitochondrial DNA mutations increase with age, thought to result in the increased production of injurious free radicals that negatively affect contractile properties of the TA muscle
- <u>Vascular changes</u>: laryngeal blood flow decreases ~50% in rats → reduced oxygenation and increased accumulation of cellular waste products

Age-Related Changes in the Supraglottic Vocal Tract

- <u>Facial musculature</u>: decreased elasticity, reduced blood supply, atrophy, and collagen fiber breakdown
- <u>Temporomandibular joints</u>: thinning of articular discs, reduced blood supply, and regressive remodeling of the mandibular condyle and glenoid fossa
- although dental structures are altered with aging, tooth loss can be prevented
- <u>Salivary glands</u>: decreased salivary function → oral dryness, dysphagia, oral discomfort, increased susceptibility to oral infection
- <u>Oral cavity and oropharynx</u>: epithelial thinning, fissuring, and reduced strength of the tongue (endurance unaffected), degenerative changes in the pharyngeal and palatal muscles, thinning of oral cavity mucosa (increased risk of xerostomia)
- lingual pressure during swallowing decreases, but maximum tongue pressures during swallow remain stable into old age

Acoustic Changes in the Aging Voice

- <u>Voice changes</u>: reduced volume, vocal range, intensity and endurance, increased breathiness, change in pitch, decreased ability to modulate pitch and intensity; highly variable
- listeners can discern accurately between young, middle, and older age groups
- older voices described as hoarse, raspy, breathy, unsteady, tremulous, shaky → more pronounced with poor physical conditioning (weak respiratory and abdominal muscles) and inadequate vocal support
- speaking fundamental frequency (f0) changes with age:
  1. <u>Men</u>: decreases through the fifth decade, and then increases, possible due to muscle atrophy and hormonal changes

2. <u>Women</u>: remains constant or decreases slightly until menopause, then gradually decreases
- changes less prominent in professional singers who maintain stable speaking f0 throughout adulthood, suggesting a role for vocal exercise
- jitter and shimmer increased relative to younger people, and associated with higher Voice Handicap Index (VHI) scores
- singers and healthy, physically fit older adults display less jitter and shimmer and sound younger than those in poor health

OTHER AGE-RELATED CHANGES

Psychology and Intellect (See Chapter 29)

- alterations in cognition, personality, and delusional disorders may impair the ability to concentrate, perform vocal tasks, and cooperate optimally with voice rehabilitation

Menopause

- estrogen deprivation causes changes in the mucous membranes that line the vocal tract, the muscles, and the body
- hormone replacement therapy may be helpful, but possible increased risk of malignancy
- avoid androgenic drugs in women unless masculinization of the voice is desired

Thyroid Dysfunction (See Chapter 23)

- may have atypical presentations, and can be challenging to diagnose in the elderly
- <u>Hypothyroidism</u>: loss of range, efficiency, muffled voice, mental slowing, loss of energy, neurotic behavior, hearing loss, weight gain, musculoskeletal discomfort, dry skin, changes in facial appearance—may be mistakenly attributed to age
- <u>Hyperthyroidism</u>: vocal tremor, muscle spasm, dysrhythmia (atrial fibrillation/flutter), proptosis
- voice changes typically resolve with treatment

Hearing Loss

- frequently coprevalent with dysphonia in older voice patients
- pitch distortion (diplacusis) and loudness distortion (recruitment) affect vocal performance
- may necessitate modifications in rehabilitation strategies

TREATMENT

Voice Optimization

- must address comorbidities and optimize physical conditioning
- age-related disuse and inactivity leads to muscle atrophy
- laryngeal, respiratory, and postural muscle tone and endurance are critical to voice quality
- <u>Additional factors</u>: good nutrition, weight control, adequate salivary quality and flow, good oral and dental hygiene, minimizing medications associated with cough, drying effects, and altered cognition, reflux management
- maximizes performance level and helps prolong careers of older singers
- voice therapy is often a necessary adjunct to optimization
- for most patients, rehabilitation improves vocal function and eliminates the perception of an "old" voice
- when therapy and medical management fail to result in a satisfactory voice, laryngeal surgery may be beneficial

Voice Therapy

- most effective, initial therapy for presbylarynx
- combining traditional voice therapy, singing training, acting voice techniques, and aerobic conditioning improve neuromuscular performance
- increased compliance correlated with degree of improvement in Voice-Related Quality of Life (VRQOL) scores
- good physical health, sound singing technique, and voice therapy reduce perception of an "old" voice, and improve stable f0, intensity range, and vocal quality at least into the seventh decade
- vocal function exercises and resonant voice therapy improve laryngeal function, muscular tone, and voice quality
- <u>Objective changes</u>: improved glottic closure, decreased breathiness, increased subglottic pressure, increased maximum phonation time
- combined voice therapy and singing exercises expedite and improve outcomes in older patients
- <u>Singing exercises</u>: increase breath support, phrase length, frequency range, vocal strength, agility, accuracy, endurance, and may eliminate tremolo
- <u>Acting voice exercises</u>: improve vocal strength and projection, control of face and body function, phonatory expression of emotion, preparation and interpretation of spoken materials

Surgery

- most will respond well to voice therapy with improved VRQOL scores post-treatment
- <u>Indications</u>: inadequate response to voice therapy, significant glottic gap, patient discontent with voice
- <u>Surgical options</u>:
  1. <u>Injection medialization laryngoplasty</u>: most substances (ie, saline, Gelfoam, hyaluronic acid, collagen) may be used in outpatient setting to evaluate treatment response in anticipation of permanent medialization or if poor surgical candidate; duration varies with substance used; calcium hydroxyapatite (CaHa) has longer duration (~18 months) but may cause permanently reduced mucosal wave
  2. <u>Lipoinjection medialization laryngoplasty</u>: may be effective as monotherapy, particularly useful for correction of persistent musculomembranous gap following type 1 thyroplasty, ~40% resorption
  3. <u>Type 1 thyroplasty</u>: permanent, unilateral or bilateral, performed under local anesthesia with conscious sedation
- manual compression of thyroid cartilage may predict results of medialization—less helpful with extensive laryngeal ossification

CHAPTER

22

Reflux Disease

Justin Ross, Mary J. Hawkshaw, and Robert T. Sataloff

INTRODUCTION

- **Gastroesophageal reflux (GER)**: reflux of stomach contents through the lower esophageal sphincter (LES) into the esophagus
- **Laryngopharyngeal reflux (LPR)**: reflux of stomach contents through the upper esophageal sphincter (UES)
- **Reflux laryngitis (RL)**: a component of LPR characterized by erythema and edema of laryngeal structures due to irritation from gastric refluxate
- high incidence of GER in patients with dysphonia (~80%)
- ~80% of patients with clinical LPR will be confirmed with pH-impedance testing

HISTOLOGY AND PATHOPHYSIOLOGY

- <u>Gastric reflux</u>: occurs when gastric or intra-abdominal pressure becomes greater than LES pressure
- **LES hypotonia** is the most significant pathophysiologic component of GERD and LPR
- causes include mechanical sphincter dysfunction, gastric or intestinal hypersecretory conditions, esophageal motility disorders, delayed gastric emptying, hiatal hernia, etc
- peristalsis, esophageal mucous, and acid-neutralizing effect of saliva protect the esophagus from acid
- no native protective mechanisms against reflux in the larynx and pharynx
- alterations in mucin gene expression in laryngeal mucosa and/or mucosal metaplasia may predispose the larynx to mucosal damage from refluxate
- proximal acid and pepsin exposure likely responsible for most laryngeal symptoms
  1. pepsin found in the esophageal and laryngeal mucosa of patients with LPR
  2. uptake of pepsin occurs after binding specific receptors on laryngeal mucosal cells
  3. pepsin remains stable in mucosal cells until acidification <6.5 pH prompts reactivation
  4. intracellular pepsin may explain symptoms due to weakly acid reflux
  5. salivary pepsin collected 30 minutes prior to breakfast is an emerging diagnostic tool for LPR, and may be more accurate than 24-hour pH monitor
- bile refluxate is an additional cause of laryngeal irritation

CLINICAL EVALUATION

History

Esophageal Symptoms

- chest pain, dysphagia, heartburn, odynophagia, regurgitation, excess saliva production
- no correlation with frequency of heartburn and GERD severity
- GERD 90% likely if heartburn and regurgitation are coprevalent
- regurgitation prominent in patients with extraesophageal symptoms
- ~80% of people with both heartburn and regurgitation have extraesophageal symptoms
- heartburn present in a minority of otolaryngologic patients with extraesophageal sx of GERD

Extraesophageal Symptoms

- wheezing, shortness of breath, chronic cough, loss of dental enamel with hypersensitivity, hoarseness, laryngitis or laryngospasm, nausea, otalgia, globus pharyngeus, halitosis, otitis media
- up to 75% of patients with chronic hoarseness, 20% with chronic cough, 45% with unexplained chest pain, and 70% to 80% of asthmatics will have associated GERD
- distal esophagitis is present in less than 10% of patients with unexplained chest pain, 30% to 40% with asthma, and approximately 20% with reflux laryngitis
- important to rule out coronary artery disease as a cause of chest pain with electrocardiogram (ECG) and/or stress test
- onset of asthma later in life without any associated allergic component may indicate GERD-induced asthma if poor dietary hygiene
- reflux is the third most common cause of chronic cough

Laryngopharyngeal Reflux

- 4% to 10% of patients seen by otolaryngologists
- etiology or significant cofactor in up to ~80% of patients with laryngeal and voice disorders
- coprevalent with GERD in ~25% of patients
- increased incidence of vocal fold polyps and Reinke's edema
- <u>Associated nonlaryngeal conditions</u>: obstructive sleep apnea, Sjögren's syndrome, chronic rhinosinusitis, poor dentition, sudden infant death syndrome (SIDS), and otitis media
- may worsen underlying chronic obstructive pulmonary disease

- may decrease success of tympanoplasty and surgical repair of laryngeal trauma and laryngotracheal stenosis
- common in singers and athletes due to compression of abdominal muscles and bodily agitation
- Reflux Symptom Index (RSI) is a subjective assessment of LPR symptom severity (Table 22–1)
- RSI is a valid and reliable tool to track LPR treatment response

Gluten Sensitivity

- celiac disease (CD) has a 0.5% to 1% prevalence in the United States
- nonceliac gluten sensitivity (NCGS) has a 0.5% to 6% prevalence in the United States
- subdivided into allergic, autoimmune, nonallergic/nonautoimmune (NA), and immune
    1. Allergic subtype: generally against wheat
    2. Autoimmune subtype: CD, dermatitis herpetiformis, gluten ataxia
    3. NA subtype: NCGS
- theories on gluten sensitivity-GERD connection:
    1. nutrient malabsorption and resultant dysmotility

TABLE 22–1. Reflux Symptom Index

Within the last month, how did the following problems affect you?	0 = no problem, 5 = severe problem					
1. Hoarseness or a problem with your voice	0	1	2	3	4	5
2. Clearing your throat	0	1	2	3	4	5
3. Excess throat mucus or postnasal drip	0	1	2	3	4	5
4. Difficulty swallowing food, liquid, or pills	0	1	2	3	4	5
5. Coughing after you ate or after lying down	0	1	2	3	4	5
6. Breathing difficulties or choking episodes	0	1	2	3	4	5
7. Troublesome or annoying cough	0	1	2	3	4	5
8. Sensation of something sticking or a lump in your throat	0	1	2	3	4	5
9. Heartburn, chest pain, indigestion, or stomach acid coming up	0	1	2	3	4	5
>13 considered positive for LPR	Total:					

Source: Adapted from Belafsky PC, Postma GN, Koufman JA. Validity and reliability of the Reflux Symptom Index (RSI). *J Voice.* 2002;16(2):274–277.

2. hormonal dysregulation resulting in decreased LES pressure and dysmotility
3. direct inflammatory effect of gluten resulting in increased mucosal permeability

- <u>Sx</u>: GERD symptoms, motility problems, and esophageal erosive lesions more common in patients with gluten sensitivity, specifically CD
- most common gastrointestinal symptoms mimic irritable bowel syndrome (IBS)
- no clear evidence linking gluten sensitivity to LPR
- <u>Dx</u>: anti-TTG IgA/IgG, DGP IgA/IgG, AGA IgA/IgG, Total IgA, wheat-specific IgE, HLA-DQ2/8
- test if refractory to antisecretory therapy or indicated by patient history
- only AGA IgG and HLA-DQ2/8 are lower in NCGS relative to general population
- <u>Tx</u>: Gluten-free diet—antisecretory tx generally not required

Helicobacter pylori

- helical, gram-negative, microaerophilic, flagellated bacteria
- associated with chronic type B gastritis, peptic ulcer disease, and gastric carcinoma
- <u>Dx</u>: IgG in serum via ELISA, urease breath test, and biopsy
- no definitive relationship between LPR-related symptoms and *H pylori*, but has been shown to be present more often in laryngeal biopsy samples of individuals with malignant and benign laryngeal disease compared with normal controls
- <u>Tx</u>: several options available
    1. **Triple therapy**: clarithromycin, amoxicillin or metronidazole, and proton pump inhibitor (PPI) for 2 weeks
    2. **Quadruple therapy**: bismuth, tetracycline, nitromidazole, and PPI for 10 to 14 days (may be used if penicillin allergy or contraindication to macrolide exposure)

Physical Exam

- comprehensive exam focusing on ears, nasal cavity, dentition, oral cavity, oropharynx, flexible laryngoscopy, and if possible rigid strobolaryngoscopy
- extraesophageal reflux occasionally associated with middle ear effusion
    1. pepsin found in 20% of pediatric patients undergoing tympanotomy tube placement compared with 1.4% of controls
    2. ~48.6% prevalence of LPR in children with otitis media

3. current guidelines do not support treatment of reflux in children with otitis media
- <u>Nasal cavity</u>: mucosal edema, turbinate hypertrophy, and/or rhinorrhea—postnasal drip (PND) is a laryngeal irritant and may increase acid sensitivity
- <u>Oral cavity</u>: lucency of the central incisors due to enamel erosion by frequent acid exposure
- <u>Oropharynx</u>: posterior pharyngeal cobblestoning indicates LPR or PND
- <u>Neck</u>: tense and tender musculature secondary to compensatory muscle hyperactivity
- flexible and/or rigid laryngoscopy, and ideally stroboscopy, should always be performed
    1. rigid laryngoscopy is preferable due to higher resolution
    2. <u>Signs of reflux laryngitis</u>: arytenoid erythema/edema, interarytenoid pachydermia, pseudosulcus, edema of false and true vocal folds, ventricular obliteration, postcricoid edema, Reinke's edema, granulomas/granulation, interarytenoid bar, and thick endolaryngeal mucus
    3. **Reflux Finding Score** (RFS) is used to quantify severity of LPR; high intra- and interrater reliability; demonstrates pH-monitor confirmed treatment efficacy (Table 22–2)

Diagnostic Testing

Therapeutic Trial

- symptomatic resolution following medical management (PPI, H2-blocker, or prokinetics) for 8 to 12 weeks confirms a diagnosis of GERD/LPR
- **generally first step in diagnosis**
- patients with otolaryngologic symptoms require a higher dose than those with esophageal symptoms of GERD (ie, heartburn)

Imaging

- generally **low yield** in the diagnosis of GERD/LPR
- <u>Chest x-ray</u>: helpful in excluding pulmonary causes of chronic cough
- <u>Barium esophagram</u>: demonstrates esophageal strictures, perforations, diverticula, masses, hernias, and incomplete emptying
    1. double-contrast barium swallow or barium swallow with water siphonage is ideal
    2. hiatal hernia is the most common finding, nonspecific, ~9% will have reflux symptom
    3. large hernias predispose to low LES pressures

TABLE 22–2. Reflux Finding Score	
Subglottic edema	0 = absent 2 = present
Ventricular obliteration	2 = partial 4 = complete
Erythema/hyperemia	2 = arytenoids only 4 = diffuse
Vocal fold edema	1 = mild 2 = moderate 3 = severe 4 = polypoid
Diffuse laryngeal edema	1 = mild 2 = moderate 3 = severe 4 = obstruction
Posterior commissure hypertrophy	1 = mild 2 = moderate 3 = severe 4 = obstructing
Granuloma/granulation	0 = absent 2 = present
Thick endolaryngeal mucus	0 = absent 2 = present
>10 considered positive for LPR	Total:

Source: Adapted from Belafsky PC, Postma GN, Koufman JA. The validity and reliability of the Reflux Finding Score (RFS). *Laryngoscope.* 2001;111(8):1313–1317.

- Nuclear medicine gastric emptying study: noninvasive, primarily used in infants
- Esophageal scintigraphy: technetium 99m-sulfur colloid ingested and abdominal compression applied to elicit reflux

Upper Endoscopy

- useful for demonstrating strictures, erosive esophagitis, Barrett's esophagus, and malignancy
- performed in patients who **fail medical management** and have had **GERD symptoms for 5 or more years**, or patients with **alarm**

symptoms of malignancy such as odynophagia, progressive dysphagia, weight loss, night sweats, etc

- 50% to 60% with esophageal GERD symptoms will show signs of erosive esophagitis, the remainder diagnosed with nonerosive reflux disease (NERD)
- most patients with extraesophageal symptoms will not have erosive esophagitis
- patients with Barrett's esophagus will often have minimal heartburn likely due to reduced acid sensitivity in the distal esophagus
- may be appropriate in most LPR patients when classic symptoms are rare and duration of disease is difficult to establish

24-Hour pH Monitor

- gold standard for the diagnosis of GERD
- sensitivity 96% and specificity 95%
- without at least dual-probe monitoring (distal and proximal), sensitivity for LPR is ~62%
- distal and proximal probes placed 5 cm and 20 cm above the LES, respectively; proximal probe can be placed above or below the UES
  1. Triple-probe monitoring: hypopharyngeal, mid-esophageal, and distal esophageal sensors
  2. Tetra-probe monitoring: hypopharyngeal, mid-esophageal, distal esophageal, and intragastric sensors
- **pH <5 at the proximal sensor is diagnostic of LPR**
- positive reflux at the proximal sensor predicts treatment response in patients with pulmonary disease
- hypopharyngeal reflux can occur in the absence of symptomatic distal acid reflux events
- impedance monitoring cannot be used to definitively establish or rule out LPR due to variable diagnostic yield (14%–83%) but is useful in combination with therapeutic trial of PPI
- performed on antireflux therapy to assess treatment response
- useful to have professional voice users sing during testing, as this can provoke reflux events
- value of pharyngeal monitoring (Restech) is under investigation

Telemetry Capsule pH Monitoring

- a capsule is placed in the esophagus where it monitors pH for 48 hours
- valuable in the assessment of GERD, but untested in LPR
- large probe size would likely make proximal placement uncomfortable

Combined Multichannel Intraluminal Impedance

- identifies gas, liquid, and mixed refluxate, and divides them into acid (pH <4), weakly acid (pH 4.1–7), and nonacid (pH >7) events
- increases diagnostic yield for LPR when combined with 24-hour pH monitoring

Esophageal Manometry

- used in the diagnosis of motility disorders
- essential prior to Nissen fundoplication and pH monitor distal probe placement
- often invaluable after Nissen fundoplication

Erosive Esophagitis

- diagnosed with upper endoscopy, characterized by the severity of mucosal breaks in the esophagus
- **Los Angeles Criteria**
    1. Grade A: one or more mucosal breaks <5 mm in length
    2. Grade B: one or more mucosal breaks >5 mm in length, not extending across mucosal folds
    3. Grade C: one or more noncircumferential mucosal breaks extending across mucosal folds
    4. Grade D: one or more circumferential, esophageal mucosal breaks
- predicts treatment outcomes → long-term PPI therapy is required, and discontinuation of treatment results in recurrence of erosive esophagitis in ~80% of patients

MANAGEMENT

Nonmedical Management

- **dietary changes** including avoidance of large meals, citrus, tomato, spicy food, high-fat foods, low pH beverages (colas, coffee, tea), alcohol, tobacco use, and eating too close to sleep (2–3 hours) for patients with nocturnal reflux
    1. chocolate and onions can decrease LES pressure
    2. very low acid diet and consumption of alkaline water appear helpful
- **weight loss** and avoidance of tight-fitting clothes
- **elevating the head of bed** 6 to 8 inches via full-length wedge

1. bending at the waist can increase intrathoracic/abdominal pressure
2. can also sleep on left side
- avoid certain medications
    1. <u>Lower LES pressure</u>: anticholinergics, sedatives, theophylline, prostaglandins, calcium channel blockers
    2. <u>Esophageal irritants</u>: potassium, ferrous sulfate, tetracycline, NSAIDs, aspirin, bisphosphonates
- apply dietary and behavioral modifications along with any medical or surgical intervention for optimal results

Medical Management

- PPI or histamine-2 receptor antagonist (H2RA) therapy is the **first-line treatment for GERD**
- high relapse rate when treatment discontinued: ~66% of NERD, and almost all erosive esophagitis
- if symptoms continue despite medical therapy, 24-hour pH monitoring is indicated
- 24-hour pH monitoring more sensitive and specific than therapeutic trial

Proton Pump Inhibitors

- <u>Mechanism</u>: inhibits parietal cell hydrogen-potassium ATPase
- <u>Medications</u>: omeprazole, pantoprazole, esomeprazole, lansoprazole, and rabeprazole
    1. delayed release (enteric coating) or immediate release (PPI + sodium bicarbonate, no enteric coating)
    2. omeprazole/sodium bicarbonate is superior to enteric coated omeprazole when assessing time to sustained symptomatic relief
    3. eating a meal within 30 minutes of administration is recommended
    4. rabeprazole has the fastest onset
- ~70% of patients will respond clinically to a therapeutic trial of PPI
- <u>Interactions</u>: decreased absorption of aspirin (requires acidic gastric pH), decreased conversion of clopidogrel to active form (competitive inhibition of hepatic CYP-450)
- <u>Pregnancy</u>: no increased risk of major congenital birth defects, spontaneous abortions, or preterm delivery have been demonstrated
- <u>Complications</u>: headache, diarrhea, dyspepsia, long bone fracture, cardiovascular and cerebrovascular events in patients on antiplatelet therapy, acute kidney injury (AKI) chronic kidney disease (CKD),

interstitial nephritis, atrophic gastritis, hypergastrinemia, worsening of vitiligo, nutrient malabsorption, dementia, angioedema, anaphylaxis

1. PPIs increased rates of revascularization, stent thrombosis, and major adverse cardiovascular events among patients on dual antiplatelet therapy, but have no effect on all-cause mortality and are protective against gastrointestinal bleeding

2. PPI with clopidogrel monotherapy increases risk of ischemic stroke and composite stroke/myocardial infarction/cardiovascular death, primarily with omeprazole, less so with pantoprazole

3. increased risk of long bone fracture, especially hip and spine, but is independent of bone mineral density; risk related to duration of use varies in literature; smoking may increase risk of fracture, though recent research has not confirmed this

4. association between hospital acquired *Clostridium difficile* infection and PPI without clear evidence of causation, but reported in the literature inconsistenly

5. possible increased risk of community-acquired pneumonia, especially within the first 30 days of therapy, and higher rates of hospitalization, though the research supporting these findings is flawed

6. use of PPI but not H2RA associated with increased rate of community acquired pneumonia in acute stroke patients, although this is unlikely to be causal

7. PI use may be associated with AKI and acute interstitial nephritis, especially in patients older than 65 years

8. PPI use is associated with CKD, especially with twice daily dosing, and an increased risk relative to H2 antagonists

9. may increase risk of AKI and severe hepatic encephalopathy in patients with spontaneous bacterial peritonitis

10. possible increased risk of progression to cirrhosis as well as hepatocellular carcinoma and hepatic decompensation in patients with hepatitis C

11. associated with increased risk of dementia in patients 75 years of age or older, possibly due to PPI mediated β-amyloid accumulation in the brain or vitamin B12 deficiency

Histamine-2 Receptor Antagonists

- <u>Mechanism</u>: Inhibit gastric acid secretion by antagonizing H2 receptors on parietal cells
- <u>Medications</u>: **cimetidine, ranitidine, famotidine, nizatidine**
- relieve symptoms in 60% of all patients and 75% with NERD
- repair of mucosal injury <50% of cases

- symptomatic improvement >1 year seen in <50%
- treatment of LPR requires higher doses than GERD
- <u>Side effects</u>: hepatitis, platelet defects, and drug interactions due to **CYP450 inhibition** (eg, Dilantin, warfarin, theophylline)
  1. <u>Drug interactions</u>: cimetidine>ranitidine>famotidine (never)
  2. cimetidine associated with peripheral androgen antagonism, but symptoms (eg, gynecomastia, impotence) are rare except in high doses

Antacids

- alkaline salts composed of magnesium hydroxide, aluminum hydroxide, calcium carbonate, and others depending on the commercial brand
- alginate preparations create a barrier at the gastroesophageal junction, and are more effective than other antacids

Baclofen

- skeletal muscle relaxant that increases postprandial LES pressure
- useful in treatment of upright reflux, chronic cough, rumination, aerophagia/belching, and reflux-related sleep disturbance

Prokinetic Agents

- increase LES pressure and decrease time to esophageal clearance; no prokinetic agents have been studied in patients with LPR
- <u>Cisapride</u>: not available in United States due to cardiac toxicity
  1. <u>Side effects</u>: diarrhea, nausea, QT prolongation and ventricular arrhythmias (if concurrently treated with macrolides)
  2. does not cross blood-brain barrier
- <u>Metoclopramide</u>: utility limited by extrapyramidal side effects

Surgical Management

- <u>Indications</u>: symptoms refractory to medical management, patient intolerance to medications; patient unwillingness to undergo long-term medical therapy; patients presenting with severe complications such as Barrett's esophagus, stricture, or ulceration
- <u>Preoperative evaluation</u>: H&P, upper endoscopy, barium esophagram, 24-hour pH monitoring, esophageal manometry, ± pulmonary function testing and voice objectives
- <u>Procedures</u>: Nissen fundoplication, partial fundoplication, Hill posterior gastropexy

1. Nissen fundoplication: laparoscopic, and transabdominal or transthoracic
2. Partial fundoplication: Thal (anterior wrap, 270°), Belsey (transthoracic anterior wrap, 270°), Dor (anterior wrap, 180°–200°), Lind (posterior wrap, 300°), and Toupet (posterior wrap, 270°)

- choice of procedure depends on esophageal motility and length
  1. normal or dysfunctional motility: Nissen fundoplication
  2. absent motility (scleroderma, achalasia, etc): partial fundoplication
- improvement of symptoms in ~90% patients
- <u>Complications</u>: mortality (~0%), infection, herniation, splenic injury, bleeding, pulmonary embolism, hypercapnia, pneumothorax, pneumomediastinum, dysphagia, gastroparesis, esophageal or gastric perforation

COMPLICATIONS OF REFLUX DISEASE

GERD

- **Stricture:** occurs in 2% to 10% of patients with long-term, untreated GERD
- **Ulceration:** commonly presents as odynophagia, and may result in bleeding
- **Iron deficiency anemia:** only occurs in patients with ulcerative esophagitis secondary to blood loss
- **Barrett's esophagus:** occurs in 10% to 15% of patients with long-term GERD (*see* Chapter 36)
- **Esophageal carcinoma:** GERD is a proven risk factor, and those with long-term LPR symptoms should be evaluated by esophagogastroduodenoscopy

LPR

- **Laryngeal granuloma:** generally resolves with treatment of GERD/LPR
- **Delayed wound healing**
- **Laryngeal stenosis:** present in >90% of patients with laryngeal stenosis
- **Laryngospasm:** involuntary vocal fold adduction most commonly at night
- **Muscle tension dysphonia:** chronic irritation → hyperfunctional laryngeal musculature → true vocal fold lesions (nodules, Reinke's edema, hematoma, ulcers, granuloma, etc)

- **Reinke's edema**: may be comorbid with smoking, hypothyroidism, and phonotrauma
- **Laryngeal carcinoma**: insufficient evidence for causal link; possible co-carcinogen in alcohol and tobacco users

REFLUX IN PEDIATRIC PATIENTS

- <u>Presentation</u>: dysphonia, halitosis, laryngospasm, laryngomalacia, asthma, recurrent pneumonia, sudden infant death syndrome, sleep apnea, regurgitation, otitis media
- <u>Evaluation</u>: physical examination, laryngoscopy, bronchoscopy, 24-hour pH monitor
- <u>Tx</u>: H2RAs, PPIs (omeprazole, lansoprazole, and esomeprazole approved for use in United States) , fundoplication in refractory cases with life-threatening complications
- **Sudden infant death syndrome (SIDS)**: association shown in an animal model, but not in humans
- **Otitis media**: presence of pepsin and pepsinogen found in effusions of children with otitis media, but cause-and-effect relationship remains unclear; current research does not support antireflux therapy for otitis media

ESOPHAGOPHARYNGEAL REFLUX

- exposure of laryngopharyngeal structures to undigested food, regurgitated from the proximal esophagus, likely secondary to dysmotility
- mechanism of injury not related to acid or pepsin
- only 50% benefit from diet modification or medication

CHAPTER

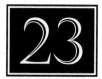

23

Thyroid-Related Disorders of the Larynx

Paul M. Papajohn, Nicholas C. Cameron, Mary J. Hawkshaw, and Robert T. Sataloff

INTRODUCTION

- the thyroid gland regulates protein synthesis and tissue metabolism through the production of thyroid hormones under control of thyrotropin (TSH) and thyrotropin-releasing hormone (TRH)
- disorders of the thyroid gland can cause laryngeal dysfunction through hormone effects, local effects on the recurrent laryngeal nerves, or iatrogenic nerve injury
- thyroid disorders are extremely common in clinical practice and should be considered in patients with laryngeal complaints including hoarseness, globus, vocal fatigue, muffling of voice
- iatrogenic injury to the recurrent laryngeal nerves should be considered in patients with true vocal fold (TVF) paresis/paralysis and/or postoperative hoarseness

ANATOMY

- **thyroid gland**: butterfly-shaped gland composed of two lateral lobes, isthmus, pyramidal lobe
- each lobe typically measures 4 × 1.5 × 2 cm with a total gland weight of 20 g
- located in the anterior neck at the level of the second through fourth tracheal cartilages, but can extend further superior
- spans between vertebral levels C5 and T1
- <u>Arterial supply</u>: **superior thyroid artery** (external carotid artery), **inferior thyroid artery** (thyrocervical trunk), thyroid ima artery (1.5%–12%)
- <u>Venous drainage</u>: superior, middle, and inferior thyroid veins
- lobes lie in close proximity to the **recurrent laryngeal nerve** (RLN) and **superior laryngeal nerve** (SLN)

Recurrent Laryngeal Nerve (RLN)

- RLN → motor innervation to all intrinsic laryngeal muscles of the larynx except the cricothyroid muscle; sensation to the TVF, subglottic larynx, upper esophagus, and trachea; parasympathetic innervation
- right RLN travels superiorly in an oblique path (lateral to medial), crossing the inferior thyroid artery into the tracheoesophageal groove
- left RLN travels in a linear path to the tracheoesophageal groove
- right and left RLN enter the larynx between the inferior cornu of the thyroid cartilage and arch of the cricoid cartilage

Nonrecurrent Inferior Laryngeal Nerve (NRILN)

- rare (0.5%–1% of population) anomaly in which RLN branches from the vagus nerve at the level of the larynx; occurs almost **exclusively on the right side**
- associated with vascular anomalies such as aberrant right subclavian artery (RSCA)
- <u>Innervation pattern:</u>
    1. type I NRILN arises from the vagus nerve and courses with the vessels of the superior thyroid peduncle
    2. type IIA NRILN arises from the vagus nerve at the level of the inferior thyroid artery
    3. type IIB courses beneath the trunk of the inferior thyroid artery

Superior Laryngeal Nerve (SLN)

- SLN divides into internal (iSLN) and external (eSLN) branches approximately 2 to 3 cm above the superior pole of the thyroid gland
- iSLN parallels the superior thyroid artery → pierces thyrohyoid membrane → sensory innervation to lower pharynx, supraglottic larynx, portions of TVF, base of tongue
- eSLN parallels the superior thyroid artery → motor innervation to **cricothyroid muscle**
- anatomical course of the eSLN varies and is classified in numerous ways (*see* Table 23–1 and Figure 23–1)

TABLE 23–1. Anatomic Variations of eSLN

Classification	Type and Criteria			
Cernea	Type 1: crossing the STA ≥1 cm above superior pole	Type 2a: crossing the STA <1 cm above superior pole	Type 2b: crossing below the upper border of thyroid	Type Ni: not identified
Kierner	Type 1: crossing the STA ≥1 cm above superior pole	Type 2: crossing the STA <1 cm above superior pole	Type 3: crossing below the upper border of thyroid	Type 4: descending dorsally until termination at CTM
Friedman	Type 1: descends superficial to IPC	Type 2: neural penetration of IPC	Type 3: descends deep to IPC	

Note. CTM, cricothyroid muscle; IPC, inferior pharyngeal constrictor; STA, superior thyroid artery.
Source: Adapted from Wang et al, *World Journal of Surgery,* 2017

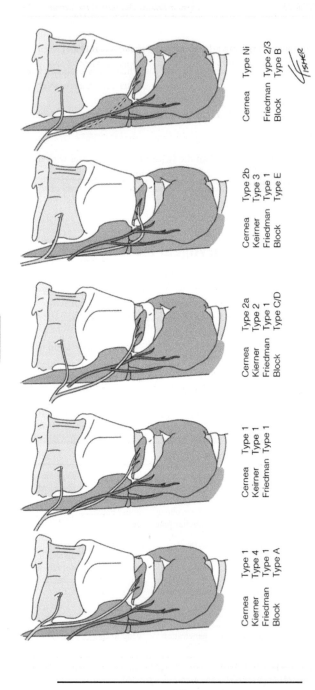

Cernea	Type 1		Cernea	Type 1		Cernea	Type 2a		Cernea	Type 2b		Cernea	Type Ni
Kierner	Type 4		Keirner	Type 1		Kierner	Type 2		Keirner	Type 3			
Friedman	Type 1		Friedman	Type 1		Friedman	Type 1		Friedman	Type 1		Friedman	Type 2/3
Block	Type A					Block	Type C/D		Block	Type E		Block	Type B

FIGURE 23–1. Anatomical variations of the course of the eSLN (illustration by Casey Fisher, DO). Used with permission from Sataloff et al., *Professional Voice: The Science and Art of Clinical Care* (4th ed.). San Diego, CA: Plural Publishing; 2017.

- parathyroid glands: attach to posterolateral surface of thyroid gland, responsible for calcium homeostasis via production of parathyroid hormone (PTH)

Parathyroid Glands

- **Superior parathyroid**: most commonly found at level of cricothyroid joint, about 1 cm above the intersection of RLN and inferior thyroid artery
- **Inferior parathyroid**: typically found 1 to 2 cm from inferior thyroid artery insertion into lower pole of thyroid
- each gland typically weighs 20 to 40 mg
- Vascular supply: inferior thyroid artery, occasional contributions from superior thyroid artery

PHYSIOLOGY

- **hypothalamus** → thyrotropin-releasing hormone (TRH) → **anterior pituitary** → thyroid-stimulating hormone (TSH) → **thyroid** → increased production of T4 (primarily) and T3
- T4 is transported by thyroxine-binding globulin (TBG, binds 75% of T4), transthyretin (binds 15% of T4), and albumin (binds 5% of T4)
- T4 is converted into the more active T3 by 5′-monodeiodinase in the liver, kidneys, and muscle
- T3 is four times more active than T4 and binds to TBG with higher affinity
- only unbound thyroid hormone is active
- **Regulation**: elevated T4 inhibits release of TRH and TSH; decreased T4 stimulates release of TRH and TSH
- **Effects**: thyroid hormone binds to intracellular receptors that bind directly to DNA, altering gene expression
    1. elevated metabolic rate (thermogenesis, increased oxygen consumption), neural and skeletal development, increased sympathetic activity, and regulation of protein synthesis
    2. laryngeal thyroid hormone receptors (TR-α and TR-β) are found within the fibrous lamina propria, cartilage, and glandular elements

HYPOTHYROIDISM

- Etiology:
    1. Primary: congenital (thyroid dysgenesis: *PAX8*, *FOXE1*, TSH receptor mutations), autoimmune (Hashimoto thyroiditis),

iatrogenic (thyroidectomy, radioiodine therapy, or external irradiation), thyroid hormone resistance syndrome (*THRB* mutation), medications (lithium, iodides, *p*-aminosalicylic acid), iodine deficiency

2. Secondary: pituitary failure, hypothalamic failure

- <u>Pathophysiology</u>: dysphonia possibly due to increased production of submucosal mucopolysaccharides
- <u>Presentation</u>: lethargy, muscle weakness, weight gain, cold intolerance, dry skin, brittle hair, constipation, menstrual irregularities, muscle cramps, neurological dysfunction, globus sensation, dysphonia (~**up to 80%**)
- rapid symptom onset in the setting of acute hypothyroidism—may occur 36 to 48 hours post-thyroidectomy
- nasal congestion, rhinorrhea, and or pharyngeal dryness may be evident, especially in the professional voice user
- <u>Voice characteristics</u>: lowered pitch and decreased voice clarity despite relatively normal laryngeal examination, vocal fatigue, muffled voice, loss of range
- <u>Dx</u>: ↑ TSH, ↓ free T4 (primary hypothyroidism); antithyroid peroxidase antibody (anti-TPO) and antithyroglobulin antibody (anti-Tg) in Hashimoto thyroiditis; ultrasound ± biopsy if indicated; strobovideolaryngoscopy if voice-related complaint
- <u>Stroboscopic findings</u>: diffuse, usually mild laryngeal edema similar to Reinke's edema and other causes, impaired mucosal wave
- **Laryngeal myxedema**: production of mucopolysaccharides increases fluid content of the lamina propria via an osmotic effect → increased vocal fold mass and decreased vibratory function
- in severe hypothyroidism, myxedema can produce profound dysphonia due to decreased muscle strength and even vocal fold paresis (rarely paralysis)
- even in the setting of low-normal range thyroid function tests, this diagnosis should be considered, especially if TSH levels are in the high-normal range or are elevated
- thyroid replacement therapy (eg, levothyroxine) associated with improvement in vocal fundamental frequency

HYPERTHYROIDISM

- <u>Etiology</u>:
  1. Primary: diffuse hyperplasia associated with autoimmune cause (Graves' disease), hyperfunctioning ("toxic") multinodular goiter, hyperfunctioning ("toxic") adenoma, granulomatous (de Quervain) thyroiditis, subacute lymphocytic thyroiditis, iodine-

induced hyperthyroidism, neonatal thyrotoxicosis associated with maternal Graves' disease

2. <u>Secondary</u>: TSH-secreting pituitary adenoma, pituitary resistance to thyroid hormone

3. <u>Miscellaneous</u>: struma ovarii (ovarian teratoma with ectopic thyroid), hCG-secreting tumors (eg. choriocarcinoma), factitious thyrotoxicosis (exogenous thyroxine intake)

- <u>Presentation</u>: heat intolerance, sweating, palpitations, weight loss, tremors, weakness
- <u>Voice characteristics</u>: laryngeal muscle weakness, dehydration, vocal tremor
- dysphonia uncommon in mild hyperthyroidism
- <u>Dx</u>: ↓ TSH (except in TSH-secreting tumors), ↑ free T4; antithyroid stimulating immunoglobulin (anti-TSI) in Graves' disease; radioactive iodine uptake (RAIU) scan to differentiate diffuse versus focal hyperfunction; strobovideolaryngoscopy if voice-related complaint
- severe hyperthyroidism and toxic goiter, even when treated preoperatively, are often associated with negative voice outcomes after surgery

EVALUATION

- clinical evaluation of every thyroid disorder or nodule should begin with a thorough history and physical exam
- the American Thyroid Association (ATA) has provided recommendations regarding indications for biopsy and additional workup

History and Physical Exam

- factors that raise suspicion of malignancy include rapid rate of thyroid lesion growth, hoarseness, childhood history of head and neck radiation, family history of thyroid cancer or familial syndrome associated with thyroid cancer (eg, multiple endocrine neoplasia syndromes) in a first-degree relative
- inquire about presence of pain, dysphagia, and symptoms of hypo- or hyperthyroidism
- physical exam red flags include cervical lymphadenopathy, fixation of the thyroid gland to surrounding structures (eg, skin, thyroid cartilage, trachea), vocal fold paresis or paralysis
- assessment and documentation of vocal fold motion by use of videostroboscopy, flexible laryngoscopy, 70° or 90° rigid oral endoscope, or laryngeal mirror examination

Radiologic Imaging

- **thyroid ultrasound:** should be considered in all patients who present with a suspected thyroid nodule on physical exam or as an incidental finding on head and neck imaging for another indication
- Ultrasound features predictive of malignancy: hypoechogenicity, irregular margins, microcalcifications, rim calcifications with extrusive soft tissue component, extrathyroid extension
- Computed tomography (CT)/magnetic resonance imaging (MRI): may consider if concern of substernal extension, compressive symptoms present, or bulky nodal disease

Overview of ATA Guidelines for Thyroid Nodule

- **serum TSH and ultrasound** should be obtained after finding a nodule
- nodules with low TSH should have a thyroid scan (Iodine 123 or Technetium 99m)
- cold nodules and nodules with normal or elevated TSH results should have a neck ultrasound that involves thyroid and cervical lymph nodes assessment
- **fine needle aspiration** (FNA) is the procedure of choice in diagnosing thyroid cancer (consider ultrasound guided)

Bethesda System for Thyroid Cytology (Table 23–2)

- Nondiagnostic cytology: repeat FNA, ultrasound guided, with preference to have on-site cytology interpretation (strong recommendation); repeatedly nondiagnostic with high-suspicion ultrasound, clinical risks for malignancy or growth in size of nodule requires surgical excision, otherwise close observation can be considered (weak recommendation)
- Benign cytology: no treatment or further immediate investigations (strong recommendation); follow-up with ultrasound and FNA in 1 year for high-suspicion group, ultrasound only in 1 to 2 years for intermediate-suspicion group, and ultrasound only in more than 2 years for low-suspicion group; if repeated ultrasound/FNA is benign, then no further follow-up will be required; adequate dietary iodine intake advised
- Atypia of undetermined significance/follicular lesion of undetermined significance (AUS/FLUS): surveillance, molecular testing or surgery can be considered on a case-by-case basis (strong recommendation)

TABLE 23–2. American Thyroid Association Sonographic Patterns of Thyroid Nodules and Recommendations for Fine Needle Aspiration (FNA)

Sonographic Pattern	Sonographic Features	Risk of Malignancy	Recommendation for FNA
High suspicion	Solid hypoechoic nodule or solid hypoechoic component of a partially cystic nodule with one or more of the following features: irregular margins, microcalcifications, taller than wide shape	70%–90%	FNA of nodules more than 1 cm in largest dimension otherwise repeat ultrasound in 6–12 months
Intermediate suspicion	Hypoechoic solid nodule without high suspicion features	10%–20 %	FNA of nodules more than 1 cm, otherwise repeat ultrasound in 12–24 months
Low suspicion	Isoechoic or hyperechoic solid nodule, or partially (>50%) cystic nodule, with eccentric solid area without high suspicion features	5%–10%	FNA of nodules more than 1.5 cm, otherwise repeat ultrasound in 12–24 months
Very low suspicion	Spongiform or partially cystic nodules without high or intermediate suspicion features	<3%	FNA or observe nodules more than 2 cm in largest dimension 1–2 cm nodules need repeat ultrasound in 2 years Less than 1 cm nodules require no intervention and no follow-up
Benign	Purely cystic nodules	<1%	No FNA required but consider aspiration for comfort or cosmesis

Source: Adapted from the 2015 American Thyroid Association guidelines.

- <u>Follicular neoplasm/suspicious for follicular neoplasm</u> (FN/SFN): surgery or molecular testing in low-suspicion groups and carefully selected low-risk patients (weak recommendation)
- <u>Suspicious for malignancy</u> (SUSP): surgery is strongly recommended; consider molecular testing only if it may change decision-making regarding surgery (weak recommendation)
- <u>Malignant</u>: surgical approach is strongly recommended

PATHOLOGIC DISORDERS OF THE THYROID

- both structural and inflammatory disorders of the thyroid can lead to changes in voice
- <u>Structural disorders</u>: mass effect on RLN/SLN leading to paresis/paralysis, invasion of trachea/larynx (impaired motion)
- <u>inflammatory disorders</u>: may cause RLN/SLN neuropraxia

Hashimoto's Thyroiditis

- most common cause of hypothyroidism in the United States
- associated with other autoimmune conditions (ie, systemic lupus erythematosus, Sjögren syndrome, scleroderma, others)
- increased risk of papillary thyroid carcinoma and non-Hodgkin's lymphoma
- <u>Pathophysiology</u>: antithyroglobulin and antimicrosomal Ab stimulate anti-TSH receptor leading to transient hyperthyroidism then hypothyroidism
- <u>Histopathology</u>: fibrosis, lymphocytic infiltration
- <u>Presentation</u>: slowly enlarging gland, painless, symptoms of hypothyroidism, may be subclinical
- <u>Dx</u>: antithyroid peroxidase (anti-TPO) antibodies, erythrocyte sedimentation rate (ESR), thyroid function tests (TFTs), FNA for prominent nodules
- <u>Tx</u>: long-term thyroxine therapy with TFT monitoring, consider surgical resection if compressive symptoms

Granulomatous (de Quervain) Thyroiditis

- most common cause of painful thyroid
- <u>Pathophysiology</u>: may be viral or postviral inflammatory response
- <u>Presentation</u>: **painful**, mild thyroid enlargement, self-limiting, flu-like symptoms

- <u>Dx</u>: history, TFTs
- <u>Tx</u>: nonsteroidal anti-inflammatory drugs (NSAIDs), steroids, observation

Subacute Lymphocytic Thyroiditis

- painless thyroiditis
- usually self-limiting
- common in postpartum women

Diffuse and Multinodular Goiters

- <u>Pathophysiology</u>: iodine deficiency (endemic) or dyshormonogenesis leads to increased TSH causing chronic thyroid hyperplasia with nodule formation
- <u>Presentation</u>: multiple nodules, thyroid fullness, compression symptoms (hoarseness, dysphagia, dyspnea), may extend substernally; hyperthyroid symptoms in setting of toxic multinodular goiter
- <u>Dx</u>: thyroid ultrasound, consider CT neck and chest if compressive symptoms present, TFTs
- <u>Tx</u>: hormonal suppression with levothyroxine, iodine replacement, radioactive iodine therapy, surgical excision

Graves' Disease

- <u>Pathophysiology</u>: autoimmune formation of thyroid-stimulating immunoglobulins (TSIs) bind and active TSH receptor leading to gland hyperplasia and increased T3 and T4 secretion
- <u>Risks</u>: female > male (5:1), radiation exposure, family history, age 20 to 40 years
- <u>Histopathology</u>: hyperplasia, increased colloid, papillary projections
- <u>Presentation</u>: hyperthyroid symptoms, goiter, **exophthalmos,** optic neuropathy, pretibial myxedema, dermopathy
- <u>Dx</u>: decreased TSH, increased T4/T3, TSI antibodies, RAIU
- <u>Tx</u>: control of adrenergic excess (β-blockers, ie, propranolol); restoration of euthyroid state (propylthiouracil, methimazole); **radioactive iodine ablation**; subtotal thyroidectomy (failed medical therapy/compression); ophthalmology evaluation

Malignant Thyroid Disease

Papillary Thyroid Carcinoma

- most common thyroid cancer ~75%

- best prognosis
- indolent natural history; slow growing
- <u>Histopathology</u>: single layers of thyroid cells arranged in avascular projections or papillae, large pale nuclei, intranuclear inclusion bodies, **psammoma bodies** (laminated calcified spheres)
- <u>Variants</u>: tall cell, columnar cell, diffuse sclerosing, follicular variant are associated with higher risk of recurrence
- <u>Treatment</u>: lobectomy versus total thyroidectomy ± central neck dissection, postoperative radioactive iodine ablation, suppressive levothyroxine therapy
- definitive surgical treatment is controversial and depends on clinical factors, age of patient, clinical staging

Follicular Thyroid Carcinoma

- second most common thyroid cancer ~16%
- cannot rely on FNA for diagnosis; surgical specimen required
- more aggressive than papillary
- <u>Histopathology</u>: small follicles containing small, cuboidal cells with poor colloid formation; distinguish between adenoma and carcinoma based on **capsular or vascular invasion**
- <u>Treatment</u>: similar to papillary thyroid carcinoma

Medullary Thyroid Carcinoma

- ~5% of thyroid cancers
- neuroendocrine tumor that involves the parafollicular or C cells
- associated with MEN 2a, MEN 2b, RET proto-oncogene; must screen for associated endocrinopathies
- must screen for pheochromocytoma with urine metanephrines prior to surgery
- more aggressive than papillary and follicular carcinoma
- <u>Histopathology</u>: sheets of cells with abundant, interspersed amyloid that stains Congo red
- <u>Treatment</u>: total thyroidectomy, central node dissection ± ipsilateral node dissection if clinically positive nodal disease
- monitor for recurrence using serum calcitonin and/or carcinoembryonic antigen (CEA)
- family members should be screened for RET

Anaplastic Thyroid Carcinoma

- ~1% to 2% of thyroid carcinoma

- typically seen in older patient with sudden rapid growth of thyroid gland
- very poor prognosis; highly aggressive; death within 6 to 36 months typically
- <u>Histopathology</u>: undifferentiated follicular cells
- <u>Tx</u>: tracheostomy, isthmusectomy, **palliation**, radiation therapy, doxorubicin

SURGICAL CONSIDERATIONS

Introduction

- prior to any thyroid or parathyroid surgery, a thorough voice assessment should be performed to identify any preexisting vocal fold dysfunction
- preoperative discussion with the patient on potential risks and voice outcomes of the procedure is essential for informed consent
- possible risks associated with voice outcomes in thyroid and parathyroid surgery include:
  1. vocal fold paresis/paralysis
  2. intubation-related vocal fold trauma
  3. retraction-related laryngeal trauma
- even with confirmed integrity of the RLN intraoperatively, transient changes in the voice quality are common after thyroid or parathyroid surgery
- negative voice outcomes unrelated to nerve injury can include infection, hemorrhage, soft tissue trauma, intubation-related vocal fold and/or arytenoid trauma, integrity of the laryngeal cartilages, and impairment of the extrinsic strap muscles or fixation of skin to trachea limiting vertical laryngeal movement
- the larger the thyroid gland being removed, the more likely the patient is to report negative voice outcomes
- all patients with postoperative voice changes should undergo a thorough evaluation with acoustic analysis, strobovideolaryngoscopy, and/or laryngeal electromyogram (EMG) to assist early recognition and proper treatment

Post-Thyroidectomy Vocal Fold Paresis and Paralysis

Recurrent Laryngeal Nerve Injury (*See* Chapter 18)

- RLN injuries may cause substantial social and professional impact

- RLN injury prevalence is decreasing with advances in medical technology and surgical experience
- rates 0.9% to 4.7% for transient paresis; 0% to 1.7% for permanent injury
- rates of RLN are higher for low-volume thyroid surgeons as compared to high-volume surgeons
- historically thyroid surgery was the main cause of iatrogenic RLN injury; however, other head and neck procedures including carotid endarterectomy and anterior cervical fusion have higher rates of injury
- the volume of thyroid surgery still makes it the most common cause of iatrogenic RLN injury
- intraoperative nerve monitoring systems (**NIMS**): aid in identification of RLN but have **no effect on preservation of neural integrity (controversial)**
- understanding of anatomy and **careful exposure of** RLN improve preservation of neural integrity

External Branch of the SLN Injury

- eSLN is also vulnerable to injury, especially near the superior pedicles of the thyroid gland
- injury results in signs and symptoms that can be subtle and nonspecific but include vocal fatigue, hoarseness, breathiness, loss of projection, and loss of range, especially at higher pitches
- stroboscopy findings may include ipsilateral glottal rotation, absence of brisk adduction and abduction, vocal fold bowing, vocal fold lag, inferior displacement of the affected TVF, decreased or increased mucosal wave

TREATMENT OF THYROIDECTOMY-RELATED VOCAL FOLD PARESIS AND PARALYSIS

Voice Therapy

- most patients with unilateral RLN paresis/paralysis will obtain satisfactory voice and airway with voice therapy alone, but success depends on several factors including the severity of the paresis/paralysis
- helpful to establish preoperative baseline, increases patient compliance, and improves psychological readiness for surgery
- usually first-line therapy, unless aspirating or severe vocal dysfunction

Surgical Management (See Chapter 33)

Indications

- nerve transection (eg, s/p thyroidectomy): reanastomosis at time of injury unless excised intentionally or other prohibitive factors
- nerve injury (crush, stretch, thermal, etc): observation with temporary injection TVF medialization
- aspiration: early TVF medialization; consider barium swallow or fiberoptic endoscopic evaluation of swallowing (FEES) to assess for aspiration or penetration once the injury is discovered
- desire for increased voice quality and volume

Injection Laryngoplasty

- medialization technique during which a material is injected lateral to the thyroarytenoid muscle
- goals of therapy include improved glottic closure and voice quality, reduced aspiration
- can be performed awake or under general anesthesia
- Materials: saline, voice gel, Gelfoam, fat, fascia, collagen, AlloDerm, hyaluronic acid, calcium hydroxylapatite
- temporary therapy to reduce symptoms of TVF paresis or assess potential improvement from thyroplasty

Type I Thyroplasty

- technique in which autologous cartilage or synthetic materials (eg, Gore-Tex, Silastic) are implanted medial to the thyroid cartilage to permanently medialize the vocal fold
- consider after trial of voice therapy, injection laryngoplasty, and adequate time (6 to 12 months) to allow for nerve recovery
- occasionally appropriate earlier than 6 months (eg, after known transection with severe dysphonia and aspiration), but revision likely to be necessary

Reinnervation

- goals of therapy are to prevent atrophy and increase/maintain bulk of laryngeal muscles
- improved vocal quality and mucosal wave, as well as decreased aspiration have been reported
- RLN reinnervation can improve long-term (>3 years) voice quality and adduction over injection medialization alone in patients with total denervation

- ideally, severity of denervation should be established by LEMG
- should be performed at time of primary surgery if nerve transection occurs and is recognized
- usually performed in combination with injection laryngoplasty or thyroplasty to provide early symptom relief

CHAPTER

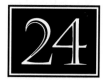

Autoimmune and Rheumatologic Disease

Jason E. Cohn, Jacob Burdett, Mary J. Hawkshaw, and Robert T. Sataloff

PATIENT EVALUATION

History

- persistent unexplained changes in the voice
- cough (dry versus productive)
- pain
- dysphagia/odynophagia (may be associated with neoplastic lesions)
- existence of personal or familial allergic, infectious, or systemic disorders

Physical Examination

- assess for atypical breathing and vocal characteristics
- general inspection and palpation of the nose, oral cavity, throat, and neck
- evaluate for nasal, mucosal, skin lesions
- when safe, **direct visualization** of the laryngeal complex via flexible and rigid endoscopy preferably with stroboscopy
- vocal fold dysfunction, mucosal alterations, purulent infections of the larynx, mass lesions, structural abnormalities, and occasionally subglottic lesions may present
- Always consider: pulmonary, renal, otologic and other manifestations of autoimmune/rheumatoid disease

AUTOIMMUNE/INFLAMMATORY CONDITIONS OF THE LARYNX

Sarcoidosis

- *inappropriate immune response* to an unknown antigen resulting in the *formation of granulomas*
- affects 10 per 100,000 individuals in the United States
- 70% of cases affect patients 25 to 45 years of age with female preponderance (~3:1)
- heritage propensity: Black > Northern European > Others
- classically affects pulmonary system, can affect larynx (usually supraglottic)
- Etiology: inappropriate immune response to an unknown antigen leads activated macrophages to activate immunologic pathways
- Histopathology: characterized by noncaseating granulomas without necrosis; duration of granulomas is variable

- <u>Presentation</u>: most common presenting complaints: hoarseness, dyspnea, dysphonia, and stridor; may display a "honking" vocal quality
- <u>Dx</u>: pink, edematous, turban-like supraglottic edema on laryngoscopy; glottis and subglottis tend to be spared
- definitive diagnosis requires tissue biopsy with noncaseating granulomas
- <u>Tx</u>: first-line treatment is oral steroids, topical or inhaled steroids for dermatologic and pulmonary manifestations, respectively
- azathioprine if steroids are unsuccessful
- surgical debulking in refractory cases or acute airway compromise

Relapsing Polychondritis

- episodic, progressive inflammatory disease, leading to destruction of cartilaginous structures
- incidence is 3.5 cases per million
- 3:1 female-to-male predominance
- onset typically between the ages of 40 and 60
- approximately one-third have coexisting autoimmune, connective tissue, or vasculitic conditions
- <u>Etiology</u>: T-cell-mediated reaction against type 2 cartilage; cartilage high in glycosaminoglycans
- <u>Presentation</u>: typically painful swelling of the cartilages of the auricles and nose, can affect any cartilaginous structure; ± arthritis, visual change and ocular dryness/discomfort, hearing loss, vertigo
- chronic disease can lead to saddle nose deformity
- <u>Laryngeal involvement</u> (50% of cases): nonproductive cough and hoarseness
- <u>Tracheobronchial involvement</u>: dyspnea and stridor; may increase the risk of general anesthesia
- <u>Dx</u>: **McAdam's Criteria** (requires 3/6 manifestations)
  1. bilateral auricular chondritis
  2. nonerosive inflammatory polyarthritis
  3. nasal chondritis
  4. ocular inflammation (conjunctivitis, scleritis, uveitis)
  5. respiratory tract chondritis (laryngeal and tracheal cartilages)
  6. vestibulocochlear dysfunction (hearing loss, tinnitus, and vertigo)
- <u>Tx</u>: nonsteroidal anti-inflammatory drugs (NSAIDs), systemic or injected corticosteroids, methotrexate, cyclophosphamide, anti-TNF-α agents, potassium-titanyl-phosphate (KTP) laser (if localized disease)
- tracheotomy may necessary for obstruction secondary to diffuse inflammation or destruction of laryngeal skeleton

- long-term prognosis is poor—morbidity and mortality related to respiratory involvement, coronary artery disease, or corticosteroid side effects

Systemic Lupus Erythematosus

- multisystem inflammatory disease caused by the presence of circulating autoantibodies
- incidence 1:1000 with a significant female-to-male predominance (9:1)
- ethnic populations (African or Asian) are at greatest risk. all populations to some degree
- upper airway disease can affect up to 30% of those diagnosed with SLE
- <u>Histopathology</u>: variable findings with few specific characterizing manifestations; connective tissue and blood vessel inflammation with superficial, perivascular, and deep lymphocytic infiltration; fibrinoid deposits
- <u>Presentation</u>: vocal fold thickening or immobility with or without cricoarytenoid joint arthritis. subglottic stenosis (30% of cases); progressive sore throat, cough, hoarseness, dysphagia, dysphonia, foreign-body sensation, strained respirations, rarely airway obstruction
- **Mechanisms of laryngeal symptoms**: poor vascular supply to nerves supplying the larynx, compression of laryngeal nerves due to pulmonary hypertension (subsequent left atrial enlargement), mucosal edema, ulceration of mucosal surfaces
- <u>Dx</u>: direct laryngoscopy (edema of aryepiglottic folds, vocal fold paralysis, and upper airway obstruction), computed tomography, laryngeal electromyography, and serology (ANA, anti-dsDNA)
- <u>Tx</u>: antimalarials and corticosteroids either as monotherapy or in combination with other immunosuppressive agents: cyclophosphamide and azathioprine

Rheumatoid Arthritis

- rheumatoid arthritis (RA) is a systemic inflammatory joint disease that leads to the destruction of cartilage and erosion of bone
- the prevalence is 3% of the adult population with female preponderance (2:1)
- affected ages are most commonly between 40 and 50 years
- the larynx is involved in approximately 25% of cases
- cricoarytenoid joint (CAJ) most commonly affected in larynx
- <u>Etiology</u>: systemic inflammatory joint disease primarily affecting synovial joints notoriously in the wrists and hands

- <u>Histopathology</u>: inflammation of CAJ synovial lining → articulating surfaces affected → fibrosis → ankylosis
- <u>Presentation</u>: dysphonia, dysphagia, foreign-body sensation, odynophagia, sore throat, change in voice quality (eg, decreased pitch and mean phonation time), referred otalgia, inspiratory stridor
- typically begins as pain and arytenoid mucosal erythema; progresses to normalization of laryngeal mucosa with (CAJ) dysfunction and/or submucosal nodules on the true vocal folds (rheumatoid nodules)
- CAJ dysfunction/ankylosis → rapidly progressive dyspnea and airway obstruction from fixed vocal fold adduction
- <u>Dx</u>: laryngoscopy, CT scan, antirheumatoid factor, anticyclic citrullinated protein
- may find submucosal (rheumatoid) nodules on the true vocal folds (TVFs) and/or CAJ deformity/immobility on laryngoscopy
- <u>Tx</u>: voice therapy, oral steroids, NSAIDs, leflunomide, and other cytotoxic agents; may require TVF lateralization procedures, tracheotomy

Scleroderma

- <u>Etiology</u>: autoimmune disease characterized by chronic inflammation and progressive, systemic fibrosis
- onset is normally between 35 and 40 years of age with female preponderance
- <u>Histopathology</u>: genetic susceptibility versus an unknown external stimulus leads to production of profibrotic cytokines and fibrosis of multiple organ systems
- <u>Presentation</u>: vocal deterioration, dysphagia, dyspnea, and airway obstruction in severe cases
- patients may have history of gastroesophageal reflux disease, Raynaud's disease, and sclerodactyly
- <u>Dx</u>: serological testing for ANA, anticentromere, antitopoisomerase I, and anti-RNA polymerase I/III autoantibodies; strobovideolaryngoscopy (vocal fold hemorrhage, scarring, hypervascularity, and varicosities are suggestive)
- <u>Tx</u>: resection of laryngeal nodules with triamcinolone injections

Granulomatosis With Polyangiitis (Wegener's Granulomatosis)

- <u>Etiology</u>: unknown—multisystem inflammatory disorder characterized by necrotizing vasculitis and granuloma formation within the upper and lower respiratory tracts and glomerulonephritis

- primarily involves the subglottis due to presence of ciliated respiratory epithelium—16% develop subglottic stenosis
- Histopathology: necrotizing, small vessel granulomatous vasculitis with multinucleated giant cells
- Presentation: subglottic granulomatous tissue with varying degrees of obstruction (respiratory distress), bleeding, and pain; most commonly presents with nasal manifestations (eg, crusting, atrophic rhinitis, septal perforation, saddle nose deformity)
- Dx: positive antiproteinase 3 antibody (C-ANCA), erythrocyte sedimentation rate (ESR), C-reactive protein (CRP), flexible laryngoscopy
- Tx: **oral steroids and immunosuppressants (first line)**; occasionally requires resection, dilation, laryngotracheoplasty with anterior and posterior cricoid splits with or without stents, microvascular free flaps, tracheotomy
- complete remission in ~75% of patients, ~50% relapse rate

Pemphigus Vulgaris

- autoimmune bullous disease affecting mucous membranes of the larynx and oropharynx
- affects males and females equally most commonly between 40 and 60 years
- patients typically Mediterranean, Middle Eastern, and Jewish descent
- Etiology: autoantibodies targeting epidermal tight-junction protein desmoglein leading to sloughing and separation of cells
- Histopathology: subepithelial inflammation with acantholysis and bullae formation in the epidermis; IgG and complement (particularly C3) deposits on immunohistochemistry
- Presentation: vesicles and bullae most prevalent on pressure points that rupture easily, persistent aphthous ulcers. most common laryngeal symptom is hoarseness
- Dx: characteristic bullae that rupture easily—denuded area reveals fibrinous white exudate, biopsy is diagnostic
- Tx: **systemic corticosteroids**, evidence lacking for other immunomodulating agents, antibiotics for superimposed infections

Other Inflammatory Disorders That Affect the Larynx

- Reiter's disease, gout, Crohn's disease, and ankylosing spondylitis

CHAPTER

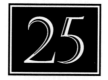

Allergy

Austin T. Baker, Sarah Christine Nyirjesy, Justin Ross, and Brian J. McKinnon

IMMUNOLOGY OF THE ALLERGIC RESPONSE

Hypersensitivity Reactions (See Table 25–1)

Innate Immunity

- <u>First-line defenses capable of rapid response</u>: barrier mechanisms (skin, mucus), bioactive molecules (complement proteins, lysozyme), toll-like receptors (TLRs)
- TLRs recognize pathogen-associated molecular patterns (PAMPs) on microbes resulting in cytokine generation, complement activation, and phagocytic responses

Adaptive Immunity

- complex mechanism of immunity specific to distinct antigens and based on immunologic memory
- cell-mediated (T-cell) and humoral responses (B-cell)

TABLE 25–1. Hypersensitivity Reactions

Type	Mediator	Mechanism	Example
Type I: Immediate	IgE	• Ag binds to IgE bound to mast cells and basophils leading to vasoactive mediator release.	• Systemic and localized anaphylaxis (urticaria, angioedema, itching, wheeling, bronchospasm, rhinorrhea, sneezing)
Type II: Cytotoxic	IgG, IgM	• Ab binding to cell surface antigens leading to phagocytic or complement mediated destruction	• Transfusion reactions • Goodpasture's syndrome • Hemolytic anemia • Myasthenia gravis
Type III: Immune Complex	IgG, IgM, IgA	• Ag-Ab complexes deposit in various tissue leading to complement activation and neutrophil migration	• serum sickness • glomerulonephritis • SLE
Type IV: Cell-Mediated	T-Cell	• delayed-type hypersensitivity • sensitized Th1 cells mediate direct cellular damage	• Contact dermatitis • Graft rejection

Cells and Components of the Allergic Response

T-Lymphocytes

- produced in bone marrow and mature in thymus
- recognize protein fragments bound to major histocompatibility complex (MHC) presented by other cells
  1. MHC I: presented by all cells in the body
  2. MHC II: found on antigen-presenting cells
- Helper T-cells (CD4+): recognize antigens presented on MHC II molecules; differentiate into Th1 or **Th2 cells**
  1. Th1: involved in phagocyte-mediated defense against intracellular microbial infections
  2. Th2: involved in the allergic response; secrete cytokines IL-4, IL-5, IL-10, and IL-13
- Cytotoxic T-cell (CD8+): catalytic cells that recognize antigens on MHC I molecules

B Lymphocytes

- mature in bone marrow and are responsible for humoral immunity
- produce all major classes of antibodies
- naive B cells produce IgM and IgD and undergo isotype class switching when stimulated by Th2 cells or other signals

Antigen-Presenting Cells

- monocytes, macrophages, dendritic cells
- process antigens and present peptides via MHC II molecules to be recognized by helper T cells

Mast Cells

- **major effector in type I hypersensitivity**
- IgE cross-linking leads to rapid degranulation of contents responsible for the majority of allergic symptoms

Cytokines

- proteins secreted by immune cells in response to antigen stimulation that facilitate immune reactions and specific cell function; includes interleukins (IL), tumor necrosis factor (TNF), colony-stimulating factors, interferons
- **IL-2**: produced by T cells; involved in T-cell clonal expansion
- **IL-3**: produced by CD4+ T cells; plays a role in development of mast cells and eosinophils in the bone marrow

- **IL-4**: produced by CD4+ T cells; stimulates and sustains the transformation of CD4+ cells into Th2 cells; primary signal involved in plasma cell maturation from B cells with isotype switching to IgE production
- **IL-5**: produced by CD4+ T cells; activates and recruits eosinophils to areas of inflammation
- **IL-10**: produced by macrophages and CD4+ T cells; plays a role in immune system regulation; can inhibit antigen-presenting cells and cytokine synthesis
- **IL-13**: aids in immune cell recruitment to areas of allergic inflammation by increasing adhesion molecules at inflammatory sites
- **TNF-α**: produced primarily by activated macrophages; induces fever, apoptosis and inflammation, and inhibits viral reproduction and tumorigenesis

The IgE-Mediated Allergic Response

Sensitization

- <u>Atopy</u>: susceptibility to allergic reactions to normally harmless antigens; likely due to a genetic predisposition; skewed amount of CD4+ T cells responding along the Th2 pathway and overproduction of IgE antibodies
- allergens such as pollens, grasses, and mold are deposited on mucosal surfaces
- antigen-presenting cells process the antigen, migrate to lymph nodes, and present peptides to helper T cells via the antigen MHC-II complex
- naïve CD4+ T cells then differentiate into Th2 cells and release IL-4, IL-5, and IL-13
- IL-4 stimulates B lymphocytes to differentiate into plasma cells with isotype switching to produce IgE antibodies; IgE antibodies bind to the Fc receptors of mast cells and basophils leading to sensitization

Early Response

- mast cell and basophil dependent; occurs in a sensitized host **within minutes** to antigen exposure
- antigen cross-links to specific IgE antibodies on mast cells resulting in release of some preformed mediators and de novo synthesis of mediators
- edema, urticaria, nasal congestion, rhinorrhea, and sneezing are immediate results of this reaction
- **Histamine**: primary mediator; causes vasodilation, vascular permeability, bronchoconstriction, mucus secretion

- **Heparin**: anticoagulant, enhances phagocytosis
- **Tryptase**: proteolytic enzyme
- **Leukotrienes**: formed via metabolism of arachidonic acid; cause bronchoconstriction, vasodilation, chemotactic recruitment of inflammatory cells
- **Prostaglandins**: formed via metabolism of arachidonic acid; causes bronchoconstriction, vasodilation, platelet aggregation
- **Platelet-activating factor**: recruits eosinophils and causes further cytokine release
- **Additional mediators**: TNF, colony-stimulating factors

Late Response

- occurs **4–12 hours** after initial exposure
- chemotactic properties of IL-4, IL-5, IL-13 and leukotrienes (LTB4 and LTC4) recruit eosinophils, neutrophils, and basophils to amplify and sustain the inflammatory state without additional allergen exposure
- may occur after an initial resolution of symptoms but ultimately results in persistent allergy symptoms lasting 24 hours or longer
- results in **priming** (additional production of allergen-specific IgE) and **hypersensitivity** (increased response to subsequent allergens)
- symptoms include worsening congestion, increased rhinorrhea, and wheezing

ALLERGY THERAPIES AND TREATMENTS

Nonmedical Treatment

- acaricide-based pesticide to kill dust mites
- impermeable bed covers
- high-efficacy particulate air (HEPA) Filters
- removal of pets from home
- clean linens
- frequent dusting/vacuuming
- nasal saline irrigation removes mucus and helps with mucociliary clearance

Pharmacotherapy: Symptomatic Control

- **Intranasal corticosteroids**: most effective class of medication; local reduction of inflammatory process; mild side effects of epistaxis, nasal dryness, and irritation

- **Oral antihistamines**: mainstay treatment; quick onset and are effective in treating sneezing, rhinorrhea, itching, and ocular symptoms; less effective for nasal congestion
  1. First-generation side effects: sedation and anticholinergic drying side effects; may interfere with singing or speaking by interfering with vocal fold lubrication
  2. Second-generation side effects: less sedation and drying side effects
- **Nasal antihistamines**: fast onset; effective for sneezing, itching, rhinorrhea; mildly effective for nasal congestion; does not treat ocular symptoms
- **Oral decongestants**: commonly combined with antihistamines for improved control of nasal congestion and to counteract sedation; the improved drying effects may further exacerbate the vocal quality side effects seen with antihistamines; stimulatory side effects (insomnia and tachycardia) may be seen
- **Oral corticosteroids**: used as a **last resort** for short-term control of severe disease; long-term use is inappropriate due to serious side effect profile
- **Oral antileukotrienes**: symptomatic control comparable to antihistamines and function well in combination with antihistamines; can cause less mucosal dryness than other agents
- **Nasal mast cell stabilizers**: mildly efficacious for prophylactic therapy, minimal side effect profile
- **Mucolytic agents**: liquefy mucus and increase output of thin respiratory tract secretions, may be combined to counteract drying effects of antihistamines and decongestants
- **Fluticasone proprionate/azelastine combination therapy**: multiple studies have shown improvements with combination therapy over monotherapy, current guidelines recommend reserving this for patients who have failed monotherapy, Dymista is a combination intranasal spray (often cost-prohibitive)
- differing combinations may need to be tried for success, especially when considering side effects on the professional voice

Immunotherapy

- allergy **desensitization** that allows for tolerance through titrated exposure to allergens
- **Subcutaneous immunotherapy (SCIT)**: proven method that decreases allergy symptoms and decreases development of new inhalant allergies; two phases, **escalation phase** which involves gradually increasing allergen concentration, and **maintenance**

phase where a set dose is given at increasing intervals; risk of anaphylaxis

- **Sublingual immunotherapy (SLIT):** Drops of allergen extract placed under the tongue; research **suggests similar efficacy and improved safety benefits** compared to SCIT; commercially available for allergies to ragweed, timothy grass, and dust mites, but can be used for other inhaled allergens; is a viable alternative for children
- Alternate routes of administration:
    1. **Epicutaneous (EIT):** delivered through patches; thought to improve activation of and antigen presentation by dendritic cells in the epidermis without systemic absorption of allergen; aims to improve compliance in children
    2. **Intralymphatic (ILIT):** injection of allergen directly into lymph nodes; thought to enhance antigen presentation and subsequent generation of immune cell responses without increasing Th2 immunity; preliminary studies show significantly fewer required doses to achieve similar results compared to SLIT and SCIT; **lack of anaphylaxis** provides large safety benefit

Alternative and Developing Therapies

- **Surgical therapy:** does not directly affect allergic inflammation and is an adjunct therapy for nasal congestion after failed medical management; surgical options include submucosal resection of inferior turbinate, nasal valve repair, septoplasty, and removal of nasal polyps
- **H3 and H4 antihistamines:** H3 and H4 receptors may have higher affinity for histamine than H1 and H2 receptors leading to increased eosinophil activation, currently under investigation
- **Omalizumab:** monoclonal IgE antibody inhibitor, currently not approved by the U.S. Food and Drug Administration (FDA) for allergic rhinitis, increased efficacy as a therapy for resistant seasonal allergic rhinitis with comorbid asthma, high cost and potential side effects limit use, combination with immunotherapy may decrease side effects caused by immunotherapy and decrease the duration of the escalation and maintenance phases, additional monoclonal antibodies are currently being studied and developed
- **Toll-like receptor agonists:** specific bacterial ligands developed to bind and activate toll-like receptors on antigen-presenting cells inducing a Th1 response via innate and adaptive immunity; preliminary studies have been undertaken to determine efficacy as an adjuvant to current immunotherapy
- **Allergoids:** physically or chemically modified allergens reducing their ability to cross-link IgE and cause allergic inflammation

ALLERGIC RHINITIS (AR)

- IgE-mediated inflammation of nasal mucosa resulting in bilateral rhinorrhea with postnasal drip, nasal congestion, sneezing, and/or nasal itching in response to an inhaled allergen
- <u>Etiology</u>: genetic (eg, HLA-DR loci), environmental (eg, heavy maternal smoking in first year of life, start of daycare/group education after age 3, early exposure to pet dander, oldest in birth order)
- <u>Pathophysiology</u>: Type I IgE-mediated hypersensitivity reaction to extrinsic proteins of normally harmless substances; possibly due to abnormally high levels of IgE or inappropriate IgE production to benign substances causing mast cells to release mediators → mediators cause vasodilation and stimulation of mucus-secreting glands → recruitment of other inflammatory cells, especially **eosinophils**
- common inhaled allergens:
  1. <u>Seasonal</u>: pollens from **grasses (spring)**, **trees (summer)**, and **weeds (fall)**
  2. <u>Perennial</u>: dust mites, cockroaches, molds (worse in humid weather), pet dander (cats, dogs, birds)
- More common in children (mean age of onset 8–11 years): ~80% of cases present before the age of 20; in children, more boys than girls are affected but sex difference equalizes by adulthood
- <u>Comorbidities</u>: **asthma** (correlation between severity of AR and severity of asthma), atopic dermatitis, allergic conjunctivitis, nasal polyposis, otitis media with effusion, and rhinosinusitis
- <u>ARIA (Allergic Rhinitis and its Impact on Asthma) Classification</u>:
  1. <u>Mild</u> (includes all of the following): normal sleep, no impairment of daily activities, sport, leisure, no impairment of work and school, no troublesome symptoms
  2. <u>Moderate-severe</u> (one or more): abnormal sleep, impairment of daily activities, sport, leisure, impaired work and school, troublesome symptoms
  3. <u>Intermittent</u>: <4 days/week or for <4 weeks
  4. <u>Persistent</u>: >4 days/week and >4 weeks
- <u>Seasonal-perennial classification</u>
  1. <u>Seasonal AR</u>: disease caused by an IgE-mediated inflammatory response to seasonal aeroallergens; length of seasonal exposure to these allergens is dependent on geographic location and climatic conditions
  2. <u>Perennial AR</u>: disease caused by an IgE-mediated inflammatory response to year-round environmental aeroallergens; may include dust mites, mold, animal allergens, or some occupational allergens

3. <u>Episodic AR</u>: disease caused by an IgE-mediated inflammatory response that can occur if an individual is in contact with an exposure that is not usually a part of the individual's environment
- <u>Presentation</u>: **bilateral** clear rhinorrhea, postnasal drip, itchy nose, nasal congestion, conjunctival erythema or epiphora, sneezing, **pale-pink or blue discoloration of nasal mucosa**, swelling of nasal turbinates, frequent throat clearing, allergic shiners (dark discoloration below eyelids from venous pooling), persistent adenoids, allergic crease (across nasal bridge from nose rubbing), adenoid facies (from mouth breathing), malaise and fatigue (more common in children), hyposmia, headache, facial pain, or ear pain
- commonly have family history of atopic or allergic disease
- <u>Complications</u>: fatigue, decreased quality of life, sleep disordered breathing, depression, learning and attention impairment
- <u>Dx</u>: avoidance trial of allergens supports diagnosis of AR; confirm with IgE-mediated response to a specific allergen detected through cutaneous or blood testing; imaging not typically recommended—obtain sinus computed tomography (CT) if comorbidities of AR are suspected (eg, chronic rhinosinusitis, nasal polyposis, etc)

Treatment Options

- **Nonmedical**: allergen avoidance/environmental controls, acaricide-based pesticide to kill dust mites, impermeable bed covers, high-efficacy particulate air (HEPA) filters, removal of pets from home
- **Intranasal steroids: first-line treatment**, efficacy reached after 1 week of therapy, continuous use is more effective than intermittent, oral steroids are *not* recommended—similar efficacy as intranasal, but with significant side effects, if insufficient control of symptoms with intranasal steroids add daily intranasal antihistamine or short course of oxymetazoline (3 days or less)
- **Intranasal antihistamines:** include azelastine and olopatadine, more rapid onset of action than intranasal steroids (~15 minutes), useful in patients with episodic nasal symptoms or pretreatment prior to nasal allergen exposure
- **Oral antihistamines:** useful in patients with concurrent ocular symptoms and pruritus, but have minimal effect on nasal congestion, maximum benefit with continuous use
- **Leukotriene receptor antagonists (montelukast):** not a first-line therapy for allergic rhinitis except if comorbid with asthma, efficacy similar to oral antihistamines but more expensive

- **Immunotherapy**: Indicated in patients with inadequate response to treatment with pharmacologic therapy; subcutaneous or sublingual
- **Surgical Tx**: inferior turbinate reduction indicated for persistent nasal airway obstruction and enlarged inferior turbinates in patients who have failed medical management; performed via submucous resection with outfracture of bony remnant
- **Other approaches**: acupuncture shows limited benefit, no role for herbal therapy

CHRONIC RHINOSINUSITIS

- defined as symptoms of rhinosinusitis lasting ≥12 weeks
- subtypes include chronic rhinosinusitis with nasal polyps (CRSwNP) and chronic rhinosinusitis without polyps (CRSsNP)
- <u>Etiology</u>: commonly multifactorial; infection, mucociliary dysfunction, structural abnormalities, environmental factors (smoking, allergy, pollution)
- <u>Presentation</u>: facial pain/pressure, nasal obstruction, nasal/postnasal discharge, hyposmia/anosmia, fever, headache, halitosis, dental pain, fatigue, cough, ear pain/pressure/fullness; symptoms are commonly less severe than acute rhinosinusitis.
- <u>Dx</u>: ≥12 weeks of 2 or more of the following symptoms— mucopurulent drainage, nasal obstruction, facial pain/pressure, hyposmia/anosmia, as well as one documented finding suggestive of inflammation on endoscopy or imaging (eg, purulent mucus or edema of middle meatus, polyps, sinus mucosal thickening)
- <u>Tx</u>: oral/topical antimicrobials (typically macrolides), intranasal corticosteroids, short course of oral steroids (CRSwNP), allergy treatment, high-volume, low-pressure nasal lavage, mucolytic agents, surgical therapy reserved for those who fail medical management

ALLERGY TESTING

AAO Skin Testing Guidelines

- screening panels should not include more than 14 relevant antigens and their controls; test for both seasonal and perennial allergens
- <u>Seasonal</u>: pollens from grasses, weeds, and trees that are most common in that geographic region
- <u>Perennial</u>: dust mites (*Dermatophagoides pteronyssinus*, *D. farinae*), animal dander, cockroach, molds (poor cross-reactivity, include several in screening panel)

- follow screening panel with single dilutional intradermal tests for selected antigens that are negative on prick testing
- if screening is positive and immunotherapy is considered, no more than 40 antigens for confirmatory test
- intradermal testing should always be preceded by prick testing to minimize adverse events
- if patient is started on immunotherapy, follow-up skin testing to quantify degree of sensitivities is required

Skin Testing Methods

- **Skin prick or puncture technique**: drop of allergen onto patient's skin → insertion of fine needle through droplet into skin → introduction of specific allergen into patient's skin → activation of IgE-sensitized cutaneous mast cells → histamine release from mast cell granules → wheal and flare appears in ~20 minutes
  1. <u>Advantage</u>: high sensitivity and specificity (>80%)
  2. <u>Disadvantage</u>: may decrease sensitivity in population >50 years
- **Intradermal technique**: create bleb via percutaneous needle insertion of allergen; used to identify IgE-specific allergens; best when skin prick test is negative but high clinical suspicion
  1. <u>Advantage</u>: more sensitive than skin prick
  2. <u>Disadvantage</u>: uses higher concentration of antigen so greater risk of anaphylaxis
- **Intradermal Dilutional Testing (Serial Endpoint Titration)**: introduce serially increasing concentrations of antigen into skin → endpoint is concentration at which the wheal size increases
  1. <u>Advantages</u>: useful to titrate concentrations for immunotherapy; highly sensitive, quantitative analysis
  2. <u>Disadvantage</u>: time consuming
- **Scratch testing**: scratch patient's skin and insert allergen; rarely used, poor sensitivity and specificity; included for historical purposes
- <u>Contraindications</u>: coexistent severe or uncontrolled asthma, atopic dermatitis (relative contraindication), dermatographism (in vitro testing required), patients at risk for compromised survival if anaphylaxis occurs due to other conditions including severe unstable cardiovascular disease or required use of β-blockers
- <u>Adverse Effects</u>: pain, erythema, local swelling, pruritus, anaphylaxis, death (only reported cases with intradermal testing when not preceded by prick testing)
- <u>Considerations</u>: variability in the allergen extract concentrations used, skin testing devices, number of skin tests performed, interpretation and documentation of results

- use standardized allergen extracts when available, record measurements of wheal and erythema for allergen positive and negative controls at 15 to 20 minutes after placement
- Medications to avoid:
  1. **Oral H1-blockers (antihistamines)**: inhibit wheal-and flare responses for 24 hours or more (avoid for 48–72 hours before skin testing), loratadine and desloratadine can inhibit response for 7 days
  2. **Tricyclic antidepressants**: doxepin, desipramine can suppress wheal for 2 to 4 days
  3. **β-blockers (eg, propranolol, metoprolol)**: want to avoid up to 72 hours prior to skin testing in case epinephrine is required to treat anaphylaxis—unopposed α-adrenergic agonism can lead to hypertensive crisis and arrhythmias
- H2-blockers, systemic corticosteroids, and leukotriene modifiers do not affect skin response
- <u>Pros</u>: more sensitive than blood testing, less expensive
- <u>Cons</u>: possible anaphylaxis, affected by patient medications

Radioallergosorbent Test (RAST)

- immunoassay of patient's serum for allergen-specific IgE
- <u>Method</u>: (1) incubate serum with suspected allergen absorbed on a solid phase (plastic disc or bead); (2) add anti-IgE antibody for this allergen labeled with fluorescing agents (radiolabeling is rarely used, making RAST a misnomer)
- <u>Advantages</u>: measure sensitivity to specific antigens without concern for adverse reactions, no need to stop medications, can use with dermatographism or severe eczema
- <u>Disadvantages</u>: less sensitive, more expensive
- detection of sensitization to an allergen does *not* diagnose an allergy without presence of clinical symptoms

Other Tests for Allergic Rhinitis With Inconclusive Evidence

- acoustic rhinometry
- olfactory testing
- microarray testing
- nasal nitric oxide measurements
- testing for food allergy
- nasal allergen challenges
- nasal smears for eosinophilia

ALLERGIC LARYNGITIS

- acute or chronic laryngitis with dysphonia due to exposure to allergen with associated **thick-viscous endolaryngeal secretions** and reactive vocal fold hyperemia and edema due to **throat clearing** and coughing
- difficult to differentiate from laryngopharyngeal reflux (LPR) due to similar symptoms
- Etiology: likely similar to AR; "unified airway concept" suggests this is due to concomitant mediator responses of upper and lower airways via shared epithelium
- Pathophysiology: suspected IgE-mediated type I hypersensitivity affecting upper airway, usually related to the late-phase eosinophilic infiltration and mediator release (not early mast cell degranulation); controversial since mast cells and eosinophils are not typically found in high numbers in the squamous epithelium of the vocal folds
- Most common allergen: dust mite antigen sensitivity
- Presentation: chronic symptoms with acute exacerbations; **dysphonia** (raspy voice quality; limited volume and range of pitch), chronic overactive **cough**, globus sensation, postnasal drip, **repeated throat clearing**, odynophagia, itching of larynx, vocal fold hyperemia and edema, shimmering pale edematous arytenoid mucosa
- viscous mucus within the larynx from the lungs and/or nasal cavity with simultaneous increased **endolaryngeal mucus production**
- Dx: suspect from history and physical (H&P); diagnosis of exclusion; requires positive allergy test or history of allergy; flexible laryngoscopy (nonspecific hyperemia or viscous endolaryngeal mucus);
- Additional testing: 24-hour pH monitor or LPR medical treatment failure, pulmonary function tests, chest x-ray, sinus imaging
- patients should avoid dust, pollen, smoke, chemical pollutants, use of steroid inhalers or systemic decongestant medications, whispering, throat clearing
- benefit from adequate hydration, steam inhalation, sugar-free throat lozenges, cool mist humidifier, isotonic saline sprays, vocal rest, voice therapy
- Medical Tx: Nasal steroid and nasal antihistamine (patients with chronic cough due to allergy-associated postnasal drip); immunotherapy if refractory
- If voice improvement required immediately: short course of oral steroids or steroid injection to superficial lamina propria of vocal folds
- Surgical Tx: indicated only in severe cases of unresolved Reinke's edema, edematous nodules, or hemorrhagic polyps—mini-microflap resection of lesions or Reinke's evacuation

CHAPTER

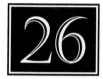

Respiratory Dysfunction

Haig Panossian, Mary J. Hawkshaw, and Robert T. Sataloff

ANATOMY

Anatomy of Tracheobronchial Tree

- trachea: C-shaped cartilaginous rings with posterior membranous wall
- main bronchi: right and left, divide from trachea at carina
- lobar bronchi
- segmental bronchi
- bronchioles
- terminal bronchioles
- acinus: respiratory bronchioles, alveolar ducts, alveolar sacs, and alveoli

Respiratory Musculature

- muscles of inspiration: diaphragm, external intercostals
- diaphragm: contraction increases volume of thoracic space and resulting vacuum causes expansion of lungs and inspiration
- accessory muscles of inspiration: pectoralis major and minor, serratus anterior, sternocleidomastoid, scalenes, latissimus dorsi
- muscles of active expiration: internal intercostals, abdominal muscles (external oblique, internal oblique, rectus and transversus abdominis), subcostals, serratus posterior inferior, quadratus lumborum
- active contraction of abdomen and back muscles important to provide "support" while projecting speech and singing

Neural Control

- breathing at rest controlled by $PaCO_2$-sensitive central chemoreceptors in medulla
- inspiratory activity triggered by ventral and dorsal respiratory centers in medulla
- posterior cricoarytenoid muscles (innervated by recurrent laryngeal nerve, branch of CN X) activate just before inspiration to abduct vocal folds
- phrenic nerve (originates from spinal roots C3–C5) controls diaphragm
- voluntary inspiration important for voice production, strenuous exercise; controlled by primary motor cortex

Inspiration

- **Functional residual capacity (FRC):** volume of air in lungs at rest
- ~40% of total lung capacity (TLC)
- thorax has passive tendency to expand

- active inspiration via contraction of diaphragm to increase thoracic volume
- external intercostal muscles elevate ribs to increase thorax diameter

Expiration

- generally passive during breathing at rest; active during projected speech, singing, and strenuous exercise
- elastic recoil of alveoli combined with active muscular compression of airway
- force of recoil has direct correlation to volume of inspiration
- equal pressure point (EPP)—airway pressure equal to active expiratory pressure (not including elastic recoil)
    1. normally reached in cartilaginous airway, avoiding airway collapse during phonation
    2. alveoli and bronchioles may collapse fully during expiration (no cartilaginous support)
- active expiration using internal intercostal, abdominal, and back muscles
- controlled, efficient expiration is hallmark of trained vocalists

EVALUATION

Pulmonary Function Testing (See Chapter 5)

- FEF_{25-75} ("midflow") may reveal underlying pulmonary abnormality in patient who presents with dysphonia
- spirometry generates **flow-volume loops** (Figure 26–1)
- plot of flow (liters/second) against volume (liters) during forced expiration
- abnormal inspiratory loop: flattening (ie, vocal fold paralysis, paradoxical vocal fold motion, variable extrathoracic obstruction—laryngeal tumor)
- abnormal expiratory loop
    1. <u>flattening</u>: dynamic intrathoracic obstruction (tracheomalacia, tracheal mass)
    2. <u>concave upward</u>: obstructive pulmonary disease
    3. <u>narrowing</u>: restrictive lung disease
- flattening of both loops: fixed airway obstruction (ie, tracheal stenosis, tumor, extraluminal tracheal obstruction)
- reversible obstructive pulmonary disease evaluated with spirometry before and after administration of inhaled bronchodilator
- **Methacholine challenge**: assists in diagnosis of suspected asthma with inconclusive spirometry
- methacholine dose increased until FEV1 drops by 20% (PD20FEV1)

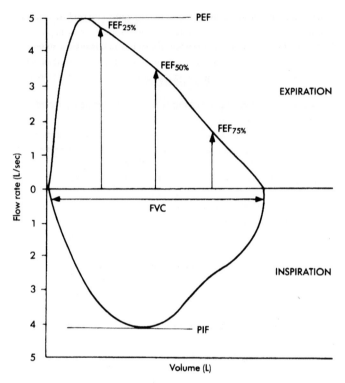

FIGURE 26–1. Flow Volume Loop. (FEF, forced expiratory flow; FVC, forced vital capacity; PEF, peak expiratory flow.) Used with permission from Sataloff et al., *Professional Voice: The Science and Art of Clinical Care* (4th ed.). San Diego, CA: Plural; 2017.

- PD20FEV1 in normal subjects >8 mg/mL
- **Diffusing capacity**: relative ability of oxygen to diffuse across arteriole-alveolar membranes
- tested using diffusion of inhaled carbon monoxide in blood (DL_{CO})
- diagnostic of interstitial lung disease

PATHOPHYSIOLOGY

Asthma

- reversible bronchial inflammation causing obstruction
- mediated by CD4+ T lymphocytes, eosinophils, interleukin (IL)-4 and IL-5

- bronchospasm leads to increased airway resistance caused by smooth muscle contraction of bronchioles causing distal airway collapse
- <u>Presentation</u>: paroxysmal dyspnea, characteristic expiratory wheeze, chest tightness, cough, dysphonia in professional speakers and singers (ineffective support leading to compensatory muscle tension dysphonia)
- equal pressure point (EPP) shifts to distal airway, may lead to air trapping and hyperinflation
- lowered subglottic pressure from decreased expiratory airflow rate, can affect phonation
- may be exacerbated by allergy, cold weather, exercise (including singing), uncontrolled reflux
- <u>Dx</u>: history, PFTs with obstruction reversible with bronchodilators; may require methacholine challenge testing (see previous discussion); often elevated serum eosinophil count
- dysphonia in a patient with long-term inhaled steroid (ICS) use should prompt evaluation for *Candida* overgrowth, laryngeal muscle atrophy
- use of inhaled ciclesonide and beclomethasone dipropionate seem to result in a lower prevalence of dysphonia relative to other ICSs

Intermittent

- symptoms occur less than twice per week with no restriction in activity between exacerbations, one or no exacerbations requiring oral glucocorticoids per year, or only with certain circumstances (exercise)
- FEV1 within normal range
- <u>Tx</u>: short-acting β-2 agonist (SABA) bronchodilators for acute attack or prior to exercise, control of exacerbating diseases (reflux, allergic rhinitis, chronic sinusitis, etc)

Mild Persistent

- symptoms more than twice per week but not daily, mild interference with normal activity, two or more exacerbations requiring oral glucocorticoids per year
- FEV1 within normal range (greater than 80% of predicted), normal FEV1/FVC ratio
- <u>Tx</u>: daily low-dose inhaled glucocorticoid; alternatively theophylline; oral leukotriene antagonists (montelukast, zafirlukast); mast cell stabilizer (cromolyn)

Moderate Persistent

- daily symptoms, need for daily SABA, some limitation in normal activity

- FEV1 60% to 80% of predicted, FEV1/FVC ratio below normal
- <u>Tx</u>: daily low-dose inhaled glucocorticoid with addition of long-acting inhaled β-agonist (LABA)

Severe Persistent

- daily symptoms, nightly nocturnal awakening, need for SABA for symptoms relief more than once per day, severely limited normal activity
- FEV1 less than 60% of predicted, FEV1/FVC ratio below normal
- <u>Tx</u>: add leukotriene antagonist to regimen, may require daily or alternate-day oral glucocorticoids; anti-IgE monoclonal antibody if concurrent allergy; anti-IL-5 monoclonal antibody for eosinophilic asthma

Exacerbations

- SABA q20 minutes via nebulized or metered-dose low-dose inhaler at home
- if incomplete response, addition of oral glucocorticoids at home based on previously determined action plan
- if need for urgent medical attention and presentation to emergency department, addition of supplemental oxygen, nebulized SABA, systemic glucocorticoids, IV magnesium sulfate

Aspirin-Exacerbated Respiratory Disease (AERD)

- formerly known as Samter's triad
- combination of asthma, chronic rhinosinusitis (CRS) with nasal polyps, and exacerbations due to aspirin or COX-1 inhibiting nonsteroidal anti-inflammatory drugs (NSAIDs)
- etiology not fully understood, related to dysregulation of arachidonic acid metabolism and overproduction of leukotrienes
- <u>Dx</u>: clinical diagnosis; aspirin challenge
- <u>Tx</u>: asthma treatment including leukotriene inhibitor, management of CRS, avoidance of aspirin/NSAIDs
- aspirin desensitization therapy indications:
    1. refractory nasal polyposis despite adequate medical and surgical therapy
    2. atherosclerotic disease requiring daily aspirin use
    3. chronic inflammatory disease requiring NSAID therapy

Chronic Obstructive Pulmonary Disease

- typically seen in adults with greater than 40 pack-year smoking history
- <u>Presentation</u>: dyspnea on exertion (early), chronic cough, and sputum production
- <u>Pathology</u>: increased levels of CD8+ T lymphocytes, neutrophils, CD68+ macrophages
- <u>Dx</u>: spirometry demonstrates decreased FEV1/FVC (<0.7) with severity inversely correlated to FEV1, administration of bronchodilator causes no or limited improvement; DLCO; pulse oximetry; arterial blood gas
- <u>Physical findings</u>: audible expiratory wheeze, crackles at base of lung or decreased breath sounds, increased A-P diameter of chest
- imaging may demonstrate increased lung volume due to air-trapping
- <u>Tx</u>: smoking cessation; short-acting anticholinergic; long-acting muscarinic agents; long-acting β-2 selective agonists; inhaled glucocorticoid; pulmonary rehabilitation; severe disease may require supplemental oxygen; exacerbations may require systemic steroids ± antibiotics

Emphysema

- **Centrilobular**: affects proximal acinus, specifically respiratory bronchiole; classically in smokers
- **Panacinar**: enlargement or destruction of all parts of acinus; more common in α-1 antitrypsin deficiency
- alveolar destruction leads to decreased elastic recoil and alveolar pressures
- EPP shifts distally as in asthma
- chronic hypoxic vasoconstriction of small pulmonary arteries results in intimal hyperplasia and smooth muscle hypertrophy and/or hyperplasia

Chronic Bronchitis

- productive cough for at least 3 months in 2 consecutive years
- other causes of cough must be ruled out
- increased mucus-producing goblet cells in airway
- hypoxia and respiratory acidosis
- may develop right heart failure

Bronchiectasis

- abnormal dilation of airways leading to impaired clearance of secretions
- thick airway secretions provide medium for bacteria growth and airway inflammation, causing progressive airway dilation and inflammation
- <u>Etiology</u>: genetic (primary ciliary dyskinesia, cystic fibrosis); asthma/chronic obstructive pulmonary disease; rheumatic disease; immunodeficiency; recurrent infections/pneumonia; chronic or foreign-body aspiration; aspergillosis; mycobacterial infection; idiopathic
- <u>Presentation</u>: daily cough productive of thick, tenacious sputum; dyspnea
- exacerbations characterized by change in color of sputum, fatigue, pleuritic chest pain, possible fevers, night sweats
- <u>Dx</u>: history, crackles on auscultation, lab tests (CBC, immunoglobulin counts), spirometry with obstructive pattern (decreased FVC, FEV1)
- imaging: chest x-ray and computed tomography demonstrate airway dilation (parallel "tram tracks"), bronchial wall thickening, linear atelectasis, irregular opacification
- <u>Tx</u>: treatment of underlying disease, bronchial hygiene therapy, exacerbations require antibiotics, severe disease may require surgical resection of affected portion of lung or transplantation

Allergic Rhinitis (See Chapter 25)

- environmental antigens may elicit type I allergic reaction
- immediate response mediated via immunoglobulin E (IgE)
- causes release of mediators from mast cells and basophils
- late-phase reactions mediated via prostaglandins and leukotrienes
- <u>Presentation</u>: nasal congestion, rhinorrhea, sneezing, postnasal drip, watery, itchy eyes, throat soreness
- <u>Dx</u>: history, skin testing (prick, intradermal), serologic radioallergosorbent test (RAST) or enzyme-linked assays for antigen-specific IgE
- <u>Physical findings</u>: transverse crease of nasal dorsum ("allergic salute"), boggy nasal turbinates (may shrink with application of topical decongestant), nasal polyps, periorbital ecchymosis ("allergic shiner"), posterior pharyngeal cobblestoning, and other lymphoid hypertrophy
- <u>Tx</u>: avoidance of allergen, intranasal steroid spray, intranasal antihistamine spray, oral antihistamines (may cause drying of mucosal surface and dysphonia), nasal decongestant (short term), oral

leukotriene antagonists, mucolytic agents, interleukin monoclonal antibody, immunotherapy injection

Restrictive Pulmonary Disease

- etiologies include:
    1. weakened musculoskeletal support, including myasthenia gravis, multiple sclerosis, amyotrophic lateral sclerosis
    2. physical restriction, including morbid obesity, kyphosis
    3. parenchymal disease, including pulmonary fibrosis, congestive heart failure, pulmonary edema, pneumonia, neoplasm
- <u>Dx</u>: spirometry demonstrates decreased volumes with normal flow (FEV1 and FVC both decreased, but may have increased FEV1/FVC ratio)

Paradoxical Vocal Fold Motion
(See Chapter 19)

CHAPTER

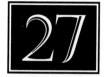

Cough and the Unified Airway

Kevin Tie, Kenneth W. Altman, and Rupali N. Shah

INTRODUCTION

- cough is the fifth most common reason for which patients seek medical care in the United States
- cough is defined as a respiratory reflex that aids in respiratory clearance
- the cough reflex is a coordinated release of air with intrathoracic pressures as high as 300 mm Hg and air velocities up to 500 miles per hour
- cough is stimulated by inflammation and irritation of the airway and is mediated by sensory afferents of the vagus nerve
- cough can be categorized by duration of symptoms
    1. <u>Acute cough</u>: <3 weeks
    2. <u>Subacute cough</u>: 3 to 8 weeks
    3. <u>Chronic cough</u>: >8 weeks (patients seek medical attention most often)
- the unified airway refers to the close relationship of the upper and lower airways and is integral to understanding and treating cough
- cough is an indicator of underlying disease and is a truly interdisciplinary issue

CLINICAL EVALUATION

History

- characterization of cough based on duration of symptoms helps narrow the differential diagnosis and aids in management
- <u>"Red flag" signs and symptoms</u>: syncope, rib fracture, pneumonia, hemoptysis, stridor, and palpitations
    1. patients may need acute care—bypass chronic cough algorithm
- recent illnesses
    1. upper respiratory tract infections (URTI)
- timing
    1. postprandial cough may indicate reflux
    2. cough associated with choking may indicate aspiration
- quality
    1. productive cough may indicate an infectious etiology
    2. dry cough may indicate an allergic etiology
- social history
    1. living or occupational environments and recent changes
    2. exposures including pets and irritants: dust, chemicals, debris, and tobacco smoke

- medication side effects or changes
    1. sitagliptin, angiotensin-converting enzyme inhibitors (ACEIs)
- patient-reported quality of life measures
    1. Cough Severity Index
    2. Leicester Cough Questionnaire
    3. Newcastle Laryngeal Hypersensitivity Questionnaire

Physical Examination

- comprehensive exam for patients with chronic cough includes a full head and neck exam, lung auscultation, looking for signs of systemic disease, and laryngoscopy
- ear exam for manifestations of allergies, retracted tympanic membranes, or serous otitis media
    1. ear pathology occasionally can cause referred cough through stimulation of cranial nerves IX or X
- neck exam for lymphadenopathy that may suggest infection or malignancy
- upper airway assessment should be performed with a flexible endoscope
    1. "bird's-eye view" of the laryngeal environment
    2. evaluation of the sinonasal, nasopharyngeal, and hypopharyngeal cavities
    3. evaluate for signs of infection or tumor
    4. note the color, vascularity, and presence of edema on the mucosal lining from the nasal cavity to the larynx
    5. chronic inflammation can lead to lymphoid hyperplasia and cobblestoning or significant mucus secretion
    6. evidence of pooled secretions or laryngeal penetration may be warning signs of aspiration
    7. mobility, symmetry, and closure of the true vocal folds should be assessed
    8. the subglottis may be inspected in a cooperative patient with proper positioning and local anesthesia
- for adult patients with a history of occupational or environmental exposures, perform appropriate objective tests
    1. methacholine challenge for work-related or other asthma/ eosinophilic bronchitis
    2. sputum or induced sputum cytology for eosinophilia
    3. before and after exposure testing to demonstrate potential causality (eg, perform both at the end of a regular work week and, if positive, repeat at the end of a period off work to document any work-related changes)

- immunologic tests for hypersensitivity guided by specific exposure history
    1. skin tests, specific serum IgE antibodies, specific serum IgG antibodies for suspected hypersensitivity pneumonitis, beryllium lymphocyte proliferation tests for chronic beryllium disease

Differential Diagnosis

- duration of cough will guide the differential
- most patients seen in the otolaryngology office will present with chronic cough
- most cases of acute cough or subacute cough often resolve prior to medical assessment or are addressed by a primary care physician

Exclusionary Diagnosis: Angiotensin-Converting Enzyme Inhibitors

- otolaryngologic side effects include angioedema and cough
- incidence of cough has been reported anywhere from 0.2% to 33%
- cough is usually described as "dry" or "tickly" and is not dose dependent
- cough can begin anywhere from the first dose to years after initiation of treatment
- median time for resolution of the cough is 26 days after discontinued use

ACUTE AND SUBACUTE COUGH

Acute Cough

- duration less than 3 weeks

Upper Respiratory Tract Infection

- most common cause of acute cough
- most common viral pathogens: influenza, parainfluenza, adenovirus, rhinovirus, and respiratory syncytial virus
- cough associated with a URTI is most prevalent (83%) in the first 48 hours and diminishes to 26% over the course of the next 2 weeks
- Presentation: nasal obstruction, rhinorrhea, sneezing, increased lacrimation, fever
- Physical exam:
    1. nasal examination commonly shows clear watery discharge with edematous mucosal lining of the turbinates

    2. green, yellow, thick, or foul-smelling drainage may indicate a bacterial infection

    3. mild edema and erythema in the posterior glottis may be seen secondary to coughing

    4. auscultation of the lungs is usually normal

- Tx:

    1. hospital admission or further workup for URTI-associated cough is not commonly required unless the patient is immunocompromised

    2. symptomatic control with over-the-counter preparations such as antihistamines and decongestants

    3. central modulation of the cough reflex can be accomplished with agents including dextromethorphan, morphine, and codeine

    4. mucolytics also may aid the symptomatic relief of cough

Acute Sinusitis

- <u>Most common pathogens:</u> *Streptococcus pneumoniae, Haemophilus influenzae, Staphylococcus aureus,* and some anaerobes
- <u>Tx:</u> **Antihistamines** and **decongestants**

    1. if no resolution, begin culture-directed antibiotic therapy with intranasal steroid and short-term nasal decongestant

    2. if medical therapy has failed, consider functional endoscopic sinus surgery in patients with chronic rhinosinusitis (CRS, see pags 290, 313) or allergic fungal sinusitis (AFS)

Other Causes of Acute Cough

- Exacerbation of chronic diseases (asthma, chronic obstructive pulmonary disease [COPD], allergies), the initial catarrhal stages of *Bordetella pertussis*, pneumonia, congestive heart failure, and pulmonary embolism

Subacute Cough

- Duration between 3 and 8 weeks

Postinfectious Cough

- Classified as a cough lasting between 3 and 8 weeks, with a chest x-ray ruling out pneumonia
- Due to extensive disruption of epithelial integrity and widespread airway inflammation of the upper and/or lower airways with or without transient hyper-responsiveness

- Increased secretions produced secondary to inflammation continue to stimulate the cough reflex

Bordetella pertussis

- pertussis or "whooping cough" is a highly contagious, unique cause of postinfectious cough
- timeline:
    1. incubation period of 1 to 3 weeks
    2. catarrhal period that may include conjunctivitis, rhinorrhea, fever, and cough
    3. paroxysmal period of worsening cough including characteristic "whoop"
- <u>Dx</u>: recent infections in the community, contact with a known case, biphasic cough, characteristic "**whoop**," or cough-vomit syndrome
- <u>Prevention</u>: **DTaP vaccine**
- <u>Tx</u>: **erythromycin** or **trimethoprim/sulfamethoxazole** (for patients who cannot tolerate macrolides)
    1. do not delay for confirmation with diagnostic testing
    2. treatment initiated during the paroxysmal stage has limited benefit
    3. symptomatic control of the paroxysmal cough with β-agonists, corticosteroids, and antihistamines has shown no benefit and is not recommended
    4. patients should isolate themselves during the first 5 days of treatment to avoid infectious spread

Other Causes of Subacute Cough

- exacerbation of underlying diseases such as asthma, COPD, upper airway cough syndrome (UACS)
- gastroesophageal reflux may also play a role in subacute cough
    1. repeated forceful cough causes an increase in abdominal pressure that may aggravate preexisting reflux disease

CHRONIC COUGH

- duration greater than 8 weeks
- often multifactorial in etiology
- most common etiological factors in immunocompetent, nonsmoking patients with normal chest radiograph findings
    1. upper airway cough syndrome (UACS)
    2. asthma and related syndromes

    3. gastroesophageal reflux disease and laryngopharyngeal reflux (*see* Chapter 22)
- exclude chronic systemic diseases and tumors
  1. sarcoidosis
  2. granulomatosis with polyangiitis (GPA)
  3. laryngeal and bronchogenic tumors may cause postobstructive pneumonia
  4. abdominal tumors may cause diaphragmatic irritability
  5. large gastric stromal tumors may increase reflux by acting as a gastric outlet obstruction
  6. tumors resulting in vagal irritability
- obtain chest x-ray and consult a pulmonologist to address any findings, including but not limited to:
  1. interstitial lung disease
  2. bronchiectasis
  3. bronchogenic carcinoma
- diagnoses of exclusion
  1. neurogenic cough
  2. somatic cough syndrome
  3. tic cough
- multifactorial treatment often necessary
- *see* Figure 27–1 for chronic cough management algorithm

Upper Airway Cough Syndrome (UACS)

- also known as cough attributable to postnasal drip
- most common cause of chronic cough
- <u>Presentation</u>: sensation of nasal passage secretions draining into the nasopharynx, nasal congestion and discharge, and increased throat clearing

Irritant Etiology

- <u>Pathology:</u>
  1. inflammatory effects lead to mediator release, increased edema, and mucus production along the entire respiratory tract, including the nose, sinuses, pharynx, and lungs
  2. increased mucus is transported throughout the respiratory tract, notably at the larynx
  3. irritation of the larynx and pharynx leads to compensatory behaviors (eg, throat clearing and coughing)
  4. anatomic and histologic changes of the laryngeal mucosa observed as laryngeal edema and irregularities, and occasional mucosal tear, submucosal hemorrhage, and other vocal fold pathology

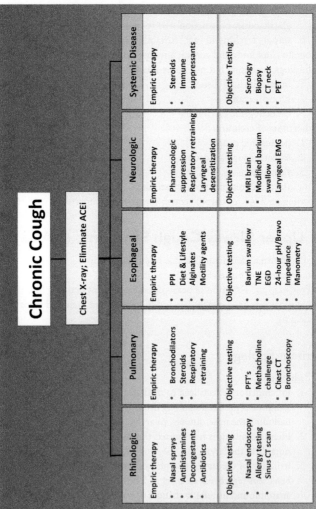

FIGURE 27–1. Management algorithm including empiric therapies and diagnostic testing associated with different cough-related disease states and anatomic sites. (ACEi, angiotensin-converting-enzyme inhibitor; CT, computed tomography; EGD, esophagogastroduodenoscopy; EMG, electromyography; MRI, magnetic resonance imaging; PET, positron emission tomography; PFT, pulmonary function testing; PPI, proton pump inhibitor; TNE, transnasal esophagoscopy.)

- <u>Dx</u>: history and physical, flexible laryngoscopy, radiographic studies
- nasopharynx or oropharynx may show mucoid or mucopurulent secretions with cobblestoning of the mucosa from chronic inflammation
- computed tomography (CT) scan may show paranasal sinus disease when inflammation has resulted in obstruction and postobstructive infectious drainage
- appropriate therapy with resolution of cough is often the key to diagnosis

Allergic Etiology

- allergenic triggers
    1. <u>Spring</u>: tree, grass, and pollen
    2. <u>Fall</u>: weeds and molds
    3. <u>Perennial</u>: dust mites, animal dander, cockroach, and indoor molds such as aspergillus and penicillium
- <u>Presentation</u>: nasal obstruction, clear to yellow rhinorrhea, postnasal drip, nasal pruritus with paroxysms of sneeze, conjunctival pruritus, and clear discharge
- <u>Physical exam</u>: pale, boggy nasal mucosa with clear to yellow rhinorrhea
- <u>Tx</u>:
    1. intranasal corticosteroids, antihistamines, and/or cromolyn
    2. immunotherapy for desensitization (does not give immediate relief)
    3. avoidance of allergen

Chronic Rhinosinusitis

- objective evidence of sinus disease (endoscopically or radiographically) with at least 12 weeks of 2 or more of the following symptoms: mucopurulent drainage, nasal obstruction, facial pain, or decreased olfaction
- most common pathogens: coagulase-negative *Staphylococcus*, *Staphylococcus aureus*, and gram-negative rods (*Pseudomonas aeruginosa, Stenotrophomonas maltophilia, Escherichia coli,* and *Serratia marcescens*)
- Less well-defined etiologies include viral infections, fungal infections, and osteitis
- <u>Tx</u>:
    1. antibiotics dictated by culture or broad-spectrum coverage
    2. saline irrigation has proven to be beneficial

3. oral or topical intranasal steroids are effective in modulating inflammation
4. if medical therapy has failed, consider functional endoscopic sinus surgery

Asthma, Cough Variant Asthma, and Nonasthmatic Eosinophilic Bronchitis

- etiology of asthma and NAEB is unknown but may be associated with exposure to inhaled aeroallergens or an occupational sensitizer

Asthma and Cough Variant Asthma

- hyperresponsive bronchi leading to reversible bronchoconstriction that causes dyspnea, wheezing, chest tightness, and prolonged expiratory phase
- may be associated with triggers such as viral URIs, allergens, and stress
- accounts for 24% to 29% of chronic cough in nonsmoking adults
- **Cough variant asthma (CVA)**
    1. asthma in which cough is the dominant or only symptom
    2. compared to asthma, patients have a stronger cough reflex and less hyperresponsiveness to methacholine
- Dx: history and physical, PFTs (*see* Chapter 26)
- spirometry may demonstrate expiratory obstruction with significant $\beta 2$-adrenergic response
- methacholine inhalation challenge causing a 20% or greater decrease in lung function is highly sensitive
- Tx: inhaled bronchodilator, inhaled corticosteroids
- complete resolution may require up to 8 weeks of treatment
- avoid allergen or occupational sensitizer
- leukotriene receptor antagonist helps reduce symptoms
- refractory or severe symptoms may require oral steroids
- antibiotics should be guided by sputum culture
- some inhalers may cause laryngeal irritation

Nonasthmatic Eosinophilic Bronchitis (NAEB)

- cough with eosinophilic airway inflammation, similar to asthma, but no airway hyperresponsiveness, and with sputum eosinophilia (>3% nonsquamous sputum eosinophils)
- patients demonstrate atopic tendencies, with elevated sputum eosinophils, increased IL-5 gene expression, and increased eicosanoid production

- <u>Presentation</u>: cough may be the only symptom (transient, episodic, or persistent)
- <u>Dx</u>: presence of eosinophilia with sputum induction or bronchial wash fluid obtained with bronchoscopy, exclusion of other causes of cough
- <u>Tx</u>: **inhaled corticosteroids**
- avoid allergen or occupational sensitizer
- leukotriene receptor antagonist montelukast may provide additional benefit
- refractory or severe symptoms may require oral corticosteroids

Gastroesophageal Reflux Disease and Laryngopharyngeal Reflux

- *see* Chapter 22 for additional details
- prevalence of GERD-related chronic cough has increased from 10% in 1981 to 36% in 1998
- laryngopharyngeal reflux (LPR) refers to manifestations of the reflux of stomach contents in the pharynx and larynx
- contents such as acid, bile, and pepsin are implicated in laryngeal irritation
- reflux-associated cough should be suspected in patients who have cough in the morning, at night, after eating, or after lying down
- mechanisms hypothesized to contribute to GERD-related cough
  1. an esophageal-bronchial reflex in the mucosa of the distal esophagus may stimulate chronic cough
  2. gross aspiration usually results in immediate cough, whereas microaspiration can produce a chronic inflammatory condition that later results in cough
  3. reflux-mediated local inflammation may result in vagal sensitization and modified sensory feedback (neurogenic airway inflammation)
  4. acid or nonacid reflux may result in abnormal esophageal contractions that provide a cough stimulus

NONASTHMATIC INFLAMMATORY AIRWAY DISEASE IN ADULTS

Chronic Bronchitis

- chronic productive cough for at least 3 months in 2 consecutive years
- disease of bronchi characterized by an abnormal inflammatory response to gases and particles such as cigarette smoking

- smoke exposure is the most common irritant
- prevalence of cough is increased by 2-fold to 3-fold in active smokers and 1.3-fold to 1.6-fold in passive smokers
    1. effects are dose dependent
- prevalence of cough returns to near normal in ex-smokers
    1. when active cigarette smoking is the lone etiology of cough, 94% of patients notice symptomatic improvement after abstinence for at least 4 weeks
    2. initial short-term increase in cough sensitivity prior to resolution
- other irritants include dust, chemicals, and debris
- Pathology:
    1. mucus hypersecretion and decreased airway clearance mechanisms mediated by Th 17
    2. mucus clearance is impaired due to reduced ciliary function, occlusion of distal airways, and respiratory muscle weakness leading to ineffective cough
- Presentation: productive cough, dyspnea, and wheezing
- worse in the morning with phlegm production
- Dx: chronic productive cough for at least 3 months in 2 consecutive years
- spirometry shows obstructive pattern
- Tx: directed at underlying COPD
- Mucolytics: minor reduction in the exacerbation rate of patients with chronic bronchitis
- Antibiotics:
    1. production of green purulent sputum is highly sensitive (94.4%) and specific (77%) for a high bacterial sputum load
    2. potentially pathogenic microorganisms (eg, *Haemophilus influenzae*) that often permanently colonize the respiratory tract of symptomatically stable patients frequently are not isolated on standard sputum cultures
    3. long-term use of low-dose azithromycin has demonstrated efficacy with improved quality of life (QOL) and decreased exacerbations
- Roflumilast: phosphodiesterase type 4 inhibitor with anti-inflammatory effects; significantly improves pre-bronchodilator FEV1 and exacerbation rate

Bronchiectasis

- irreversible abnormal dilatation and thickening of the bronchi
- characterized by mucopurulent sputum from chronic inflammation and infection

- bronchial wall damage and permanent destruction can occur, causing shortness of breath
- typically recurrent and progressive
- typically affects women above age 70
- patients with immunodeficiencies such as IgG/IgA deficiency or combined variable immunodeficiency (CVID) are at risk of developing bronchiectasis over time
- may be secondary to rheumatoid arthritis, GERD, Crohn's disease, ulcerative colitis, cystic fibrosis, tuberculosis, allergic bronchopulmonary aspergillosis, and Kartagener's syndrome
- <u>Pathology</u>: vicious cycle hypothesis
    1. airway inflammation
    2. structural airway damage and resultant mucous stasis
    3. pooled mucus colonized with bacteria
    4. further inflammation
- most commonly *Haemophilus influenzae* and *Pseudomonas aeruginosa*
- <u>Presentation</u>: shortness of breath, diffuse crackles or wheezes, coarse rhonchi, chronic productive cough with purulent sputum production, digital clubbing, hemoptysis, systemic features of weight loss and fatigue
- <u>Dx</u>: high-resolution CT (HRCT) scan demonstrating a bronchus with an internal diameter wider than its adjacent pulmonary artery that fails to taper and bronchi visualized 1 to 2 cm from the pleural surface
- <u>Tx</u>: goals of therapy are to mobilize secretions, reduce inflammation, treat and prevent infection, and treat the primary condition
- spirometry and regular sputum cultures to monitor disease activity
- airway clearance techniques such as high-frequency chest wall oscillation devices and nebulized saline
- antibiotic treatment should be sputum guided
    1. attempt to eradicate *Pseudomonas* if cultured for the first time
    2. consider antibiotic prophylaxis in patients having ≥3 exacerbations per year

Bronchiolitis

- small airways affected by infectious, postinfectious, inflammatory, or idiopathic processes
- damage may be reversible or irreversible
- commonly viral, more common in children
- <u>Etiologies</u>: *Mycoplasma pneumoniae*, *Chlamydia pneumoniae*, inhalation of organic or nonorganic material, systemic lupus erythematosus, rheumatoid arthritis, Sjögren's syndrome, radiation, or medications such as amiodarone, sulfasalazine, or cephalosporins

- <u>Presentation</u>: dry or productive cough with mucus particles, dyspnea, night sweats, fatigue, chest tightness, wheezing, inspiratory crackles, manifestations of systemic disorders
- <u>Dx</u>:
    1. chest x-ray may show nonspecific findings
    2. HRCT showing centrilobular nodules, branching linear structures in the secondary pulmonary lobules, or areas of air trapping is most sensitive
    3. spirometry monitors severity and response to treatment
- <u>Tx</u>:
    1. avoidance of exposures and/or discontinuation of suspected causative medications
    2. antimicrobial agents when infectious
    3. systemic steroids or immune-modulating agents may be necessary

UNEXPLAINED CHRONIC COUGH

- also termed *idiopathic chronic cough* or **chronic refractory cough (CRC)**
- defined as a cough that persists despite guideline-based treatment
- seen in 20% to 46% of patients presenting to specialist cough clinics
- diagnosed when there is no identifiable cause of chronic cough (unexplained or idiopathic chronic cough) or when the cough persists after investigation and treatment of cough-related conditions (refractory chronic cough)

Neurogenic Cough

- hypothesized to be a result of sensory neuropathy often due to laryngeal hypersensitivity from postviral damage to the internal branch of the superior laryngeal nerve (SLN)
- <u>Proposed mechanisms</u>: temperature sensitivity, pH sensitivity, neuropeptides mediating afferent neural responses, axonal hyperexcitability, brain stem trauma, neurosis, psychosis, and tics
- **Cough-variant dystonia:** in same family of neurogenic disorders as spasmodic dysphonia and hemifacial spasm
    1. responds to botulinum toxin injected into the medial bellies of the thyroarytenoid muscles
- <u>Presentation</u>: onset after illness or surgery that puts laryngeal nerves at risk, nonproductive cough, long duration of complaint, laryngeal dysesthesias (eg, foreign-body or tickle sensations), globus, throat pain, throat clearing, dysphagia, dysphonia, dyspnea, choking, stridor

- lack of response to antibiotics, asthma medications, or reflux medications
- increased susceptibility to chemical (eg, gastric acid reflux, chemical odors), temperature (eg, breathing cold or warm air), mechanical (eg, talking, laughing, change in body position), or other stimuli
- <u>Physical exam</u>: should include thorough neurological exam and flexible laryngoscopy
- peripheral motor or sensory abnormalities associated with vagus nerve neuropathy
- <u>Signs of neurologic injury</u>: incomplete velopharyngeal closure, salivary pooling in the piriform sinus, excessive secretions at the valleculae or hypopharynx
- flexible laryngoscopy
  1. evaluation of the soft palate for motor deficits
  2. visualization of larynx in a relatively physiologic position
  3. minimizes vocal fold motion abnormalities due to the positioning, tongue tension, and stimulation of the oropharynx
- <u>Tx</u>: tricyclic antidepressants (TCAs), gabapentin, and pregabalin
- **Amitriptyline** (TCA): inhibits norepinephrine and serotonin reuptake
  1. may reduce the sensory threshold of the afferent nerves, thereby improving the cough reflex
  2. <u>Side effects</u>: appetite or weight changes, arrhythmias (torsades de pointes), gastrointestinal upset, hyperpyrexia, impotence, mouth pain, respiratory depression, sedation, serotonin syndrome
- <u>GABA analogs</u>: gabapentin has demonstrated improved cough-specific QOL and reduced cough frequency and severity, but improvements were not sustained after discontinuing treatment
- <u>Other drugs</u>: baclofen (γ-aminobutyric acid agonist), botulinum toxin, tramadol
- Nonpharmacologic interventions:
  1. respiratory muscle retraining
  2. cough suppression therapy (CST): see page 320
- <u>SLN block</u>: see page 321

Somatic Cough Syndrome and Tic Cough

- somatic cough syndrome previously referred to as psychogenic cough
- <u>Dx</u>: extensive evaluation that includes ruling out tic disorders, uncommon causes, and ensuring that the patient meets *Diagnostic and Statistical Manual of Mental Disorders* (Fifth Edition) (*DSM-5*) criteria
- tic cough previously referred to as habit cough
- core clinical features include suppressibility, distractibility, suggestibility, variability, and a premonitory sensation about whether the cough is single or one of many tics

Cough Suppression Therapy

- outpatient therapy delivered over multiple sessions
- recommended for idiopathic and refractory chronic cough that persists (>8 weeks) despite optimal medical assessment and management
- can sometimes be used as adjunctive treatment in cases of chronic cough of varying etiologies
- effective and safe for patients with a refractory chronic cough and has been shown to improve cough-related QOL, cough hypersensitivity, and cough frequency
- CST by a speech-language pathologist comprises four components: (*see* Table 27–1)

TABLE 27–1. Components of Cough Suppression Therapy

Component	Techniques
Education	- educate patients on the cough reflex and cough reflex hypersensitivity - reframe the reasons for coughing - describe the unnecessary nature of the cough - explain the potential negative effects of repeated coughing: laryngeal trauma, perpetuation of cough cycle, exacerbation of throat or laryngeal irritation - educate patients on voluntary cough control
Vocal hygiene	- increase frequency and volume of water intake - reduce caffeine and alcohol intake - avoid passive smoking or smoky environments - promote nasal breathing
Cough control strategies	- identify cough triggers - substitute cough sensations and urges with suppression or distraction techniques: forced swallow, sipping water, sucking sweets - teach breathing exercises: relaxed throat breathing, pursed lip breathing, breathing pattern retraining
Psychoeducational counseling	- set realistic goals, time frames, and outcomes - motivate patients and reiterate techniques and aims of therapy - help patients internalize responsibility for cough behaviors rather than attribute to external phenomena - manage stress and anxiety - address adverse symptoms such as incontinence

1. education
2. vocal hygiene training
3. strategies to control cough
4. psychoeducational counseling

New Treatment Modalities for Chronic Cough

Vocal Fold Augmentation

- may be effective in chronic cough refractory to pharmacologic and behavioral treatments with concurrent vocal fold paresis and/or glottic insufficiency on laryngeal videostroboscopy (64) and/or laryngeal electromyogram
- injection augmentation may influence cough production via:
  - volume effect
    1. resolves mild glottic insufficiency to prevent microaspiration and irritation that perpetuates cough and to increase cough efficiency
    2. improvement in glottic closure interrupts the positive feedback loop incited by forceful or traumatic glottic closure, repeated vocal fold trauma, and release of neuropeptides
    3. decreases shortness of breath, especially during speech
  - altered sensory signaling
    1. alteration in proprioceptive input to the reflex
    2. changes in upstream neuropeptide release as a result of decreased closing force
    3. modification of the perception of laryngeal irritants due to a change in the position and exposure of laryngeal sensory nerve endings
  - placebo effect

Superior Laryngeal Nerve Block

- therapeutic option for neurogenic cough
- effective, low-risk, and low-cost in-office treatment
- 1:1 mixture of a long-acting particulate corticosteroid and a local anesthetic
- may alter sensory feedback of the SLN, thereby disrupting the cough signaling pathway
- injections are directed at site of trigger points (eg, within the thyrohyoid space) that cause discomfort or cough upon palpation

CONCLUSION

- a systematic approach should be taken to treat patients with chronic cough
- first objective should be to rule out other diagnoses such as cancer, aspiration, and neurologic and systemic diseases, or ACEI use or smoking
- use duration of cough to narrow differential diagnosis
- consider CRC if chronic cough persists despite guideline-based treatment
- future studies are necessary to confirm the efficacies of vocal fold augmentation and SLN block in treating chronic cough

CHAPTER

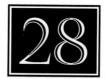

Care of the Transgender and Gender Nonconforming Patient

Justin Ross, Mary J. Hawkshaw, and Robert T. Sataloff

INTRODUCTION

- <u>Gender dysphoria</u>: conflict between a person's physical or assigned gender and the gender with which they identify
- <u>Transgender identity</u>: individuals whose gender identity and/or expression differs from their biologic sex
- <u>Sexual orientation</u>: the gender(s) an individual is attracted to and has romantic feelings toward
- **respect the patient's preferred name and pronoun**
    1. if another person accompanies the patient, they may refer to the patient with the appropriate name or pronoun—be alert to these interactions
    2. if the patient is alone, you may offer your own; for example, "Hello, I am Dr. X, and I use the pronouns he and him. What do you prefer?"
- requires addressing multiple dimensions of well-being
- alteration of fundamental frequency (f0) alone by voice-altering therapy and/or surgery is often insufficient and should be accompanied by behavioral modifications to speech-associated mannerisms
- Adult male f0 range: **80 to 165 Hz**
- Adult female f0 range: **145 to 275 Hz**
- many vocal qualities can be more important to gender identification than f0

MEDICAL AND VOICE THERAPY

Female to Male (Trans-men)

- androgen therapy produces masculinization similar to the pitch, frequency, jitter, and shimmer similar to the change experienced by biologic males during puberty
- administration of androgens causes increased vocal fold mass, but does not alter the size or superior position of the female larynx
- long-term low-dose therapy is generally sufficient to maintain a masculine fundamental frequency
- androgen therapy may result in restriction of voice function across a number of domains, particularly vocal power (projection and intensity)
- suboptimal results from medical therapy may be related to diminished androgen sensitivity and in older patients
- trans-male patients are less likely to pursue or be referred for voice therapy, but assessment by transgender voice specialists often reveals functional restrictions that can be treated

- research surrounding the application of voice therapy in trans-male patients is scant with a low level of evidence, and management is largely guided by expert opinion
- emphasis should be placed on the development of less melodic speech, with relatively down-intoned, flat syllables, without development of muscle tension dysphonia (MTD)
- additional behaviors that may negatively affect trans-male vocal quality include alcohol and tobacco use, chest binding and slouching, unstable psychosocial situation

Male to Female (Trans-women)

- estrogen therapy does not alter the structure of vocal folds or other laryngeal or resonant structures; therefore, trans-women may benefit from surgical therapy when voice therapy is inadequate
- feminine speech fundamental frequencies are generally >155 Hz
- a goal of voice therapy for trans-women is to develop a fundamental frequency high enough to allow for downglides that remain >155 Hz
- emphasis should be placed on the development of melodic speech with more frequent upglides
- melodic intonation should be matched to the emotional content of the phrase
- a soft, falsetto dominant register and modification of accompanying mannerisms (eg, smiling speech) also may improve perceptual affirmation
- jaw relaxation, flattened lips, and anteriorly positioned tongue result in alterations of resonance and articulation that produce a more feminine second formant
- maintaining laryngeal elevation and pharyngeal constriction during speech produces a more reliably feminine-sounding voice, but may result in MTD and vocal fold injury
- as with trans-men, behaviors including tobacco and alcohol use should be avoided, as they may affect vocal quality

SURGICAL THERAPY

Introduction

Preoperative Evaluation

- history should include the reason they are pursuing pitch modification, participation in voice therapy, psychosocial and medical steps taken since initiating transition

- self-evaluation of voice and goals of care including desired pitch, articulation, and nonverbal communication
- speech-language pathologist (SLP) evaluation including voice objectives and conversational and singing pitch range
- flexible and rigid strobovideolaryngoscopy
- patient should be made aware that surgical loss of range will result in overall decrease of musical frequency range

Indications

- failure of speech therapy to produce a feminine voice
- fear of potential drift into a masculine register when startled ("outing")
- desire for a feminine voice without maintaining conscious control of vocal pitch
- iatrogenic vocal fold detachment following thyroid prominence reduction
- participation in transgender transition care program

Contraindications

- unwillingness to undergo surgery due to fear of complications or inadequate voice outcomes
- inability to tolerate reduction of maximal phonatory volume
- unwillingness to comply with voice therapy

Male to Female (Trans-women)

Type IV Thyroplasty (Cricothyroid Approximation)

- lengthens the vocal folds via midline suture approximation of the thyroid and cricoid cartilages
- usually under local anesthesia to assess voice quality intraoperatively
- overelevation of pitch is ideal to offset eventual relaxation of vocal fold tension
- results in an average elevation of 7 semitones in conversational voice, though results vary and are unpredictable
- more predictably, patients lose an average of 9 semitones from their lower range
- approximately one-third will revert to their preoperative baseline within a few months, usually due to loss of vocal fold tension rather than suture failure
- <u>Cricothyroid fusion (CTF)</u>: modification of type IV thyroplasty in which surfaces of inferior-posterior thyroid and anterior-superior cricoid cartilages are denuded, and the latter is subluxed under

and then suture approximated to the former; has more long-term durability than type IV thyroplasty; less successful in older patients due to cricoid cartilage ossification
- vocal fold webbing may be a useful adjunct if greater pitch elevation is desired
- Complications: permanent falsetto, loss of falsetto control, reduced pitch control or monotonal voice, expected reduction of pitch range

Laser Vocal Fold Reduction

- thins and tightens the true vocal folds via superficial application of potassium titanyl phosphate (KTP) laser to the superior true vocal fold surface
- resulting pitch change is limited relative to other procedures, and a loss of the lowest half to one and a half semitones should be expected
- technical ease and ability to perform in office offset the mild change in pitch for some patients
- similar results are achieved by CO_2 laser incision of the superior true vocal fold surface just medial to or within the laryngeal ventricle and thyroarytenoid myomectomy can be performed simultaneously

Anterior Glottal Webbing (Wendler Glottoplasty)

- reduces functional length via de-epithelialization and microsuture approximation of the anterior one-third to two-thirds of the vocal fold vibratory margin
- requires general anesthesia and suspension microdirect laryngoscopy for adequate visualization
- preservation of true vocal fold mucosa 2 mm adjacent to the anterior commissure may increase chance of surgical reversal, should that be desired
- expected pitch elevation averages 5 to 9 semitones, but the upper pitches is unaffected

Thyroarytenoid Myomectomy

- removal of a portion of thyroarytenoid muscle via a vertical mucosal incision laterally on the superior surface of the true vocal fold
- typically performed with CO_2 laser, but cold knife can be used
- this does not affect the vibratory margin but decreases vocal fold mass and elevates pitch
- bilateral myomectomy sometimes leads to prolonged aphonia likely due to resulting true vocal fold edema and stiffness
- prolonged glottic insufficiency with soft, breathy voice is expected

Anterior Commissure Advancement

- open procedure in which an inferior-based, springboard flap is created in the thyroid cartilage overlying the anterior commissure; the segment is then advanced via placement of a cartilage, Silastic or metallic implant which lengthens the vocal folds
- often creates a laryngeal prominence that may be mistaken for an "Adam's apple"

Anterior Partial Laryngectomy

- complicated open procedure during which laryngeal structure is altered to create a more narrow larynx with shortened true vocal folds
- longer procedure with higher medical costs and risk of complications
- often combined with thyrohyoid elevation
- <u>Steps</u> (simplified):
    1. after exposing the larynx via horizontal neck incision, cuts are made bilaterally in the midsagittal plane of the thyroid cartilage, ~4 to 7 mm from midline
    2. thyroid cartilage is removed, and the anterior portion of each false vocal fold is excised
    3. the new medial edges of the thyroid cartilage are approximated, and a portion of the true and false vocals are excised based upon the new dimensions of the glottis
    4. sutures are placed anterior in the true vocal folds for later approximation to the thyroid cartilage to reconstruct the anterior commissure
    5. thyroid cartilage is then plated or approximated with sutures overlying the desired site of the anterior commissure
    6. true vocal fold sutures are passed above and below the plate/ sutures and firmly secured

Thyrohyoid Elevation

- repositions the larynx superiorly by approximating the thyroid cartilage and hyoid bone
- requires removal of the superior 10 mm of thyroid cartilage; then multiple burr holes in both hyoid bone and thyroid cartilage are created, through which suture approximation will be performed
- may be performed with anterior partial laryngectomy
- shortens the length of the vocal tract, altering formant structure

Outcomes and Comments

- cricothyroid approximation is the most commonly performed procedure in male to female voice surgery, followed by glottoplasty
- all methods raise mean fundamental frequency (f0) to varying degrees
- voice quality and range are relatively preserved with cricothyroid approximation
- outcomes are longer with the CTF variant than traditional cricothyroid approximation
- anterior glottal webbing produces the most marked increase in mean f0, but can significantly restrict vocal quality and range
- there is limited role for voice surgery in the female to male patient due to the success of androgen and voice therapy, though type III thyroplasty has been attempted

CHAPTER

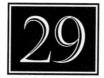

Psychological Dimensions of Voice Disorders

Deborah Caputo Rosen

INTRODUCTION

- psychological comorbidity common in voice disorders
- may be causal or reactive
- merits proactive awareness, prompt assessment, and qualified and coordinated treatment

VOICE AND EMOTION

- there is a profound mind/body linkage
- voice disturbances are distressing, particularly to professional voice users in whom voice may be "equal to self"
- <u>Parameters affected by emotional states</u>: quality, pitch, loudness, rate, vocabulary, content, syntax and patterns of muscular activity in articulatory, laryngeal, respiratory structures
- emotional stress may result in psychologic adjustment to events manifested through individual personality type
- unconscious fear of voice loss may produce defense mechanisms that block full recovery

BODY IMAGE/SELF-IMAGE

- <u>Body image theory</u>: anticipate that certain physical injuries can affect body/self-concept
- if body function has been essential to major source of self-esteem, distortion of one affects the other
- <u>Cognitive-behavioral therapy (CBT)</u>: body image-producing dysphoria results from irrational thoughts, faulty internal dialogue
- Carl Rogers: equilibrium requires that self-concept is congruent with life experience; subjective meaning and feelings attached more predictive than disability itself
- primary defense mechanisms are denial and distortion

PSYCHOLOGICAL PHASES OF VOCAL INJURY

- voice injury produces emotional responses universally, intensified for professional voice users
- phases overlap and recur (problem recognition; diagnosis—fear of the unknown; acute/rehab treatment—fear of known and outcome; acceptance—temporary = vulnerability, lasting = mourning)

- similar to grief and mourning of other losses, especially for performers
- accept reality of the loss, express emotions, live and cope in a world without the known voice, reinvest life energy in other goals, and redefine voice as product of the self, not equivalent to self

PSYCHOLOGICAL RESPONSES TO VOICE SURGERY

- surgery may elicit hospital-related phobias, pain management issues
- vocal fold surgery is elective; critical that consent is informed
- screen for personality psychopathology or unrealistic expectations pre-op
- voice rest may produce anxiety, helplessness, and disorientation
- offer counseling session to normalize fear, frustration, regression
- voice surgery for cancer diagnosis requires support for both cancer impact and voice change

PSYCHOPATHOLOGY

- recognize and coordinate treatment for voice patients with coexisting mental health disorders; essential for patient safety and effective treatment
- characteristic patterns of voicing may aid in diagnosis
- summaries reflect *Diagnostic and Statistical Manual of Mental Disorders* (Fifth Edition) (*DSM-5*) diagnostic categories

Depressive Disorders

- major depressive disorder is most common—changes in mood, affect, cognition, biological functions, lasting at least 2 weeks, which may remit, but often recurrent
- premenstrual dysphoric disorder
- substance- and medically induced depressive phenomena

Bipolar Disorders

- bridge between depressive and psychotic disorders in symptoms
- strong association with family history and genetics
- Bipolar I: classic manic-depressive disorder characterized by alternating major depressive and manic episodes
- Bipolar II: at least one major depressive episode and at least one hypomanic episode, with unstable mood and significant impairment

- <u>Cyclothymia</u>: prolonged episodes of both hypomanic and depressive episodes without meeting full criteria
- Substance/medication/medical condition–induced manic symptoms

Anxiety Disorders

- share features of excessive fear/anxiety and related behaviors, persistent fear/anxiety is disproportionate to stimulus, panic attacks are particular form of fear response
- differ in terms of stimulus and cognitive ideation
- highly comorbid
- developmental—may appear in childhood and escalate
- <u>Manifestations</u>: specific phobia, social phobia, panic disorder, agoraphobia, generalized anxiety disorder, substance-induced disorder

Obsessive-Compulsive Disorder and Related Disorders

- characterized by obsessions/compulsions, also by preoccupations and/or repetitive behavior in response to preoccupations
- important to screen for related disorders
- related disorders include body-dysmorphic disorder, trichotillomania, excoriation, substance/medication/medical condition-induced disorder, hoarding disorder
- cognitive assessment includes evaluation of range of insight

Trauma and Stress Disorders

- exposure to trauma, severe stress, childhood neglect is an explicit criterion
- <u>Manifestations</u>: reactive attachment disorder, acute stress disorder, post-traumatic stress disorder, disinhibited social disorder, adjustment disorders
- may present with anxiety symptoms or anhedonia, aggression, dissociation

Feeding and Eating Disorders

- persistent disturbance of eating-related behavior resulting in altered consumption of food that impairs health or psychosocial function
- <u>Manifestations</u>: rumination disorder, avoidant/food restriction, anorexia, bulimia, binge-eating
- similar to substance use disorders, with craving and compulsive use

- obesity has robust associations with a number of mental health disorders
- may be secondary to side effects of psychotropic meds

Substance-Related Disorders

- cluster of cognitive, behavioral, physiological symptoms indicating continued substance use despite related problems
- underlying change in brain circuitry persists beyond detox
- pathological behaviors related to use including impaired control, social impairment, risky use and pharmacologic criteria

Psychotic Disorders

- <u>Manifestations</u>: schizophrenia, other psychotic disorders, schizotypal disorder
- defined by abnormalities in five domains: delusions, hallucinations, disorganized thinking/speech, disorganized or grossly abnormal motor behavior, negative symptoms
- heterogeneous, and severity of symptoms predicts degree of cognitive or neurobiological deficits

Neurocognitive Disorders

- <u>Manifestations</u>: dementia, delirium, neurocognitive disorders (NCDs)
- major or mild NCDs caused by Alzheimer's disease, vascular, Lewy body, Parkinson's disease, frontotemporal disease, traumatic brain injury, HIV infection, substance/medication-induced, Huntington's disease, prion disease, multiple etiologies
- primary clinical deficit is cognitive, acquired not developmental

Additional Clinical Conditions

- various, including dissociative, somatic symptom, sexual dysfunction, gender dysphoria, impulse control and personality disorders; beyond scope of this chapter

PSYCHOGENIC DYSPHONIA/ CONVERSION DISORDER

- voice disorders divided into organic and nonorganic etiology
- functional refers to abnormal central nervous system function; psychogenic refers to assumed etiology

- *DSM-5*—Conversion Disorder (Functional Neurologic Symptom Disorder)
  1. symptoms of altered voluntary motor or sensory function
  2. clinical findings incompatible with recognized neurological/medical condition
  3. symptom/deficit not explained better by another diagnosis
  4. symptom/impairment causes clinically significant distress or impairment in important areas of life function
  5. does not require certainty that symptoms are feigned
  6. la belle indifference not specific to this diagnosis
  7. secondary gain not specific to conversion disorder
  8. onset frequently associated with physical or emotional trauma
  9. maladaptive personality traits common
  10. target organ often symbolically related to unconscious threat/communication conflict
- <u>Voice characteristics</u>: aphonia, whispered speech, strain-strangle, abnormal register, abnormal rhythm; involuntary vocalizations may be normal
- <u>LEMG</u>: simultaneous firing of abductors and adductors
- <u>Tx</u>: interdisciplinary treatment interventions

PERFORMANCE ANXIETY

- most research, much controversy
- prevalence high in performers
- affects and is affected by what performers do—perform
- degree of debilitation varies, some is normal and abates during performance
- *DSM-5*—Performance Anxiety
  1. marked fear about social situations during which person is exposed to scrutiny
  2. performance-only type: fear restricted to performing in public
  3. fear that behavior will demonstrate anxiety symptoms or be evaluated negatively
  4. stimulus always provokes fear/anxiety
  5. stimulus avoided or endured with intense fear
  6. fear/anxiety out of proportion to the actual threat posed
  7. fear persistent for at least 6 months
  8. fear/anxiety causes clinically significant distress or impairment in important areas of functioning
  9. fear not attributable to a substance or medical condition

- Etiology: unknown—conflicting theories (physiological, cognitive, behavioral)
- Tx: psychotherapy (cognitive, psychodynamic, behavioral), pharmacotherapy
    1. β-blockers: suppress cardiovascular response but have significant risks to health and performance, may be obtained by performers without medical supervision
    2. Benzodiazepines: significant risk of abuse, side effects, performance effects
    3. Antidepressants: indicated for underlying anxiety disorders, not useful for performance anxiety

PSYCHOACTIVE MEDICATIONS
(Table 29–1)

- should be prescribed by clinician caring for coexisting mental health diagnosis
- should be elicited during history and documented, reviewed for voice-related side effects
- ongoing treatment of patients with voice disorders taking psychoactive meds mandates coordination of care
- Antidepressants: selective serotonin reuptake inhibitors (SSRIs), selective norepinephrine reuptake inhibitors (SNRIs), dopaminergics, tricyclics, monoamine oxidase inhibitors (MAOIs)
- *Mood stabilizers*: lithium, anticonvulsants, second-generation antipsychotics
- *Anxiolytics*: benzodiazepines, antidepressants, clomipramine, antihistamines, buspirone, β-blockers
- *Antipsychotics*: haloperidol, perphenazine, fluphenazine, "atypical" (eg, risperidone, olanapine, quetiaprine, luasiadone, etc); clozapine

Psychiatric Effects of ENT Medication

- medications routinely prescribed can have psychiatric side effects (SE)
- mood, perceptual, cognitive, or behavioral disturbances
- potential drug interaction between psychoactive and ENT medications
- pre- or coexisting psychiatric disorders can be precipitated
- psychiatric symptoms may indicate organic disease (eg, thyroid, adrenal, autoimmune)

TABLE 29–1. Selected Drugs and Their Possible Psychiatric Side Effects

Drug	Side Effects
Adrenocorticosteroids	Agitation, anxiety, confusion, delirium, depression, hallucinations, mania, paranoia, psychoses, sleep disturbances
Antihistamines and decongestants	
Azatadine	Agitation, anxiety, euphoria, hallucinations, hypomania, mania, nervousness, somnolence
Loratadine	Agitation, anxiety, confusion, delirium, depression, nervousness
Fexofenadine	Somnolence
Phenylpropanolamine[a]/ guaifenesin	Agitation, anxiety, nervousness
Pseudoephedrine[b]/ guaifenesin	Hallucinations
Antisecretory agents	
Cimetidine	Confusion, delirium, depression, hallucinations, mania, paranoia
Famotidine	Agitation, anxiety, nervousness, somnolence
Lansoprazole	Hallucinations
Nizatidine	Agitation, anxiety, nervousness, somnolence
Omeprazole	Aggression, agitation, anxiety, depression, hallucinations, hostility, nervousness, violence
Ranitidine	Confusion, delirium, depression, hallucinations, mania

[a]Agents containing phenylpropanolamine can also cause confusion, delirium, depression, euphoria, hallucinations, hypomania, mania, and paranoia.

[b]Agents containing pseudoephedrine can also cause agitation, anxiety, euphoria, hypomania, mania, nervousness, and paranoia.

Source: Used with permission from Sataloff et al., *Professional Voice: The Science and Art of Clinical Care* (4th ed.). San Diego, CA: Plural Publishing; 2017.

- Risk factors—elicit:
    1. current prescribed and over-the-counter medications, including complementary or alternative remedies
    2. coexisting medical conditions with psychiatric symptoms
    3. personal/family history of psychiatric disorder
    4. age/presentation at onset
    5. history of drug or alcohol abuse

STRESS MANAGEMENT

- affects all professions
- factor in many illnesses
- psychological experience with physical consequences
- <u>Stress</u>: emotional, cognitive, and physiologic responses to psychological demands/challenges
- <u>Stress level</u>: degree of stress experienced
- <u>Stress response</u>: physiologic reaction to stress
- <u>Stressor</u>: external stimulus, internal thought, perception, emotion that creates stress
- <u>Coping</u>: managing demands appraised as exceeding the resources of the person
- physical effects neuronally and hormonally mediated
- autonomic nervous system, usually sympathetic symptoms
- chronic stress also can produce muscle tension, chronic fatigue, gastrointestinal pathology, pain syndromes, immune system alteration
- <u>Tx</u>: assess acute versus chronic
    1. <u>Acute</u>: reassurance and rest/restriction
    2. <u>Chronic</u>: psychotherapeutic (psychoeducation, cognitive behavioral therapy, time management, relaxation, hypnosis, prevention)

TEAM TREATMENT OF PSYCHOLOGICAL DIMENSIONS OF VOICE DISORDERS

- recognize comorbid psychopathology and incorporate into history taking
- psychological assessment available when indicated
- confidentiality formally extended to treatment team

Discipline-Specific Interventions

- physicians consider in differential
- SLP familiar with current models of psychological treatment, develop rapport and support disclosure
- behavioral health clinicians provide advanced assessment, offer acute treatment
- all clinicians refer to psychological professional for complex or long-term care

CHAPTER

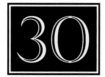

Laryngology and Medication

Marissa Evarts, Ghiath Alnouri, Mary J. Hawkshaw, and Robert T. Sataloff

continues

INTRODUCTION

- medications required commonly in voice patients including voice professionals
- side effects common and affect body through the following mechanisms, among others:
  1. <u>Bone marrow suppression</u>: anemia, leukopenia, and thrombocytopenia may lead to increased risk of infection and bleeding due to clotting abnormalities
  2. <u>GI distress</u>: nausea/vomiting may cause dehydration and mucinous secretions; acidic nature of vomit → vocal fold injury

3. <u>Neurotoxicity</u>: damage nerves that innervate laryngeal muscles, diaphragm, intercostal, abdominal and back muscles → irreversible changes in voice range and power, pitch control; may cause shortness of breath or stridor via vocal fold paresis or paralysis
4. <u>Ototoxicity</u>: due to injury to hair cells; may affect voice as a result of impaired detection of sound and pitch
5. <u>Pulmonary toxicity/fibrosis</u>: inadequate breath support for voice → may cause hyperfunction to compensate and result in vocal fold injury, scarring, and formation of vocal nodules; shortness of breath
6. <u>Stomatitis and esophagopharyngitis</u>: breakdown of mucous membranes → pain, irritation, and swelling of mouth and throat → changes in resonance of vocal apparatus, dysphagia

- biological variability makes side effects individual and unpredictable
- response to medications affected by gender, age, body size, metabolic status, and concurrent use of other medications or recreational drugs
- physician needs to optimize balance between effects and side effects

ANALGESICS

Background

- <u>Indications</u>: used for analgesia during acute or chronic illness and after surgery, anti-inflammatory properties
- <u>Important side effects</u>: risk of vocal damage due to analgesic masking of laryngeal discomfort and pain, permitting inappropriate performance
- <u>Relevant medications</u>: acetaminophen, acetylsalicylic (ASA), narcotics, NSAIDs

Acetaminophen

- often used in combination with codeine (Tylenol #3); ideal for voice patients for mild to moderate pain control and to suppress cough postoperatively (see section on Antitussives and Mucolytics)
- <u>Important side effects</u>: hepatotoxicity; constipation, which may cause abdominal discomfort and impair support

Aspirin

- <u>Important side effects</u>: interfere with clotting mechanism and may cause vocal fold hemorrhage, ototoxicity, tinnitus

Narcotics

- include oxycodone, hydrocodone, and codeine (see section on Antitussives and Mucolytics)
- Important side effects: impair intellectual function, dysarthria, voice abuse, and vocal fold injury due to sensorium change from narcotics and consequent voice misuse/abuse

Nonsteroidal Anti-Inflammatory Drugs (NSAIDs)

- include ibuprofen, ketoprofen, Toradol, and selective COX-II inhibitor, celecoxib
- Indications: see previous section "Background"
- Celecoxib: laryngeal tendonitis and other indications instead of NSAIDs that promote bleeding; may also help decrease recurrent respiratory papillomatosis (RRP) recurrence
- Mechanism of action: COX-I and COX-II inhibition
- selective COX-II inhibitors do not interfere with COX-I pathway so cause fewer dyscrasias and GI side effects than seen with NSAIDs
- Important side effects: interfere with clotting mechanism and may cause vocal fold hemorrhage, ototoxicity, GI bleeding; selective COX-II inhibitors have increased risk of cardiac events

ANTACIDS, ANTISECRETORY, AND PROKINETIC AGENTS (*See* Chapter 22)

ANTIBIOTICS

Background

- Indications: acute bacterial infection, prophylaxis to prevent infection of surgical sites
- use should be based on cultures whenever appropriate
- Important side effects: see major side effects later in chapter
- Ototoxicity: chloramphenicol, vancomycin (particularly when used with aminoglycosides)
- Relevant medications: aminoglycosides, β-lactams, fluoroquinolones

Aminoglycosides

- Mechanism of action: interfere with protein synthesis by binding to 30S and 50S ribosomal subunits; bactericidal

- <u>Important side effects</u>: renal and ototoxicity
- <u>Ototoxicity</u>: neomycin > gentamicin > tobramycin > amikacin > netilmicin

β-lactams

- includes penicillins and cephalosporins
- <u>Mechanism of action</u>: interfere with cell wall synthesis; bactericidal
- <u>Important side effects</u>: GI distress

Fluoroquinolones

- <u>Mechanism of action</u>: inhibit DNA gyrase (DNA unable to relax); bactericidal
- <u>Important side effects</u>: Black Box warning of tendonitis and tendon rupture, irreversible peripheral neuropathy, and worsening of muscle weakness in patients with myasthenia gravis
- avoid fluoroquinolones if able in children, pregnancy, and patients with myasthenia gravis

Macrolides

- <u>Mechanism of action</u>: interfere with protein synthesis by binding to 50S ribosomal subunit; may be bacteriostatic or bactericidal depending on susceptibility and concentration
- <u>Important side effects</u>: GI distress, numerous drug interactions (inhibit hepatic metabolism), cholestatic jaundice, dizziness, ototoxicity; may also cause exacerbation in patients with myasthenia gravis
- <u>Azithromycin</u>: U.S. Food and Drug Administration (FDA) warning of increased risk of fatal cardiac arrhythmias (eg, QTc prolongation) in high-risk patients (mostly females); cancer relapse with long-term use after donor stem cell transplant; azithromycin least likely to interact with other drugs

ANTIDEPRESSANTS

- drug classes include selective serotonin reuptake inhibitors (SSRIs), serotonin-norepinephrine reuptake inhibitors (SNRIs), tricyclic antidepressant (TCAs), monoamine oxidase inhibitors (MAOIs)
- <u>Important side effects</u>: anticholinergic properties associated with dry mouth and thick secretions, speech disorders, hoarseness, aphonia, restlessness, headache, gastrointestinal (GI) distress, insomnia,

palpitation, hypotension, and sexual dysfunction (with long-term use); increased suicidal thinking or behavior with initiation of treatment in people younger than 24 years
- MAOIs: hypertensive crisis when taken with tyramine-containing goods such as strong cheeses, fava broad beans, cured or smoked meats or fish, home-brewed or on-tap beer, and others

ANTIFUNGALS

Background

- Indications: treatment of acute and chronic fungal laryngitis and esophagitis, other fungal infections
- Relevant medications: fluconazole, nystatin

Fluconazole

- includes both PO and IV formulations
- Indications: laryngeal candidiasis (see section on Inhaled Corticosteroids), oropharyngeal candidiasis, esophageal candidiasis
- treatment of oropharyngeal and laryngeal candidiasis should be for at least 2 weeks to prevent relapse; treatment of esophagitis for minimum of 3 weeks and for at least 2 weeks following resolution of symptoms
- Mechanism of action: inhibition of lanosterol 14-α-demethylase; fungistatic
- Important side effects: headache, GI distress, rash
- avoid in pregnancy (category D)

Nystatin

- topical PO suspension; should be swished in mouth for 5 minutes prior to expectoration
- Indications: oropharyngeal candidiasis, prophylaxis against colonization of candidiasis in total laryngectomy patients with tracheoesophageal voice prostheses
- systemic treatment (PO fluconazole) needed to treat laryngeal candidiasis
- Mechanism of action: binds sterols in fungal cell membrane → increased permeability and leakage of cell contents
- Important side effects: GI distress; minimal to insignificant systemic effects as it is not absorbed

ANTIHISTAMINES

Background

- drug classes include first- and second-generation H1-antagonists, H2-antagonists
- see Chapter 22 on Laryngopharyngeal Reflux for in-depth description of H2-antagonists
- <u>Mechanism of action</u>: histamine H1 (or H2) receptor antagonists; have anticholinergic properties
- <u>Important side effects</u>: dryness, thick and viscous secretions worse when combined with sympathomimetic or parasympathomimetic agents, somnolence
- <u>Recommendations</u>: avoid over-the-counter antihistamine preparation for at least a couple of days prior to a performance if singer has no prior experience with the antihistamine
- oral or injected corticosteroid better option to treat acute allergic episode before professional engagement
- if no known intolerance to a specific antihistamine, no contraindication to use
- <u>Relevant medications</u>: cetirizine, chlorpheniramine, dimenhydrinate, diphenhydramine, fexofenadine, hydroxyzine, loratadine, promethazine

First-Generation H1-Antagonists

- includes chlorpheniramine, dimenhydrinate, diphenhydramine, hydroxyzine, and promethazine
- <u>Indications</u>: allergic reaction, asthma, insomnia, motion sickness, anxiety, dizziness, sedation
    1. <u>Chlorpheniramine</u>: used as antitussive in combination with hydrocodone
    2. <u>Dimenhydrinate</u>: prevention of motion sickness; off-label use in treatment of Ménière's disease
    3. <u>Diphenhydramine</u>: has vasoconstrictive properties; also used in treatment of parkinsonism; usually liquid or tablet preparation, but also available as mist; not recommended in voice users near time of performance
    4. <u>Promethazine</u>: used as antiemetic
- <u>Important side effects</u>: drowsiness, see previous section "Background"

Second-Generation H1-Antagonists

- includes cetirizine, fexofenadine, and loratadine

- <u>Indications</u>: allergic rhinitis, urticaria
- <u>Fexofenadine</u>: approved for use by pilots
- <u>Mechanism of action</u>: differ from first-generation H1-antagonists because they do not cross the blood-brain barrier, causing less sedation
- <u>Important side effects</u>: see previous section "Background," cetirizine (hepatotoxicity)

ANTIHYPERTENSIVES

- drug classes include angiotensin-converting enzyme (ACE) inhibitors, angiotensin II receptor blockers, β-blockers, and calcium channel blockers
- <u>Indications</u>: hypertension, migraine, essential tremor, others
- <u>Propranolol</u>: subjective vocal improvement in patients with laryngeal tremor
- <u>Important side effects</u>: dry cough, dryness of mucous membranes due to parasympathomimetic action, dehydration when used in combination with diuretics
- <u>β-blockers</u>: increased salivation, bradycardia, bronchospasm, may induce asthma attack; not recommended to treat performance anxiety and may cause lackluster performance

ANTIPSYCHOTICS

- drug classes include first- and second-generation antipsychotics, others (clozapine)
- <u>Mechanism of action</u>: blocks dopamine receptors
- <u>Important side effects</u>: extrapyramidal symptoms (EPSs), include acute dystonia, akathisia, Parkinson's symptoms, and tardive dyskinesia with long-term use; neuroleptic malignant syndrome
  1. may involve tongue, perioral, and laryngeal musculature and affect vocal performance
  2. <u>first-generation antipsychotics</u>: worse EPS symptoms than second generation
  3. <u>second-generation antipsychotics</u>: weight gain, hypercholesterolemia, diabetes
  4. <u>clozapine</u>: superior in efficacy to other antipsychotics with low likelihood of EPS; 1% risk of fatal agranulocytosis

ANTITUSSIVES AND MUCOLYTICS

Background

- <u>Indications</u>: antitussives are cough suppressants (may be used postoperatively to prevent cough → decrease risk of vocal fold hemorrhage); mucolytics help to dissolve thick mucus
- mucolytics may help counteract dehydrating effects of antihistamines, but should not replace adequate hydration
- <u>Relevant medications</u>: benzonatate, codeine, dextromethorphan, dornase, guaifenesin

Benzonatate

- <u>Indication</u>: antitussive
- <u>Mechanism of action</u>: suppresses cough via anesthetizing peripheral stretch receptors in the upper respiratory tract
- <u>Important side effects</u>: drying effects on vocal tract secretions worse with antihistamine combinations; hypersensitivity reactions, laryngospasm, bronchospasm

Codeine

- <u>Indication</u>: analgesic and antitussive; may be used in combination with acetaminophen postoperatively (see previous sections on Acetaminophen and Narcotics)
- <u>Mechanism of action</u>: narcotic agonist (mu receptor) analgesic; acts on central cough reflex
- <u>Important side effects</u>: same as Benzonatate, see previous section

Dextromethorphan

- <u>Indication</u>: antitussive
- <u>Mechanism of action</u>: acts on central cough reflex
- <u>Important side effects</u>: same as Benzonatate, see previous section

Dornase

- <u>Indication</u>: mucolytic; used in cystic fibrosis
- <u>Important side effects</u>: may cause temporary sore throat, hoarseness, laryngitis; subside without dose adjustment

Guaifenesin

- Indication: mucolytic; viscous secretions can be caused by dehydration and medications such as antihistamines and anticholinergic drugs
- Mechanism of action: shifts laryngeal secretions from viscous to mucinous predominance

ANTIVIRALS

Background

- Indications: prophylaxis and treatment of acute and chronic viral infections
- Relevant medications: acyclovir, amantadine, cidofovir, oseltamivir, zidovudine (ZVD, AZT)

Acyclovir

- Indications: used for treatment of herpes simplex viruses (HSV) types I and II, including recurrent herpetic superior laryngeal paresis or paralysis
- Mechanism of action: inhibits DNA polymerase
- Important side effects: GI distress, headache, lethargy, tremors, confusion, seizures
- IV formulation may cause inflammation or phlebitis at infusion site

Amantadine

- Indications: effective against influenzas, used in treatment of Parkinson's disease
- Mechanism of action: prevent attachment and penetration of the virus to host cell
- Important side effects: myoclonus of the laryngeal and pharyngeal muscles → hoarseness, dysphagia; agitation, tachycardia, extreme xerostomia and xerophonia

Cidofovir

- Indications: off-label use predominantly as an intralesional injection in the prevention and treatment of laryngeal and other respiratory papillomatosis caused by human papillomavirus (HPV)-6, 11, 16, 18, and others; IV and nebulized formulations also described in the literature
- pulmonary involvement of RRP justified indication for IV cidofovir

- cidofovir FDA approved for treatment of cytomegalovirus (CMV)-retinitis in AIDS patients
- <u>Mechanism of action</u>: cytosine nucleotide analog that inhibits DNA polymerase
- <u>Important side effects</u>: increased risk of dysplasia and adenocarcinoma controversial (similar incidence of malignant degeneration of papilloma, up to 2%–5%), local inflammatory reaction, cutaneous rash, headache, vocal fold scarring, airway obstruction
- IV formulation may cause nephrotoxicity and leukopenia; avoid in pregnancy (category C)

Oseltamivir

- <u>Indication</u>: may be effective in prophylaxis and treatment of acute influenza in adults and children older than 13 years
- <u>Mechanism of action</u>: neuraminidase inhibitor
- <u>Important side effects</u>: rash, swelling of face and tongue

Zidovudine (ZVD, AZT)

- <u>Indication</u>: used in treatment of HIV
- <u>Mechanism of action</u>: inhibits reverse transcriptase and incorporates into viral DNA
- <u>Important side effects</u>: hoarseness, cough, pharyngitis, nervousness, muscle spasm, tremor

ANXIOLYTICS

- predominant drug class is benzodiazepines
- not indicated for treatment of performance anxiety
- <u>Important side effects</u>: high addictive potential; withdrawal symptoms include seizures, dose-related sedation, dizziness, weakness, ataxia, decreased motor performance, mild hypotension, and possible impairment of performance parameters (eg, intonation and rhythmic control)

CHEMOTHERAPEUTIC AGENTS

Background

- may cause various side effects that affect voice, breathing, and swallowing when taken systemically:

1. <u>Bone marrow suppression</u>: common to almost all antineoplastic agents
2. <u>GI distress</u>: cisplatin, dacarbazine, carmustine, others
3. <u>Neurotoxicity</u>: cyclophosphamide, 5-fluorouracil (5-FU), interferon, methotrexate, tamoxifen, vinblastine, vincristine (vocal fold paresis and paralysis)
4. <u>Ototoxicity</u>: cisplatin, carboplatin
5. <u>Pulmonary toxicity/fibrosis</u>: bleomycin, methotrexate
6. <u>Stomatitis and esophagopharyngitis</u>: 5-FU, doxorubicin

- may be used for indications other than chemotherapy
    1. formulations include liquids for (intralesional) injections, topical sprays, and others
    2. <u>Relevant medications</u>: bevacizumab, 5-FU, mitomycin C

Bevacizumab

- <u>Indication</u>: off-label use as intralesional injection in the prevention and treatment of laryngeal and respiratory papillomatosis
- <u>Mechanism of action</u>: anti-VEGF antibody; thought to decrease interval of papilloma recurrence by inhibiting vascularization
- limited data regarding appropriate dosage, efficacy, and safety

5-fluorouracil (5-FU)

- <u>Indication</u>: off-label use as intralesional injection in combination with corticosteroid in the prevention and treatment of vocal fold scar
- <u>Mechanism of action</u>: pyrimidine analog that inhibits thymidylate synthase → inhibition of fibroblasts → induces apoptosis and inhibits type I collagen production
- similar to use in keloid and hypertrophic scar formation in facial plastics literature
- performed usually in series of at least three injections with subjective and objective voice improvement; unpublished data by author (RTS)
- <u>Important side effect</u>: local hematoma

Mitomycin C

- <u>Indication</u>: off-label use as topical application for adjuvant treatment of laryngotracheal stenosis
- likely delays but does not prevent recurrence of symptoms in most patients; may increase symptom-free periods of time between interventions
- improved benefit with multiple mitomycin treatments

- <u>Mechanism of action</u>: antibiotic isolated from *Streptomyces caespitosus*; inhibits DNA and RNA synthesis → partially prevents fibroblast proliferation
- <u>Important side effects</u>: deposition of fibrin → airway obstruction; no systemic side effects
- no side effects reported in studies that used a saline rinse after application
- limited data regarding timing, dosage, and application duration

CORTICOSTEROIDS

Background

- potent anti-inflammatory agents
- formulations include inhaled, intralesional, intranasal, and systemic corticosteroids
- <u>Relevant medications</u>: beclomethasone, budesonide, dexamethasone, fluticasone, methylprednisolone, mometasone, prednisone, triamcinolone

Inhaled Corticosteroids

- includes beclomethasone, budesonide, fluticasone, and mometasone
- <u>Indications</u>: asthma, reactive airway disease
- <u>Mechanism of action</u>: used to decrease inflammation in the airway
- <u>Important side effects</u>: risk of *Candida* laryngitis, dysphonia secondary to contact inflammation and atrophy of vocalis muscle; alters laryngeal microflora → increased risk of laryngeal infection, especially in immunocompromised individuals
- avoid use in professional voice users

Intralesional Corticosteroids

- includes betamethasone, methylprednisolone, dexamethasone, and triamcinolone
- topical applications (sprays) also available for similar indications
- <u>Indications</u>: sole treatment of and/or adjunct after microlaryngeal surgical removal of benign vocal fold lesions (eg, vocal nodules, polyps, cysts, granuloma) by decreasing inflammation and risk of granulation tissue, granuloma and persistent dysphonia; vocal fold scar, Reinke's edema, laryngotracheal stenosis, inflammatory laryngeal lesions such polyangiitis with granulomatosis (Wegener's granulomatosis), systemic lupus erythematosus, and sarcoidosis

- Mechanism of action: reduces level of inflammatory cytokines and growth factors → inhibits fibroblast growth → decreases collagen and glycosaminoglycan synthesis
- significant improvements in maximum phonation time and Voice Handicap Index (VHI)
- treatment benefit expected in 1 to 2 weeks after injection
- significant improvement in dyspnea and pulmonary function tests (PFTs) in patients with idiopathic subglottic stenosis shown after serial intralesional steroid injections (± surgery)
- Important side effects: local hematoma, vocal fold atrophy (usually temporary), delayed wound healing, promotion of scar, whitish plaque if steroid with suspended particles used (eg, triamcinolone), recurrence; overall, low side-effect profile and usually self-limited
- inject steroid into Reinke's space (superficial lamina propria) and not deep into vocal ligament or muscle to prevent vocal fold atrophy in treatment of benign vocal fold lesions
- prevent whitish plaque by using dexamethasone > triamcinolone (due to solution itself); usually does not have permanent effect on true vocal fold vibration; resolves spontaneously
- performed both in office (transoral or percutaneous) and operating room settings

Intranasal Corticosteroids

- includes beclomethasone, budesonide, fluticasone, mometasone, and triamcinolone
- Indication: aqueous medium used to prevent nasal dryness
- Important side effects: epistaxis; usually do not affect voice

Systemic Corticosteroids

- includes dexamethasone, methylprednisolone, and prednisone
- IV, IM, and PO formulations
- Indications: acute allergy attack, acute laryngitis, angioedema, laryngotracheal stenosis, autoimmune disease, other inflammatory conditions
- Mechanism of action: decrease inflammation and mobilize water from edematous larynx
- Important side effects: increased sugar blood levels (caution in DM patients), gastric irritation (risk of ulceration and hemorrhage, risks decreased by prophylactic use of proton pump inhibitor, H2 blocker or antacid), mood changes (euphoria, occasionally psychosis), irritability, mild mucosal dryness, increased appetite, increased energy,

blurred vision, fluid retention, muscle wasting, and fat redistribution with long-term use

- prolonged use of systemic steroids >2 weeks → systemic effects as previously stated; Clinical Practice Guidelines recommend against routine use of steroids for dysphonia prior to visualizing larynx

DIURETICS

- <u>Indications</u>: Ménière's syndrome, some premenstrual syndrome symptoms excluding dysphonia premenstrualis, heart or kidney failure, hypertension
- <u>Important side effects</u>: dehydration, decreased lubrication and thickened secretions that can affect voice, ototoxicity (loop diuretics)
- <u>Caution</u>: diuretics do not remobilize fluid effectively caused by Reinke's edema (secondary to inflammation) or hormonal fluid shifts (protein bound)

HORMONES

Background

- drug classes include androgens, estrogens, progesterones, thyroid hormones, and others
- new oral contraceptives marketed in the United States have better estrogen-progesterone balance than earlier generation drugs and voice changes are uncommon

Androgens

- <u>Indications</u>: hormonal replacement therapy, transgender procedures
- <u>Important side effects</u>: irreversible lowering of fundamental frequency in the larynx and coarsening of the voice, especially in women, through structural changes

Estrogens

- <u>Indications</u>: oral contraceptives (see previous section "Background"), hormonal replacement therapy after menopause, chemotherapy for breast cancer, transgender procedures
- estrogen replacement helpful in preventing voice changes following menopause; professional voice users should be offered this treatment under medical supervision if not contraindicated

- Important side effects: Reinke's edema during premenstrual period (increased ADH → fluid retention)

Progesterones

- Indications: oral contraceptives (see previous section "Background"), endometriosis
- Important side effects: some synthetic progesterones produce irreversible lowering of fundamental frequency in the larynx and coarsening of the voice, especially in women, through structural changes similar to those caused by androgens

Thyroid Hormones

- thyroxine will improve voice parameters by reversing effects of hypothyroidism
- *see* Chapter 23

MOOD-STABILIZING DRUGS

- includes lithium salt formulations
- Indication: alleviate manic and hypomanic episodes in patients with bipolar disorder
- Important side effects: fine tremor, thinking and memory deficit, weight gain, GI distress, tremulousness, ataxia, dysarthria, confusion, delirium, mucosal irritation, polyuria, diabetes insipidus, teratogenic effects, altered thyroid functions, and multiple drug–drug interactions; has narrow therapeutic range

NEUROLOGICS

Background

- drug classes include acetylcholinesterase inhibitors, anticonvulsants, botulinum toxin, Parkinson's medications, sympathomimetics

Acetylcholinesterase Inhibitors

- includes pyridostigmine
- Indication: used to treat myasthenia gravis
- Mechanism of action: enhances action of acetylcholine by inhibiting acetylcholinesterase

- <u>Important side effects</u>: excessive salivation, GI distress, skin rash, nervousness, confusion, weakness, cramping

Anticonvulsants

- includes carbamazepine, lamotrigine, and valproic acid
- <u>Indications</u>: seizure, trigeminal neuralgia, migraine
- <u>Important side effects</u>: may cause tremor and ataxia that affect voice
- <u>Carbamazepine</u>: agranulocytosis, aplastic anemia
- <u>Lamotrigine</u>: lethal risk of severe rash
- <u>Valproic acid</u>: teratogenic; may also cause sedation, weight gain, alopecia, elevated liver enzymes and white blood cell count

Botulinum Toxin (BT)

- neurotoxin from *Clostridium botulinum*
- includes botulinum toxin A and B
- BT type A standard of care; BT type B typically used for nonresponders, possibly due to creation of antibodies to BT type A —may be high cumulative dose or frequency related
- <u>Indications</u>: laryngeal (spasmodic dysphonia, laryngeal dystonia, laryngeal synkinesis associated with reinnervation after recurrent nerve paralysis, bilateral vocal fold paralysis, laryngeal tremor; adjunctive treatment for arytenoid dislocation and recurrent laryngeal granulomata); oromandibular dystonia, sialorrhea, cervical (spasmodic) torticollis, cosmesis, cricopharyngeus muscle spasm → dysphagia or failed voice rehabilitation in laryngectomy patients
- <u>Mechanism of action</u>: inhibits release of acetylcholine from presynaptic nerve endings at neuromuscular junction
- performed in office or operating room settings with or without electromyogram (EMG) guidance
- <u>Important side effects</u>: vary by indication depending on site of injection; mostly due to unwanted diffusion of toxin to nearby structures
  1. <u>Laryngeal indications</u>: breathiness, soft voice, dysphagia, aspiration, failure to respond, others
  2. <u>Oromandibular dystonia</u>: dysphagia and dysarthria (due to proximity of intrinsic tongue and pharyngeal muscles)
  3. <u>Cervical dystonia</u>: musculoskeletal (local and distal) and injection site pain, dysphonia, dysphagia, dry mouth, neck weakness, pruritus, nausea, flu-like symptoms, fatigue, generalized weakness; dose-dependent and may cross fascial planes

4. <u>Cosmesis</u>: no major or long-term complications following cosmetic BT
5. <u>Cricopharyngeal spasm</u>: dysphonia (weakening of laryngeal muscles) and dysphagia (weakening of pharyngeal constrictors)
- limit side effects by performing BT with endoscopy or EMG guidance

Parkinson's Medications

- include L-dopa, dopamine receptor agonists; also see section on Antivirals (amantadine)
- <u>Important side effects</u>: anticholinergic side effects
- side effects and/or course of illness may ultimately force end of a performance career

Sympathomimetics

- include methylphenidate
- <u>Indication</u>: used to treat attention-deficit disorder
- <u>Important side effect</u>: may cause slight tremor that could be audible in singing

ORAL RINSES

Background

- topical medications used to treat xerostomia, mucositis (eg, s/p chemotherapy and radiation), oropharyngeal *Candidiasis*
- <u>Relevant medications</u>: Biotene, magic mouthwash, nystatin (see section on Antifungals)

Biotene

- artificial saliva containing lactoperoxidase, glucose oxidase, and lysozyme
- oral rinse that is swished for 30 seconds and expectorated; toothpaste, gum, gel, and spray formulations also available
- <u>Indications</u>: see previous section "Background," potential prophylaxis against colonization of *Candidiasis* in total laryngectomy patients with tracheoesophageal voice prostheses
- <u>Important side effect</u>: data limited, tooth discoloration

Magic Mouthwash

- various ingredients compounded, include but not limited to diphenhydramine, viscous lidocaine, magnesium hydroxide/ aluminum hydroxide, nystatin, corticosteroids, and antibiotic
- <u>Indications</u>: see previous section "Background"
- data limited regarding efficacy and side effects

SPRAYS, MISTS, AND INHALANTS

Background

- drug classes include topically applied α-1A-adrenoceptor agonists, anticholinergics, mast cell stabilizers, and 5% propylene glycol; also see sections on Antitussives and Mucolytics, Corticosteroids

α-1A-Adrenoceptor Agonists

- includes oxymetazoline
- <u>Indications</u>: nasal decongestant used for epistaxis; also used rarely for cases of acute laryngeal edema
- <u>Important side effect</u>: nasal crusting

Anticholinergics

- includes ipratropium and tiotropium
- formulations include inhaled and intranasal
- <u>Indications</u>: rhinorrhea (vasomotor rhinitis), asthma, chronic obstructive pulmonary disease
- <u>Important side effects</u>: xerostomia secondary to decrease in mucus production and to throat irritation

Mast Cell Stabilizers

- include cromolyn
- formulations include inhaled, intranasal, and oral
- <u>Mechanism of action</u>: inhibit release of potent immune mediators from mast cells including histamine
- <u>Important side effect</u>: thickening of mucus

5% Propylene Glycol

- <u>Indication</u>: used for laryngitis sicca
- <u>Caution</u>: should be augmented by oral hydration

HERBS AND SUPPLEMENTS

Background

- many individuals, including singers, seek herbs and dietary supplements as alternatives to allopathic medications
- many herbs and some supplements have potential side effects for voice users
- some herbal medications should be avoided for 14 days prior to surgery according to the American Society of Anesthesiologists
- increased bleeding risk: ginkgo biloba, ginger, ginseng, garlic
- Relevant herbs and supplements: echinacea, Entertainer's Secret Spray, ephedra, gingko, kava, Sprout's Voice Remedy, St. John's Wort, Thayer's Cherry Slippery Elm lozenge, Throat Coat, Vita Vocal Throat and Voice Enhancer, Vocal Eze throat spray, Vocalzone pastilles

Echinacea

- used to treat upper respiratory infections and influenza
- Important side effects: may suppress the immune system; liver toxicity with long-term use
- avoid use in patients allergic to ragweed, marigolds, daisies, chrysanthemums, or chamomile

Entertainer's Secret Spray

- Contents: carboxymethylcellulose, ginger root, echinacea, aloe vera gel, glycerin
- oral spray used for lubrication of dry throat
- efficacy not supported by clinical trial

Ephedra

- used to lose weight and improve physical performance
- Important side effects: myocardial infarction, hypertension, stroke, thermogenesis, seizures

Ginkgo Biloba

- used to improve concentration, memory, and for circulation diseases such as claudication
- Important side effect: risk of spontaneous vocal fold hemorrhage particularly in combination with other anticlotting products

Kava

- used to reduce stress and anxiety
- <u>Important side effects</u>: impaired motor reflexes and unpredictable, severe liver damage; may prolong effect of anesthetics

Sprout's Voice Remedy

- <u>Contents</u>: slippery elm bark, fennel seeds, horseradish root, thyme herb, celery seeds
- oral drops used prior to performing or speaking to treat hoarseness, congestion, and inflammation
- efficacy not supported by clinical trial

St. John's Wort

- used to treat mild to moderate depression and seasonal affective disorder
- <u>Important side effects</u>: insomnia, dry mouth, GI distress, fatigue, dizziness, photosensitivity, headache; may prolong effect of anesthetics
- avoid use with other antidepressants due to increased risk of serotonin syndrome

Thayer's Cherry Slippery Elm Lozenge

- used to treat vocal irritation and hoarseness
- no risk of masking pain as does not have analgesic effects

Throat Coat

- <u>Contents</u>: licorice root and slippery elm bark
- herbal tea used to alleviate symptoms of pharyngitis
- <u>Important side effects</u>: hypertension and hypokalemia in high doses

Vita Vocal Throat and Voice Enhancer

- <u>Contents</u>: ginseng, vitamin B12, eucalyptus, wild cherry bark, osha, echinacea, slippery elm, others
- used to enhance vocal clarity, soothe throat, minimize dryness, and prevent vocal fold inflammation
- efficacy not supported by clinical trial

Vocal Eze Throat Spray

- <u>Contents</u>: marshmallow root, osha root, licorice root, propolis, aloe vera gel, other
- herbal lubricating throat spray used to enhance vocal clarity, soothe throat, and minimize dryness
- efficacy not supported by clinical trial

Vocalzone Pastilles

- <u>Contents</u>: levomenthol, peppermint oil, myrrh tincture, others
- used to relieve dry and irritated throat following voice overuse
- may mask protective physiologic response of pain

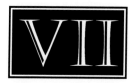

SECTION

VII

Pediatric Laryngology

CHAPTER

31

Pediatric Laryngology

David J. Lafferty, Marissa Evarts, Justin Ross, Mary J. Hawkshaw, and Robert T. Sataloff

INTRODUCTION

Pediatric Airway Anatomy

- large head and tongue, short neck, and length of mandible relative to body size increase risk of airway obstruction
- vocal folds angled anterior-inferior to posterior-superior (adult are at 90°)
- pediatric vocal folds are shorter with decreased musculomembranous-cartilaginous ratio (1:1 to 1:1.5)
- epiglottis is "U" shaped, compared to flat in adults
- calcification of the larynx and hyoid typically occur in teenage years
- flexibility of tracheal rings predisposes to dynamic obstruction during inspiration
- obligate nasal breathers until age 5 months due to relationship of esophagus and soft palate allowing simultaneous respiration and deglutition
- transition from obligate nasal breathing to nasal and oral breathing due to increased oral cavity size and inferior descent of larynx
- <u>Laryngeal descent:</u> C2–C3 (birth) → C5 (2 years) → C6 (5 years) → C6–C7 (15 years)
- pediatric airway is funnel shaped with smallest cross-sectional area at cricoid (4–5 mm), compared with glottic inlet in adults
- 1 mm of subglottic edema in a neonate reduces cross-sectional area >50%
- approximate endotracheal tube size = (age in years + 16)/4
- <u>Laryngeal chemoreflex:</u> central response to stimulation of interarytenoid cleft mucosa characterized by cough, apnea, swallowing, laryngeal closure, cardiovascular instability
  1. swallowing, apnea, and laryngeal closure are the primary responses in newborns
  2. cough becomes the primary response at 1 to 2 months of life
  3. prematurity and history of upper airway infections may increase severity

Communication Disorders

Introduction

- otolaryngologists' primarily role is treatment of underlying medical conditions
- 19% of children have some form of language delay in preschool years
- 7% of children at 5 years of age are clinically language-impaired
- *see* Table 31–1

Anatomic Anomalies

- <u>Face</u>: cleft lip
- <u>Oral cavity</u>: malocclusion, missing teeth, dental arch anomalies, unilateral or bilateral cleft palate, ankyloglossia or macroglossia
- <u>Oropharynx</u>: velopharyngeal incompetence, hypertrophy of tonsils and/or adenoids

TABLE 31–1. Stages of Speech and Language Development

Age	Milestones
Newborn	Root, suck, primitive reflexes, orients to sounds, smiles to voice, variable cries
2 months	Gurgles
4 months	Coos
6 months	Looks toward person talking to him or her, vocalizes to answer, laughs
9 months	Looks to familiar named object, inhibits to "no," vocalizes to initiate
12 months	Turns to names, understands routine commands, babbles or gestures intentionally for behavioral regulation and social interaction
18 months	Follows one-step commands, points to 5 body parts, 15 words, shakes head "no"
2 years	50 words, 2-word phrases, talks instead of gestures, 50% of speech intelligible
3 years	Follows 2-step commands, 3- to 4-word sentences, speech 75% intelligible
4 years	Speech 100% intelligible

- <u>Ear</u>: conductive or sensorineural hearing loss
- other

Assessment of Speech Disorders

- <u>History</u>: prenatal, birth, health, developmental, education, family history
- <u>Standardized measures</u>: compare speech to same-age peers using a normative curve
- <u>Nonstandardized assessment</u>: analyze speech samples to develop sound inventory and determine error type
- <u>Speech intelligibility measurements</u>: age/4 = % speech understood in conversation
    1. 2 years old = 2/4 = 50%
    2. 3 years old = 3/4 = 75%
    3. 4 years old = 4/4 = 100%
- <u>Structural-functional exams</u>: assesses the articulators (lips, tongue, jaw, velum)
- <u>Stimulability tests</u>: determine which therapeutic techniques the child will respond to

Assessment of Language Disorders

- hearing loss is routinely the first disorder excluded
- if comprehension difficulties are suspected, refer to clinical psychologist to evaluate for global disorder, autism spectrum disorder, language-specific impairment, and/or learning disorder
- U.S. federal law mandates availability of assessment and intervention via local early intervention (birth-3 years) or public schools (age 3–22 years)

Levels of Fluency Disorders (Stuttering)

- <u>Borderline</u>: difficult to diagnose, increase in disfluent words, repetitions, and prolongations
- <u>Beginning (2–8 years)</u>: rapid irregular syllable repetition, rise in pitch, blocking
- <u>Intermediate (6–13 years)</u>: onset of fear and avoidance
- <u>Advanced (≥13 years)</u>: child identifies as person who stutters

DISORDERS OF PEDIATRIC AIRWAY AND VOICE

Introduction

- prevalence of pediatric dysphonia generally 6% to 23%
- benign vocal fold lesions are most common cause of dysphonia
- <u>Common structural causes</u>: unilateral and bilateral vocal fold paresis/ paralysis, recurrent respiratory papillomatosis (RRP), laryngeal cleft, glottic web, laryngeal trauma, subglottic stenosis, nodules, cysts
- <u>Functional voice disorders</u>: functional falsetto, puberphonia, paradoxical vocal cord dysfunction, conversion-type disorders; tend to occur in mid- to late childhood
- perceptual analysis with CAPE-V (Consensus Auditory-Perceptual Evaluation of Voice) or GRBAS (Grade, Roughness, Breathiness, Asthenia, Strain) important due to limitations in acoustic and videostroboscopic analysis
- <u>Voice evaluation</u>:
  1. <u>Pitch</u>: abnormal range relative to age and gender, monotone, pitch breaks
  2. <u>Loudness</u>: too loud, too soft, monoloudness, volume lability
  3. <u>Voice quality</u>: roughness/hoarseness, breathiness, and strain/ tension
- <u>History</u>: congenital defects, systemic illnesses, gastroesophageal reflux disease (GERD)/laryngopharyngeal reflux (LPR), pulmonary disorders (eg, asthma, restrictive lung disease), hearing loss, environmental exposures (eg, tobacco, allergen, chemical), professional and avocational voice use, intubation, and surgical history
- <u>Physical exam</u>: ears and hearing, nasal obstruction, tongue position, mobility and volume, adenotonsillar hypertrophy, clefting or hypotonia of the soft palate, craniofacial anomalies
- voice assessment is best done in conjunction with a speech-language pathologist
- <u>Endoscopy/stroboscopy</u>: all efforts should be made to examine the child awake; the 2.8-mm or 4.0-mm flexible laryngoscope is capable of identifying most focal laryngeal lesions; awake rigid laryngoscopy generally is reserved for children >6 years old
- <u>High-speed video</u>: may be particularly helpful when brief phonation limits stroboscopy
- laryngeal electromyography (LEMG) most commonly used to evaluate vocal fold paresis/paralysis in order to differentiate neuropraxic from mechanical causes
- esophageal manometry and 24-hour pH impedance testing helpful to evaluate reflux refractory to therapeutic trial

Puberphonia

- persistence of adolescent voice following puberty in absence of organic causes
- also known as mutational falsetto
- more common in males than females
- incidence is 1:900,000
- rapid lowering and increase in size of the larynx occurs at puberty, which requires retraining of the voice
- Etiology: emotional stress, delayed development of secondary sex characteristics, psychogenic, nonfusion of thyroid laminae, and hypogonadism, Frohlich's syndrome, Klinefelter's syndrome
- Tx: voice therapy, psychological counseling

Vocal Fold Nodules

- reported as most common cause of dysphonia in children with 40% of children presenting with complaint of hoarseness receiving the diagnosis
- affect boys more than girls with bimodal age distribution from ages 3 to 5 years and again at 8 to 10 years; most resolve with puberty
- located in the midportion of musculomembranous portion of vocal fold and generally symmetric
- typical history consists of intermittent hoarseness that worsens with voice and improves with voice rest
- associated with muscle tension dysphonia (MTD) and possible LPR
- Tx: vocal hygiene, voice therapy, behavioral management, and proton pump inhibitors if LPR is present; surgery is rarely indicated, but the preferred technique is excision using a mini-microflap

Vocal Fold Cysts

- can either be acquired or congenital
- congenital cysts are either mucus-filled or epidermal cysts with keratinous material
- difficult to differentiate from nodules since there if often a contralateral reactive mass
- Tx: do not resolve with voice therapy, and surgical excision is generally appropriate

Anterior Glottic Web (See Chapter 12)

- mucosa that extends between the anterior segments of adjacent true vocal folds

- can interfere with airflow across musculomembranous vocal fold, preventing the mucosal wave from propagating and impairing glottic closure, can be asymptomatic
- <u>Etiology</u>: congenital or acquired
  1. <u>Congenital</u>: incomplete recanalization of embryogenic larynx; can range from anterior webbing to complete occlusion of larynx; if moderate to severe, presents with high-pitched weak cry at birth and can be associated with velocardiofacial syndrome
  2. <u>Acquired</u>: typically iatrogenic (eg, intubation, RRP excision), ingestion (caustic)
- must differentiate from mucosal bridge, which is easier to treat and has lower recurrence rate
- <u>Dx</u>: history and physical (H&P), flexible and rigid laryngoscopy with stroboscopy
- <u>Grading</u>: Cohen Classification
  1. <u>Type I</u>: involve 30% or less of the glottis and are free of subglottic extension
  2. <u>Type II</u>: involve 35% to 50% of the glottis, may involve subglottis
  3. <u>Type III</u>: involve 50% to 65% of the glottis, may involve subglottis, thick anteriorly and thin posteriorly
  4. <u>Type IV</u>: involve 75% to 90% of the glottis, uniformly thick with subglottic extension
- <u>Tx</u>: surgical excision is gold standard, high-grade webs may require laryngotracheal reconstruction
- excision is often followed by reformation; thus placement of a keel should always be considered
- **Endoscopic excision**: often successful if the web does not extend below the inferior edge of the vocal fold; techniques include endolaryngeal mucosal flap, endoscopic placement of a keel, endoscopic modification of Dedo technique, and 2-stage procedure with placement of a flanged prosthesis
- **External techniques**: laryngofissure with division of web and keel insertion or stenting and/or laryngotracheal reconstruction

Bilateral Vocal Fold Paralysis (See Chapter 18)

- <u>Pathophysiology</u>: usually congenital, associated with Arnold-Chiari malformation; vincristine toxicity, birth trauma, prolonged intubation, external trauma, cardiovascular abnormalities, peripheral neurological disease, infection
- <u>Presentation</u>: stridor (nearly all), voice typically fairly strong
- <u>Dx</u>: full neurological evaluation, computed tomography (CT) or magnetic resonance imaging (MRI) from head through aortic arch,

fiberoptic endoscopic evaluation of swallowing (FEES)/video swallow study (VSS) if aspiration suspected
- Tx: patients without aspiration, respiratory distress, failure to thrive, or significant dysphonia can be observed closely; approximately 50% of children will require tracheotomy; spontaneous recovery in 50% to 60%
    1. Initial management: watchful waiting, noninvasive positive pressure ventilation (NPPV), unilateral or bilateral cordotomy, endoscopic or external posterior cricoid split with or without grafting, tracheotomy
    2. Secondary management: cordotomy, arytenoidectomy, arytenoidopexy, laryngoplasty (endoscopic or external), laryngeal nerve reinnervation

Unilateral Vocal Fold Paralysis (See Chapter 18)

- Presentation: stridor (75%), dysphonia (50%), dysphagia (25%)
- Pathophysiology: typically iatrogenic most commonly due to cardiothoracic surgery (left sided due to patent ductus arteriosus ligation), birth trauma, prolonged intubation, external trauma, cardiovascular abnormalities, peripheral neurological disease, infection
- an estimated 80% are well compensated, 20% have persistent glottic gap and require voice therapy
- Tx: true vocal fold medialization (temporary or permanent); laryngeal reinnervation
    1. injection laryngoplasty (vocal fold augmentation), laryngeal framework surgery (type 1 thyroplasty, arytenoid adduction, arytenoidopexy), reinnervation procedures
- injection augmentation laryngoplasty can be a temporizing measure allowing for spontaneous recovery; **first line in infant with aspiration**
- medialization thyroplasty is a permanent, but partially reversible technique; **first line in adolescent** who can tolerate local anesthesia
- reinnervation (typically ansa cervicalis-to-RLN [recurrent laryngeal nerve] anastomosis) takes 3 to 6 months to show evidence of effect and negates any opportunity of spontaneous recovery

Iatrogenic Causes of Dysphonia

- Subglottic stenosis (SGS): typically following prolonged intubation; changes in subglottic pressure affect the vibrating vocal folds (see section on Chronic Airway Obstruction)
- Arytenoid dislocation: persistent dysphonia after intubation, extubation, or after trauma; often able to be reduced endoscopically

even after prolonged dislocation; LEMG helps differentiate from neuropraxic injury; prompt reduction may prevent ankylosis; older children generally can be reduced under local anesthesia; young children typically require general anesthesia; if reduction fails, options include type 1 thyroplasty, arytenoidopexy, arytenoid mobilization and repositioning, vocal fold injection, and Botox injection

- Intubation trauma: vocal fold trauma/tear, vocal process avulsion, vocal fold paresis/paralysis, arytenoid subluxation/dislocation

Functional Dystonia

- accounts for up to 7% of pediatric voice disorder referrals
- manifestations include puberphonia, aphonia, MTD, paradoxical vocal fold dysfunction
- MTD features strained voice quality, disordered pitch, reduced loudness
- Tx: manual circumlaryngeal massage and laryngeal posturing, inhalation phonation, throat focused /r/ phonation, singing/voice therapy, gargling, cough initiated phonation, resonant voice therapy, other

CONGENITAL ANOMALIES OF LARYNX AND TRACHEA

Laryngomalacia

- Definition: collapse of supraglottic structures during inspiration resulting in intermittent airflow interference and associated stridor
- **most common cause of stridor in infants**
- Etiology: immaturity or abnormal integration of peripheral nerves, brain stem nuclei, and pathways responsible for swallowing and maintenance of airway patency
- Presentation: symptoms worsen over the first 4 to 8 months of life; stridor is exacerbated by agitation, crying, feeding, upper respiratory tract infections, and supine positioning; failure to thrive (FTT)
- typically resolves spontaneously within 18 to 24 months
- Dx: H&P, flexible laryngoscopy, direct laryngoscopy and bronchoscopy (DLB)
- Laryngoscopic findings: prolapse of redundant arytenoid mucosa or cuneiform cartilage, shortened aryepiglottic (AE) folds, and/or omega-shaped epiglottis
- Comorbidities: GERD/LPR (65%–100%); synchronous airway lesions (12%–64%) including tracheomalacia, subglottic stenosis, and vocal fold paralysis

- <u>Conservative Tx</u>: indicated for mild to moderate stridor with no associated feeding difficulties
    1. monitor weight gain
    2. thickening agents for breast milk or formula
    3. slowed paced feedings in upright position
    4. medications to treat reflux
    5. may also require high-calorie diet, swallow therapy, continuous positive airway pressure (CPAP)
- <u>Surgical Tx</u>: indicated for stridor with respiratory distress, cor pulmonale, severe obstructive sleep apnea (OSA), cyanosis with feeding, aspiration pneumonia, FTT
    1. **Supraglottoplasty:** partial epiglottectomy, division of AE folds, removal of redundant mucosa, and epiglottopexy using microlaryngeal instruments, microdebrider, or CO_2 (carbon dioxide) laser
    2. **Post-op care:** aggressive antireflux therapy; head of bed elevation; short course of steroids improves efficacy; may potentially be extubated shortly after surgery; complete resolution noted in 50% to 95% of patients undergoing supraglottoplasty

Vocal Fold Immobility
(See Section on Voice Disorders)

Laryngocele

- air-filled dilations of the laryngeal saccule that communicate with laryngeal ventricle
- etiology may be congenital, increased laryngeal pressure, or mechanical obstruction
- internal laryngoceles arise in anterior ventricle and extend posteriorly and superiorly to false vocal fold and AE fold
- external laryngoceles extend cephalad through the thyrohyoid membrane
- if required, treatment is endoscopic marsupialization or open excision

Saccular Cyst

- fluid-filled and lack communication with the airway
- anterior saccular cysts are mucosal covered and protrude between false and true vocal folds
- lateral saccular cysts extend into false vocal folds
- may respond to endoscopic marsupialization but entire lining of cyst may need to be removed

Laryngeal Webs
(See Section on Voice Disorders)

Laryngeal Clefts

- incidence ranges from 0.2% to 7.6% in those undergoing DLB for recurrent respiratory symptoms
- <u>Grading</u>: Benjamin and Inglis Classification
  1. <u>Type 1</u>: extends to level of the vocal folds
  2. <u>Type 2</u>: extends below vocal folds and into cricoid cartilage
  3. <u>Type 3</u>: extends through cricoid and into cervical trachea/ esophagus
  4. <u>Type 4</u>: extends to level of thoracic trachea/esophagus
- <u>Presentation</u>: types 1 and 2 have variable rates of respiratory presenting symptoms, most commonly stridor, recurrent infections, and chronic cough; types 3 and 4 are associated with greater respiratory symptoms, recurrent pneumonia, and excessive pulmonary mucus; usually present in first few days of life
- <u>Associated syndromes</u>: Opitz Frias, Pallister Hall, VACTERL association (Vertebral defects, Anal atresia, Cardiac defects, Tracheoesophageal fistula, Renal anomalies, Limb abnormalities) association, CHARGE syndrome (Coloboma, Heart defects, Atresia choanae, Growth retardation/Genital abnormalities, Ear abnormalities)
- <u>Dx</u>: direct laryngoscopy with palpation of the interarytenoid area
- <u>Tx</u>: medical or surgical depending on extent of cleft
  1. <u>Type 1</u>: conservative measures (thickening of liquids; treatment of GERD, reactive airway disease, and food allergy), trial for approximately 6 months before reevaluation with modified barium swallow (MBS), endoscopic surgical management if conservative measures fail
  2. <u>Type 2</u>: endoscopic surgical management in addition to conservative measures
  3. <u>Type 3</u>: most require open thoracotomy and repair, unless sufficient glottic exposure for laser ablation and suture placement
  4. <u>Type 4</u>: open thoracotomy and repair
- **Endoscopic repair**: tubeless anesthesia, mucosal edges are denuded with CO_2 laser with suture closure of the cleft; tracheotomy rarely needed for types 1 and 2
- **Neck surgery and open thoracotomy**: often require tracheotomy and g-tube; crux of therapy is to re-create separate tracheal and esophageal lumen; anterior approach for greatest exposure; often performed with patient on extracorporeal membrane oxygen

(ECMO); interposition grafts utilized such as pericardium, sternocleidomastoid (SCM) muscle flaps, pleura, strap muscle, jejunum, and tibial periosteum

Congenital Subglottic Stenosis
(See Section on Chronic Airway Obstruction)

Laryngeal Hemangiomas
(See Section on Neoplasms of Larynx and Trachea)

PEDIATRIC TRACHEAL ANOMALIES
Background

- symptoms related to size of the airway
- <u>Dx</u>: bronchoscopy gold standard, imaging useful
    1. **CT/CT angiogram (CTA)**: imaging modality of choice, inspiratory/expiratory if able, assess vasculature
    2. **Chest radiograph (CXR)**: limited role, may show postobstructive hyperinflation, pneumonia, narrowing of trachea
    3. **Airway fluoroscopy**: dynamic assessment of airway, good for vascular anomalies, alternative for children who cannot tolerate bronchoscopy
    4. **Barium swallow**: esophageal anomalies
    5. **MRI/magnetic resonance angiography (MRA)**: cine MR also for dynamic assessment of airway, good for vascular anomalies
- <u>Tx</u>: expectant management, endoscopic versus open surgical repair

Tracheal Agenesis and Atresia

- rare congenital anomaly, nearly universal mortality
- <u>Presentation</u>: aphonic cry, respiratory distress, cyanosis, poor Apgar scores, tracheal rings not palpable on physical exam, other features of VACTERL association, unable to pass nasogastric tube if esophageal atresia present
- <u>Dx</u>: laryngoscopy (absence of vocal folds), can bag mask ventilate or intubate esophagus to temporize if cannot ventilate, especially if patient has tracheoesophageal fistula (TEF)
- <u>Grading</u>: Floyd Tracheal Agenesis Classification
    1. <u>Type 1</u>: proximal trachea absent, airway connects to distal TEF
    2. <u>Type 2</u>: **most common**, carina arises from lower esophagus

3. <u>Type 3</u>: main-stem bronchi originate from two separate anastomoses within the esophagus
- <u>Tx</u>: gastrostomy tube (alimentation), surgical correction
  1. esophagus and salivary fistula as neotrachea with double-barrel proximal esophagostomy
  2. fistula and neotrachea begin at superior and inferior ends of esophagostomy, respectively

Tracheal Webs

- less common than laryngeal webs
- most commonly at level of cricoid
- <u>Tx</u>: surgical correction, endoscopic versus open resection and anastomosis

Tracheoesophageal Fistula

- esophageal atresia (EA) most common congenital anomaly of the esophagus (1:3500) ± TEF
- <u>Presentation</u>: most diagnosed shortly after birth, sialorrhea, respiratory distress, cyanosis with alimentation, inability to pass 10 Fr catheter past 10 cm, other features of VACTERL and CHARGE, 50% with other congenital anomalies, mostly cardiovascular
- <u>Dx</u>: CXR (gastric bubble and air in proximal pouch); Gastrografin swallow (risk of aspiration); endoscopy preferred
- Five types of anomalies:
  1. EA with distal TEF (85%)
  2. isolated EA without TEF (8%)
  3. H-type TEF (4%)
  4. EA with proximal TEF (3%)
  5. EA with proximal and distal TEF (< 1%)
- <u>Tx</u>: immediate gastrostomy; primary anastomosis at 3 months or Foker's technique (elongate esophagus with external traction sutures prior to anastomosis)
- <u>Complications</u>: anastomotic leaks, esophageal strictures, esophageal dysmotility, tracheomalacia, GERD
- 20% of patients following repair of EA have normal pulmonary function long term

Tracheomalacia

- <u>Pathophysiology</u>: increased compliance and flaccidity of supportive anterolateral cartilaginous framework → increased collapse on

expiration when intrathoracic pressure exceeds intraluminal pressure
(most commonly in distal third of trachea)
1. Primary tracheomalacia: intrinsic weakness in the trachea itself,
   incidence higher in premature infants, EA with TEF
2. Secondary tracheomalacia: localized inflammation or breakdown
   of tracheal wall → segmental collapse of a portion of the airway,
   seen in prolonged intubation or tracheotomy, extrinsic compression
   of vascular rings, mediastinal mass, cardiac enlargement
- Sx: mild to severe respiratory symptoms depending on location,
  length, severity, degree of collapse (eg, expiratory or biphasic stridor,
  wheezing, cough, retractions, recurrent pulmonary infections,
  cyanosis, feeding difficulties, FTT, apneas, apparent life-threatening
  event (ALTE), associated with cardiovascular malformations (20%–
  58%), bronchopulmonary dysplasia (52%), GERD (50%–78%)
- Dx: bronchoscopy during spontaneous ventilation (decrease in
  luminal diameter greater than 50% at end expiration)
- Tx (mild to moderate): antibiotics for recurrent respiratory infections,
  humidified oxygen (including home oxygen), intermittent steroids,
  GERD treatment, pulmonary physiotherapy, may require frequent
  hospitalizations, CPAP
1. improvement in 6 to 12 months; resolution by 2 years due to
   cartilage maturation
- Tx (severe): surgical management
1. **Tracheotomy:** required in 12% to 62%, longer tube used to
   stent distal trachea
2. **Aortopexy:** aorta sutured to undersurface of sternum →
   increased anteroposterior (AP) tracheal diameter to stent open
   tracheal lumen; indicated for tracheomalacia associated with EA,
   TEF, or vascular rings, and severe primary tracheomalacia
3. **Tracheal stenting**: options include silicone tube (eg,
   Dumon stent or Montgomery T-tube), wire, hybrid, metal,
   or bioabsorbable stent; FDA advisory against metallic airway
   stents in benign airway disorders due to high complication rates;
   complications include infection, restenosis, granuloma formation,
   adjacent erosion of vasculature
4. **Splinting**: extraluminal, does not disrupt mucosa, may resist
   external compression to allow for tracheal growth

Tracheal Stenosis (See Chapter 14)

- Congenital stenosis: O-shaped complete cartilaginous rings;
  commonly associated with pulmonary artery sling, cardiac defects,
  lower airway arborization

- Acquired stenosis: endoluminal scarring or collapse due to prolonged intubation, tracheotomy, other previous surgery, inhalational chemical burn injury, trauma, infection, inflammatory disorders (eg, granulomatosis with polyangiitis [Wegener's granulomatosis], polychondritis)
- Presentation: symptoms depend on diameter of obstructive segment; respiratory distress, stridor, cyanosis, cough, ALTEs, intermittent wheezing, exercise intolerance
- Dx: **rigid bronchoscopy** (gold standard) to evaluate length and diameter of stenosed tracheal segment; echocardiogram and contrast chest CT often obtained to assess vascular anatomy; CT should not replace bronchoscopy for diagnosis as CT may underestimate degree and length of airway stenosis
- Grading: Cantrell and Guild Structural Classification
  1. Type 1: generalized hypoplasia of the entire trachea
  2. Type 2: funnel stenosis: normal proximal trachea with distal narrowing to carina
  3. Type 3: segmental stenosis with up to 3 rings involved
- Tx: medical versus surgical, based on length and degree of stenosis, location of stenosis, presence of previous scarring or cartilage loss, comorbidities
- **Observation**: monitored with serial bronchoscopies or high-resolution imaging, may experience "catch-up" growth and achieve normal tracheal diameter with time (~10% can be managed conservatively)
- **Endoscopic CO_2 laser**: star-shaped radial incisions followed by dilation or trapdoor flap; relative contraindications include stenosis >1 cm, cicatricial scarring, cartilage loss or deformity, and lesions at the carina; limited success in treatment of complete rings
- **Dilation**: endoscopic technique used mostly for acquired stenosis and in postoperative patients, often need repeat procedures, topical mitomycin C used to decrease scar formation; best avoided in first 3 to 4 weeks after open tracheal surgery; complications include tracheal rupture, laceration, pneumomediastinum, and pneumothorax
- **Cryotherapy:** efficacy evidence limited, but thought to cause less scarring than heat thermal energy due to preservation of extracellular matrix, may also treat granulation tissue that arises from wire or silastic stents and eliminates risk of airway combustion
- **Topical medications**: intralesional steroids, topical Mitomycin C, topical dexamethasone and fluoroquinolone
- **Open surgical repair**
  1. patch tracheoplasty, segmental resection and reanastomosis, wedge resection, tracheal autograft, slide tracheoplasty, transplanted tissue (autografts or allografts)

2. Indications: when conservative or endoscopic therapies have failed or are no longer indicated
3. will likely need intermittent distal tracheal intubation, ECMO, cardiopulmonary bypass
4. Complications: granulation tissue (most common), restenosis, excessive tension on suture lines may lead to anastomotic breakdown → catastrophic rupture of the airway, mediastinitis, pneumomediastinum, pneumothorax, death

VASCULAR RINGS

Introduction

- minimal compression to complete collapse of trachea
- extrinsic compression may result in tracheomalacia
- Sx: depend on severity; asymptomatic to chronic cough, cyanosis, stridor, recurrent bronchopneumonia, FTT
- Dx: **bronchoscopy** showing characteristic areas of compression, CTA, MRI if compression less than or equal to one-third tracheal length or right AP compression (*right* suggests double aortic arch, complete vascular ring, or pulmonary artery sling, which all warrant surgical correction)
- Tx: surgical correction of complete vascular rings, left pulmonary artery sling; may observe incomplete vascular rings depending on symptoms

Complete Vascular Rings

Double Aortic Arch

- **most common complete vascular ring**
- Pathophysiology: distal right fourth branchial arch fails to involute → development of paired aortas; right arch larger and more cephalad, passes behind esophagus before joining left arch to form left-sided descending aorta
- Dx: bronchoscopy → pulsatile compression of right anterior and posterior distal trachea (fishmouth deformity)
- Tx: surgical correction, division of vascular ring via limited left thoracotomy or video-assisted thoracic surgery
- mild respiratory symptoms persist for months to years in 30% to 50% of surgical patients

Right Aortic Arch With Aberrant Left Subclavian Artery and Left Ligamentum Arteriosum

- <u>Pathophysiology</u>: mid-left fourth arch involutes → left subclavian artery and left ligamentum arteriosum arise from *Kommerell diverticulum* (remnant outpouching of distal left fourth arch within descending aorta)
- milder symptoms than double aortic arch
- <u>Dx</u>: bronchoscopy → pulsatile compression of right lower third of trachea on right anterior wall and of right main-stem bronchus at takeoff posterolaterally (by diverticulum of Kommerell in the descending arch)
    1. lateral view of angiogram shows "hairpin" aorta at apex of chest and location of diverticulum of Kommerell
- <u>Tx</u>: surgical correction

Incomplete Vascular Rings

Aberrant Innominate Artery

- <u>Pathophysiology</u>: arises from abnormal distal takeoff from aortic arch, ascends over anterior trachea approximately 1 to 2 cm from carina
- <u>Dx</u>: bronchoscopy → anterior midtracheal pulsatile compression
- <u>Tx</u>: surgical correction depending on symptomatology
    1. aortopexy if patient experiences ATLEs or reflex apnea; resolves respiratory symptoms in 80% of patients, mild residual malacia may take months to resolve
    2. may also reimplant innominate artery into distal aorta (does not have benefit of splinting open airway from suspension)

Left Pulmonary Artery Sling

- <u>Pathophysiology</u>: develops when left pulmonary artery arises from right pulmonary artery and passes between trachea and esophagus to cause compression of right main-stem bronchus and distal trachea
- <u>Dx</u>: bronchoscopy → pulsatile compression of right anterior distal trachea and right main-stem bronchus
- complete tracheal rings and long-segment tracheal stenosis seen in 50% of patients
- <u>Tx</u>: surgical correction

MANAGEMENT OF FOREIGN BODIES

Foreign-Body Aspiration

Background

- toddlers 2 to 4 years old, males > females (2:1)
- Pathophysiology: no full posterior dentition or mature neuromuscular mechanisms for swallowing/airway protection
- Most common: organic (peanuts, beans, seeds)—may absorb water and swell → rapid complete obstruction; inert (plastic toys)—may be radiolucent and undetectable on CXR

Clinical Presentation

- symptoms vary depending on size, location, composition, degree of obstruction, etc
- Acute symptoms: gagging, choking (50% unwitnessed)
- Chronic symptoms: nonspecific pulmonary complaints (intermittent coughing or wheezing, even in absence of acute history)
- must have high degree of suspicion (may be treated for asthma, allergies, or presumed pulmonary infection prior to arriving at diagnosis)
- seven times more likely to have a delay in diagnosis than esophageal foreign bodies

Diagnosis

- Chest auscultation: decreased breath sounds ± wheezing on obstructed side
- CXR: inspiratory/expiratory views (coin usually in sagittal plane), lateral decubitus view (dependent lung remains inflated when obstruction present)
- normal CXR + suspicious history → bronchoscopy
- CT chest: high sensitity, decreases delay in diagnosis and negative bronchoscopies

Treatment

- follow Airway Foreign Body Algorithm following ERC (European Resuscitation Council) and AHA (American Heart Association) guidelines

- removal with rigid bronchoscopy (success rate 95%–99%)
- reintroduce endoscope after removal into trachea to search for additional foreign body (5%) and trauma to tracheal mucosa
- avoid manipulating foreign body to reduce further trauma and dislodgement to more distal location
- postintubation airway edema → treat with IV dexamethasone and nebulized epinephrine
- if rigid bronchoscopy with retrieval unsuccessful → use Roth net, endoscopic basket, Heimlich's maneuver in tandem with bronchoscopy; consider more invasive tracheotomy, thoracotomy, or bronchotomy (remaining 0.3%–4%)

Foreign-Body Ingestion

Background

- 1500 people die each year from complications related to foreign-body ingestion (most commonly children)
- Most common: coins, toys, disc batteries, fish bones, food
- Most commonly fatal: segment of a hot dog
- Sites of obstruction:
    1. level of upper esophageal sphincter/cricopharyngeus muscle (60%–70%)
    2. level of aortic arch in mid esophagus (10%–20%)
    3. level of lower esophageal sphincter (20%)
    4. if elsewhere → consider underlying anatomic abnormality (eg, congenital esophageal stricture)

Clinical Presentation

- symptoms depend on size of foreign body, location, site of impaction, etc
- Acute symptoms: respiratory distress (extreme compliance of party wall between esophagus and trachea → mass effect)
- Chronic symptoms: dysphagia, drooling

Diagnosis

- CXR: anteroposterior and lateral views → if coin in esophagus, face in coronal plane
- can usually differentiate coin aspiration from ingestion → face in sagittal plane

Treatment

- ABCs (airway, breathing, circulation); may need emergent tracheotomy
- removal with rigid esophagoscopy
- Timing: depends on symptoms and object
  1. **Emergent esophagoscopy**: unable to tolerate secretions, respiratory distress, disc battery/button battery, sharp object with potential to perforate esophagus (eg, open safety pin)
  2. **Observation**: if asymptomatic may postpone esophagoscopy for 12 to 24 hours, repeat CXR to see if foreign body is still there or has passed into stomach

Disc Battery/Button Battery

Background

- highest harm potential of all esophageal foreign bodies, increasing incidence
- Poison Control reported ~2000 disc batteries in 1998 versus ~10,000 in 2007
- Mechanism of injury: low-voltage electrical discharge (eg, electrical burn), leakage of battery contents (may be alkaline or acidic depending on type of battery), pressure necrosis; injury may occur as early as 1 hour after ingestion
- negative battery pole causes most severe, necrotic injury (narrowest side on lateral neck XR)

Diagnosis

- must have high index of suspicion
- if ingestion witnessed → check AP XR as described later in chapter for characteristic signs
- if ingestion not witnessed → suspect if patient has airway obstruction or wheezing, drooling, vomiting, chest discomfort, dysphagia, decreased PO intake, refusal to eat, coughing, choking, or gagging with eating or drinking
- Radiograph (neck, esophagus, abdomen): AP view for battery's double-rim or halo-effect, lateral view for step off; absence of finding does not exclude
- immediately call the 24-hour National Button Battery Ingestion Hotline at 202-625-3333

Treatment

- refer to Poison Control's *National Capital Center Button Battery Ingestion Triage and Treatment Guideline*
- parents should administer honey or sucralfate if ≤12 hours after ingestion, prevents local generation of hydroxide, reduces morbidity and mortality
- remain NPO otherwise, do not delay esophagoscopy and removal if patient has eaten
- **emergent endoscopy for removal within 2 hours of ingestion**, even if patient asymptomatic
- assess extent of injury, location, direction negative pole faces, etc
- if no perforation → irrigate injured areas with 50 to 150 mL 0.25% sterile acetic acid to neutralize residual alkali
- if substantial erosion → bronchoscopy to evaluate for tracheal wall fistula, post-op CXR and esophagram to evaluate for perforation

Delayed Complications

- TEF, esophageal perforation, mediastinitis, vocal fold paralysis, tracheal stenosis or tracheomalacia, aspiration pneumonia, empyema, lung abscess, pneumothorax, spondylodiscitis, exsanguination from perforation into large vessel, esophageal strictures
- perforations and fistulas usually delayed (98% diagnosed by 48 days after battery removal)
- higher risk of TEF if negative battery pole is facing anterior esophageal wall
- esophageal strictures delayed weeks to months

ACUTE AIRWAY OBSTRUCTION (AAO)

Introduction

- <u>Etiology</u>: laryngotracheal bronchitis (LTB), acute supraglottitis, bacterial tracheitis, adenotonsillar hypertrophy, deep neck space infection, anaphylaxis, spasmodic croup, airway foreign body, trauma, congenital anomalies, neoplasia
- <u>SSx</u>: dyspnea, voice changes, cough, dysphagia, sore throat
- <u>General appearance</u>: overall appearance will determine urgency of initial actions; restlessness, anxiety, diaphoresis indicate air hunger; initially will be tachycardic; cyanosis and bradycardia are late signs; substernal retractions, sniffing position, and use of intercostal muscles indicate increased work of breathing

- Voice characteristics: range from normal voice to hoarseness to complete aphonia; indicates inflammation of true vocal folds or subglottis; supraglottic obstruction typically does not affect the quality of voice, but may cause muffling or "hot potato voice"
- **Stertor**: snoring or snorting sound that is produced by turbulence in the pharynx
- **Stridor**: high-pitched sound produced by turbulent flow within the laryngeal or tracheal airway
    1. inspiratory stridor → supraglottic
    2. expiratory stridor → subglottic, tracheal
    3. biphasic stridor → glottic
- drooling indicates supraglottic pain and/or swelling
- accessory respiratory muscle use (eg, suprasternal and substernal retractions, nasal flaring, intercostal muscle use)
- subcutaneous emphysema result of rupture of respiratory or digestive tracts

Diagnostic Evaluation

Ventilation Assessment

- children have much higher metabolic rate than adults and thus less reserve
- pulse oximetry and transcutaneous monitoring of CO_2 provides ongoing record of ventilation
- ABGs (arterial blood gas) may not be a true reflection since children often cry and struggle while they are drawn

Radiographic Assessment

- Lateral neck XR: best initial study in AAO when emergent airway intervention is not warranted
- AP neck XR: may see steeple sign in LTB and other conditions that cause subglottic edema
- CXR: tracheal air shadow altered, radiopaque foreign bodies, pulmonary infections

Endoscopic Evaluation

- flexible laryngoscopy used to assess airway from nares to true vocal folds with local anesthesia
- examination distal to glottis is performed under general anesthesia
- can evaluate true vocal fold motion in nonparalyzed patients under general anesthesia

- rigid bronchoscope has the advantage of superior optics and ability to establish and maintain an airway

Management of AAO

Nonsurgical Intervention

- **Observation**: intervening can often make a stable airway unstable; typically monitored in ICU setting
- **Oxygen and humidity**: liquifies secretions and aids in clearance
- **Racemic epinephrine**: α-agonist properties decrease mucosal edema; lasts 30 to 60 minutes; effective in croup and decreases need for intubation and tracheotomy; due to rebound effect patients should be monitored for 4 to 6 hours
- **Corticosteroids**: suppressed cycle of inflammation that leads to edema of injured tissue; dexamethasone is most commonly used in airway due to long half-life, high anti-inflammatory potency, and low mineralocorticoid effect; dose of dexamethasone is 1.0 to 1.5 mg/kg/day with first half given in first dose and remainder given at 6 to 8 hour intervals; max daily dose is 10 mg to 30 mg; use in LTB controversial; beneficial in postintubation trauma, adenotonsillar hypertrophy secondary to EBV, allergic edema, prior to extubation of patients with epiglottitis
- **Antibiotics**: appropriate for patients with group A streptococcus (GAS) pharyngitis, epiglottitis, pertussis, diphtheria, and bacterial tracheitis
- **Heliox**: low density of helium-oxygen mixture leads to less turbulence and less gas resistance; can be used as temporizing measure in AAO
- **Nasal and oral airways**: nasal airways are tolerated better than oral airways; distal end of a nasal airway should bypass the soft palate
- **Intubation**: subglottis dictates the size of the ETT (endotracheal tube); tube should have leak around it at <30 mm Hg
  1. 0 to 3 months—3.5 mm
  2. 3 to 9 months—4.0 mm
  3. 9 months to 2 years—4.5 mm
  4. after 2 years—18+ age (years)/4
- **Translaryngeal or transtracheal ventilation**: form of emergency ventilation used as temporizing measure only until surgical airway is established
  1. 16-gauge needle inserted through cricothyroid membrane or directly into trachea and O_2 is delivered
  2. bag ventilate if the patient is <5 years old (risk of barotrauma with jet ventilation)
  3. jet ventilate if the patient is >5 years old

Surgical Intervention

- <u>Endoscopy</u>: standard laryngoscope and appropriately sized pediatric ventilating bronchoscope can be used to secure airway; if pathologic condition can be treated, child may be intubated or tracheotomy can be performed with bronchoscope controlling the airway
- <u>Open tracheotomy</u>: ***preferred* to cricothyrotomy**; emergent tracheotomy has a high incidence of complications; percutaneous tracheotomy contraindicated in children as airway is difficult to localize and stabilize due to collapsible and mobile nature of pediatric trachea
- <u>Cricothyrotomy</u>: *relative contraindications for cricothyrotomy* include age younger than 10 years, severe neck trauma with inability to palpate landmarks, and expanding neck hematoma, may perform needle cricothyrotomy in children <10 years old; higher risk of laryngeal stenosis and injury to surrounding structures due to anatomy of pediatric larynx

CHRONIC AIRWAY OBSTRUCTION

Pediatric Subglottic Stenosis (SGS)

Etiology

- <u>Congenital SGS</u>: results from abnormality during embryogenesis; membranous type is generally circumferential and is 2 to 3 mm below the TVF; cartilaginous type is more variable; most common pattern is lateral shelving appearing as an elliptically shaped cricoid cartilage
- <u>Laryngeal atresia and glottic web</u>: variant of acquired SGS where the vocal folds are involved; glottic webs are associated with velocardiofacial syndrome; most severe form is complete laryngeal atresia with fusion of true vocal folds, which presents as congenital high airway obstruction syndrome (CHAOS), diagnosed by prenatal ultrasound
- <u>Acquired SGS</u>: initially associated with laryngeal infections such as diphtheria, now predominantly due to prolonged intubation for respiratory support of neonates; factors include size of ETT, duration of intubation, traumatic intubation, presence of infection while intubated, and GERD/LPR

Diagnosis

- <u>History</u>: birth injury, history of intubation, prematurity, onset and duration of stridor (inspiratory, expiratory, biphasic), voice quality, feeding abnormalities; if presenting with extubation failure, exclude nasal obstruction, glossoptosis, and tracheobronchomalacia; in intubated patient, gather information pertaining to reason for initial intubation, size of the ETT, and presence of an air leak

- <u>Imaging</u>: airway films may show steepling or complete tracheal rings; FEES and VSS if there is suspicion for aspiration
- <u>Preoperative optimization</u>: surgery on inflamed larynx is likely to fail; inflammation may relate to GERD/LPR or eosinophilic esophagitis (EE); 30% are colonized with methicillin-resistant *Staphylococcus aureus* or pseudomonas; screen for colonization with culture of nares and tracheal aspirate; if present, treat preoperatively and postoperatively
- laryngotracheal endoscopy is the gold standard for airway evaluation
- <u>Grading</u>: Myers-Cotton Scale
  1. <u>Grade 1</u>: <50%
  2. <u>Grade 2</u>: 50% to 70%
  3. <u>Grade 3</u>: 71% to 99%
  4. <u>Grade 4</u>: 100% (no detectable lumen)

Scar Excision and Balloon Dilation

- endoscopic technique
- has reduced need for open airway surgery by 80%
- ideal in children with grade 1 or 2 stenosis with thin or weblike and soft stenosis consisting of immature scar tissue
- patients with firm or mature scar tissue, cartilaginous airway narrowing, and structural problems of the airway exoskeleton are less likely to respond
- scar division may be performed utilizing sickle knife, microlaryngeal scissors, or laser (CO_2 or Nd:YAG); scar may be divided prior to balloon dilation

Laryngotracheal Reconstruction

- division of anterior cricoid and first 2 tracheal rings and/or posterior cricoid followed by placement of cartilage graft
- <u>Single stage</u>: decannulated at end of procedure, ETT left in place as a stent for ~7 days
- <u>Double stage</u>: tracheotomy remains in place with long-term stent, may instead use a Montgomery T-tube in certain circumstances
- costal cartilage most widely used graft material
- <u>Anterior cricoid split with graft</u>: indicated in milder grades of SGS that have failed endoscopic management; typically single stage
- <u>Posterior cricoid split with graft</u>: indicated in severe SGS, posterior glottic stenosis, or bilateral vocal fold immobility

- in infants younger than 9 months, a single-stage anterior graft can be performed with a posterior cricoid split, generally left intubated for 7 to 10 days

Congenital Tracheal Stenosis
(See Section on Pediatric Tracheal Anomalies)

TRAUMATIC INJURIES TO LARYNX, TRACHEA, ESOPHAGUS, AND NECK

Introduction

- ~83% blunt, ~17% penetrating
- median age of ~13 years
- >75% have associated multisystem trauma
- pediatric neck trauma rare relative to incidence in adults
- children have shorter necks; larynx at C2–C6 depending on age, which allows for better protection by the mandible
- pediatric larynx more soft and pliable than adult larynx, thyroid cartilage does not ossify until about 20 years of age → makes the pediatric larynx more resistant to fracture from compression of cartilage against cervical vertebrae
- submucosal tissues of pediatric larynx attached loosely to underlying perichondrium → increases risk of significant edema and avulsion injuries
- children more susceptible to airway compromise from edema because airway resistance increases by power of 4 with any decrease in radius of airway lumen

Pediatric Blunt Neck Trauma

- <u>Etiology</u>: bicycle accidents, sports injuries, falls in which anterior neck strikes an object, clothesline injuries, strangulation, abuse
- <u>Initial assessment</u>: follow Advanced Trauma Life Support (ATLS) protocol, ensure secure airway first, stabilize patient, identify and treat any imminent life-threatening injuries, obtain history from patient, parent, or other witness (including mechanism of injury)
- gently palpate laryngeal framework to assess for fracture
- must have high suspicion for blunt laryngeal trauma, physical exam findings often correlate poorly with degree of injury unless patient is in acute respiratory distress
- <u>Presentation</u>: hoarseness/dysphonia, aphonia, odynophagia, dysphagia, cervical tenderness, cervical crepitus, hemoptysis, stridor, respiratory distress

Evaluation: Stable Patient

- perform flexible laryngoscopy (FL) initially when no signs of impending airway collapse
- consider CT for occult laryngeal fracture after FL if has potential for altering management
- if patient has significant endolaryngeal injury (eg, exposed cartilage) ± airway compromise, fracture, or progression of symptoms, edema, airway distress, or crepitus → panendoscopy ± tracheotomy
- if no fracture or CT not performed → observation with serial FL exams for 24 to 48 hours; if no progression of edema, OK to discharge with follow-up
- perform contrast esophagram prior to initiating PO intake

Evaluation: Unstable Patient

- if patient presents with acute airway distress → panendoscopy ± tracheotomy
- attempt gentle mask ventilation initially; avoid aggressive positive pressure to prevent worsening cervical emphysema, which may compromise ventilation
- intubation increases risk of laryngeal injury and should be performed fiberoptically in the operating room with a small endotracheal tube and good visualization of the larynx; avoid laryngeal mask airway (LMA); emergent surgical airway if needed
- if intubated in the field prior to arrival, must be suspicious for potential laryngeal injury and confirm placement of ETT
- intubation prior to airway evaluation may result in delayed diagnosis of laryngeal trauma and/or complications (eg, extubation failure, laryngotracheal stenosis)
- if emergent surgical airway indicated open tracheotomy preferred
- consider cricothyrotomy and translaryngeal or transtracheal ventilation in rare circumstances
- cricothyrotomy contraindicated if unable to palpate continuity of cricoid cartilage with tracheal rings to rule out laryngotracheal separation

Schaefer Classification System for Severity of Laryngeal Injuries

- *Grade I*: minor endolaryngeal hematoma without detectable fracture
- *Grade II*: edema, hematoma, minor mucosal disruption without exposed cartilage, nondisplaced fractures
- *Grade III*: massive edema, mucosal disruption, exposed cartilage, vocal fold immobility, displaced fracture

- *Grade IV*: grade III with 2 fracture lines or massive trauma to laryngeal mucosa
- *Grade V*: complete laryngotracheal separation

Treatment

- **Observation (grade I and select grade II injuries)**:
    1. elevate head of bed, voice rest, humidified air, acid suppression medication, antibiotics, corticosteroids
    2. tracheotomy tray should be kept at bedside, monitor with serial FL exams for 24 to 48 hours as previously discussed
    3. beware of worsening airway edema prior to resolution
    4. if subcutaneous emphysema → serial XR indicated with serial exams
- **Indications for Open Surgical Repair**: laryngeal cartilage fractures, exposed cartilage, significant mucosal lacerations, lacerations involving the free edge of the vocal folds or anterior commissure, vocal fold avulsion, cricoarytenoid dislocation, vocal fold paralysis, cricotracheal or laryngotracheal disruption
- **Surgical (select grade II, grades III to V injuries)**: secure airway first (*tracheotomy preferred*), repair of laryngeal injuries secondary; open repair standard approach for severe cases, some injuries amenable to endoscopic repair; goal to preserve anatomy and function of larynx (eg, phonation, airway patency, protection against aspiration, swallowing); endolarynx may be exposed via existing thyroid fracture, midline or paramedian thyrotomy or laryngofissure; miniplates in children more technically challenging due to nonossified thyroid cartilage, and the author (RTS) recommends figure-of-eight sutures; consider stent placement if patient at risk of developing synechiae or subsequent stenosis (eg, anterior commissure injury, significant lacerations of opposing mucosal surfaces); perform rigid esophagoscopy at time of surgery to evaluate for esophageal injury

Pediatric Penetrating Neck Trauma

- rarer than pediatric blunt neck trauma, pediatric penetrating neck trauma has prevalence of 0.28% of pediatric trauma
- <u>Etiology</u>: gunshot, fall on a sharp object, dog bite, stabbing
- <u>Initial assessment</u>: see Pediatric Blunt Neck Trauma
- <u>Presentation</u>: "hard and soft signs" as reported by Tessler et al (2017), as well as those mentioned in Pediatric Blunt Neck Trauma section
- "hard and soft signs" can predict need for selective neck exploration
- **Hard signs**: active hemorrhage, airway compromise, air bubbling wound, expanding/pulsatile hematoma, hematemesis, hemiparesis,

massive subcutaneous emphysema, pulse deficit, respiratory distress, shock; sensitivity 100%, specificity 94.4%

- **Soft signs**: neck bruit, chest tube air leak, dysphagia, dyspnea, hemoptysis, laceration >2 cm, minor hemoptysis, nonpulsatile/nonexpanding hematoma, paresthesias, stridor, venous oozing, voice changes; sensitivity 100%, specificity 75.5%
- **neck laceration >2 cm** and **venous oozing** from injury are **pediatric-specific soft signs**
- Management: data in pediatric population sparse—historically, management in adults focused on addressing three anatomic neck zones to better characterize injuries and dictate management
  1. Zone 1: below level of clavicles
  2. Zone 2: level of clavicles to angle of the mandible
  3. Zone 3: superior to angle of the mandible to skull base
- adult practice now focuses on selective neck exploration based on physical examination and use of CT angiogram in stable patients (WTA 2013 Algorithm)
- panendoscopy and esophagram indicated if relevant tissue planes are violated
- Tx: selective neck exploration if positive for hard/soft signs of injury or positive CTA
- bullet removal indicated in child with documented elevated lead levels, usually months after injury (extremely rare)

Tracheal Injury

- ranges from minor laceration to complete transection of trachea
- Presentation: cervical emphysema, respiratory distress (must have high index of suspicion)
- Tx: secure airway (if severe, tracheotomy required); may require intubation to bypass injury → perform under bronchoscopic guidance to avoid extending tracheal injury; if minor injury, may extubate or decannulate when stable and subcutaneous emphysema resolves; surgical management if significant laceration or separation of cricoid/larynx and trachea
- Cricotracheal or laryngotracheal disruption: repair with primary anastomosis of disrupted segments ± stent placement; may create stoma with distal segment of trachea if unable to perform primary anastomosis; laryngectomy or laryngotracheal separation with a permanent tracheostoma reserved as option for severe laryngeal injuries (eg, complete laryngeal crush injury); laryngeal transplant may be considered after
- Postoperative care: similar to conservative management as above for grade I injuries; tracheotomy kept until patient can be decannulated

safely; drain placed intraoperatively and removed when output is low and when risk of subcutaneous air is decreased; VSS and/ or esophagram obtained prior to initiating PO intake; serial FLs as outpatient, airway endoscopy prior to decannulation

Esophageal Injury (*See* Section on Laryngeal Trauma, Caustic Ingestion)

Airway Fire/Inhalation Injury (*See* Section on Laryngeal Trauma)

NEOPLASMS OF LARYNX AND TRACHEA

Juvenile Recurrent Respiratory Papillomatosis (JRRP)

- JRRP defined as onset prior to 12 years old
- most common benign neoplasm of the larynx of the pediatric population
- Risk factors: boys and girls affected equally, 75% diagnosed by fifth birthday, 75% affected are first born (long time spent in second stage of delivery in birth canal), vaginally delivered infants of primigravid women of low socioeconomic status
- Presentation: progressive dysphonia, inspiratory or biphasic stridor, dyspnea
- Pathophysiology: majority HPV types 6 and 11; malignant transformation rare but more common with HPV types 16 and 18; change in viral type can occur over time; usually transmitted vertically; preference for the squamociliary junction of aerodigestive epithelium; most common locations are upper and lower ventricles, undersurface of vocal folds, and laryngeal surface of epiglottis; tracheotomy may accelerate distal spread
- Complications: pulmonary involvement, hemorrhage and abscess, respiratory compromise
- consider chest imaging to evaluate pulmonary involvement
- Tx: mainstay is surgical debulking; important to only remove superficial layer of laryngeal mucosa, protect the underlying vocal ligament
- **CO$_2$ laser:** associated with development of anterior and posterior glottic scars and webs, risks muscle damage, permits deep extension of papillomatosis

- **Microdebrider**: preferred instrument, especially with exophytic and pedunculated lesion; linked with quicker voice improvement, reduced cost, shorter operative time
- Criteria for adjuvant therapy: ≥4 surgeries per year, rapid return of aggressive disease, and distal airway spread; options include cidofovir, interferon, retinoids, acyclovir, photodynamic therapy, bevacizumab, indole-3-carbinol, other

Airway Hemangiomas

- Etiology: true tumors derived from neural crest cells that exhibit features of neoplasia but have capacity to involute with age
- 2:1 female preponderance
- associated with PHACE syndrome (Posterior brain malformations; large, segmental facial Hemangiomas often in V1, V2, V3 distribution; Arterial anomalies; Cardiac anomalies and aortic coarctation; Eye anomalies)
- characterized by proliferative and involuting phases
- Pathophysiology: tumor growth regulated by the renin-angiotensin system; increased renin levels during first year of life cause proliferation; as tumor proliferates, fibrous septae separate tumor into lobular compartments; involution phase occurs between 12 and 24 months of age due to presence of antiangiogenic factors; fibrous tissue and fat deposited in place of shrinking vessels
- Presentation: biphasic stridor with barking cough in absence of dysphonia; majority present within 6 months (80%–90%); respiratory symptoms resolve slowly beginning at 9 to 12 months once proliferative phase is complete; normal swallowing
- 50% of those with airway hemangioma will have cutaneous hemangioma
- 1% to 2% with cutaneous hemangioma will have airway hemangioma
- *"beard distribution"* of cutaneous hemangioma is predictor of airway hemangioma
- symptomatic hemangiomas typically involve the subglottis
- Dx: FL → CTA if diagnosis of hemangioma is likely (some prefer immediate DLB); left-sided predominance has been reported; stain positively for GLUT1, biopsy not advised
- Tx: watchful waiting in cases with minimal symptomatology, propranolol, surgery
    1. **Propranolol**: initial dose of 0.5 to 1 mg/kg/day increased to goal dose of 2 mg/kg/day over course of days to weeks; other options include intralesional steroids and interferon α-2A
    2. **Surgical excision**: subtotal endoscopic approach or by total excision through a laryngofissure; laser is most popular

endoscopic surgical modality with CO_2, KTP (potassium titanyl phosphate), Nd:YAG (neodynium:yttrium-aluminum-garnet) lasers all demonstrate equivalent efficacy

PEDIATRIC GASTROESOPHAGEAL REFLUX AND LARYNGOPHARYNGEAL REFLUX

Introduction

- physiologic reflux is the retrograde passage of contents into the esophagus with or without regurgitation and vomiting → normal process
- pathologic reflux, or GERD, involves troublesome symptoms and/or complications secondary to reflux of gastric contents
- LPR refers to reflux occurring outside of the esophagus and reaching the pharynx and larynx, sometimes with aspiration into the subglottis, trachea, and lungs
- two primary theories:
    1. gastric contents contact the pharynx and larynx and cause direct tissue injury having bypassed multiple anatomical boundaries including the lower esophageal sphincter, esophageal reflexes, upper esophageal sphincter, and esophagoglottic closure reflex
    2. acidification of the distal esophagus causes vagally mediated arc, which results in chest pain and cough

Clinical History

- Nonverbal infant: crying, apnea, bradycardia, poor appetite, weight loss, vomiting, recurrent pneumonitis, irritability, failure to thrive, hiccups, sleep disturbance, Sandifer syndrome (see later in chapter)
- Older children: cough, epigastric pain, vomiting, dental problems
- Differential diagnosis: *eosinophilic esophagitis* is characterized by dense eosinophilic infiltration with symptoms indistinguishable from GERD that do not resolve with reflux therapy; *Sandifer syndrome* consists of spastic torticollis and dystonic upper body movements along with GERD, esophagitis, or a hiatal hernia
- Laryngeal manifestations: findings on laryngoscopy include supraglottic and posterior glottic edema, erythema, ventricular obliteration, laryngomalacia, SGS, others
- GERD is linked to laryngomalacia, vocal fold masses and scar, chronic cough

Diagnostic Testing

Laryngoscopy

- *Reflux Finding Score for Infants* (RFS-I) provides validated objective measure of reflux based on laryngoscopy; modified to have a measure of signs of extraesophageal reflux based on laryngoscopy
- low specificity—similar to adults, laryngoscopy diagnoses pediatric LPR correctly less than 40% of the time when verified with impedance testing

Esophagoscopy

- routine use is not indicated unless there are concerning symptoms such as hematemesis or unintentional weight loss
- useful in patients unresponsive to medical therapy for diagnosis of peptic ulcer disease, *Helicobacter pylori* infection, peptic esophagitis, and eosinophilic esophagitis
- visible breaks of distal esophageal mucosa are highly reliable indicator of GERD when present; however, erythema, pallor, and vascular changes are nonspecific

pH Probes

- 24-hour pH-impedance probe monitoring is the gold standard
- continuous esophageal pH probe in the distal esophagus documents the severity and the frequency of reflux
- dual pH probe monitoring can be used to assess distal and proximal reflux to correlate with laryngeal and pulmonary symptoms
- abnormal values do not correlate with severity of disease, but "normal" monitoring may indicate diagnosis other than GERD; definition of normal is controversial for LPR
- disadvantage is that child may pull out probe
- pH-impedance testing is superior; records acid, weak acid, and nonacid events
- symptom index is key in children old enough to report systems

Impedance Testing

- by measuring changes in electrical impedance along length of esophageal catheter, it detects passage of liquid, gas, solids, and mixed boluses
- shown to have greater validity and reliability than pH probe in adult studies

- has not been validated and normal values have not been established in pediatrics

Esophageal Manometry

- neither sensitive nor specific for GERD, but detects esophageal motility disorders, stasis, and others
- gastric emptying studies are useful in select cases

Imaging Studies

- barium contrast, nuclear scintigraphy, esophageal and gastric ultrasound have more limited use in diagnosing GERD

Treatment

- two-thirds of healthy infants spit up and have simple gastroesophageal reflux rather than true GERD; according to North American Society for Pediatric Gastroenterology, Hepatology and Nutrition (NASPGHAN), these infants should be managed with lifestyle modifications
- Dietary/conservative measures: thickening of formula (cereal-thickened formula is more efficacious than postural therapy in decreasing regurgitation in infants); small, frequent meals; avoidance of greasy, acidic and spicy foods, caffeine, chocolate, citrus, and tomato products; positional strategies such as prone positioning during postprandial awake periods (>6 months old)
- Pharmacologic therapy: guidelines from the NASPGHAN (North American Society for Pediatric Gastroenterology, Hepatology and Nutrition) recommend step-up and step-down therapy (diet/lifestyle modification ↔ H2 receptor blockers ↔ PPI)
    1. H2 receptor antagonist (ranitidine, nizatidine): other extrapolated data from adult studies suggest they are safe in pediatrics; drug of choice in young pediatrics
    2. proton pump inhibitors (omeprazole, lansoprazole, rabeprazole, other): superior to H2 blockers due to inhibition of meal-induced acid secretion; none approved for age <1 year; indicated in patients who require more complete acid suppression
    3. prokinetics such as cisapride, metoclopramide, domperidone, bethanechol, and erythromycin (for delayed gastric emptying) do not have sufficient evidence to support use in children
    4. Surgical therapy: laparoscopic fundoplication shown to improve extraesophageal manifestations of GERD; heartburn with and without regurgitation and pH < 4 for more than 12% of

24-hour period are both significant predictors of extraesophageal symptom improvement following surgery; predictors for LPR less clear; endoscopic procedures work better for heartburn than for extraesophageal reflux

CAUSTIC INGESTION

Alkali Injuries

- most dangerous
- serious injury rare if pH 9 to 11, severe burns when pH > 11
- Ingestion: odorless and tasteless → large volumes
- Mechanism of injury: mucosa disintegrates causing penetrating injury and **liquefactive necrosis**, granular—more adherent, higher rate of injury
- Examples: sodium hydroxide, sodium phosphate (lye, drain and oven cleaner, dishwashing detergents, laundry detergents, hair relaxer)

Acidic Injuries

- Ingestion: bitter taste → smaller volumes, low viscosity cause rapid transit to stomach
- Mechanism of injury: causes **coagulation necrosis** of mucosa, limiting deep injury
- Examples: sulfuric acid, hydrochloric acid, hydrofluoric acid (drain cleaner, toilet bowl cleaner, metal cleaner)

Bleaches

- neutral pH, large series have shown no significant morbidity and mortality, extensive workup not indicated

Clinical Presentation

- child <6 years old (most 12 to 48 months old)
- Most common symptoms: dysphagia, drooling, food avoidance, vomiting
- Severe retrosternal or thoracoabdominal pain, tachycardia, hypotension → GI injury
- dysphonia or stridor → airway obstruction
- oral injury unreliable predictor of distal injury

Diagnosis

- #1—Airway, Breathing, Circulation, call poison control to identify pH and specific recommendations
- CXR: screen for free mediastinal or subdiaphragmatic air from esophageal or gastric perforation, aspiration pneumonia/pneumonitis
- stridor or drooling → emergent laryngoscopy
- severe laryngopharyngeal injuries (edema, burns, necrosis) → emergent tracheotomy to protect airway (versus intubation), leave tracheotomy in place until injuries have evolved and stabilized
- Endoscopy: direct visualization with esophagoscopy 12 to 48 hours following injury; if outside window, increased risk of iatrogenic perforation; endoscopy performed earlier than 12 hours may underestimate injury; avoid advancing scope beyond areas of transmural or circumferential injury; unclear if rigid versus flexible endoscopy increases risk of perforation; if injury occurred greater than 72 hours prior → radiographic water-soluble contrast studies (avoid endoscopy)

Zargar Grading of Caustic Esophageal Injury

- Grade 0: no evidence of injury
- Grade I: mucosal erythema and edema
- Grade IIa: superficial, noncircumferential erosion, ulcers, hemorrhage, or exudate
- Grade IIb: deep or circumferential erosion
- Grade IIIa: multiple scattered ulcerations with patchy necrosis (brown, black, gray)
- Grade IIIb: extensive necrosis

Treatment

- Grade 0–IIa: NPO 24 to 48 hours, IV fluids, advance diet as tolerated, antireflux medication, discharge from hospital if stable
- Grade IIb–IIIa: NPO 7 to 10 days, nutrition enteral versus parenteral, contrast swallow study prior to advancing feedings
- place nasogastric tube in operating room under direct vision or fluoroscopy, blind insertion should be avoided due to increased risk of iatrogenic perforation
- emergent surgery may be required (esophagectomy, gastrectomy)
- **neutralizing agents not recommended** due to increased risk of thermal injury
- **induced vomiting with emetics contraindicated** due to increased caustic exposure and risk of perforation

- steroids controversial, studies have shown increased risk of perforation and worse stricture rates arguing against routine use
- antibiotics not recommended unless patient develops signs/symptoms of hollow viscus perforation or infection
- antireflux medications recommended to prevent secondary reflux-associated esophageal injury
- consider oral nystatin suspension to prevent delayed wound healing and stricture formation from fungal overgrowth
- requires long-term follow-up

Complications

- <u>Acute</u>: esophageal perforation (can occur any time within first 2 weeks), tracheoesophageal fistula, gastric perforation, mediastinitis, peritonitis, pneumonia, sepsis, death
- <u>Chronic</u>: esophageal strictures, hiatal hernia, reflux esophagitis, esophageal cancer
- <u>Most common</u>: esophageal strictures (treatment with balloon catheter dilation, topical mitomycin C)
- <u>Late complication</u>: esophageal carcinoma (risk 1000 times higher with caustic injury, arises within scar tissue, metastasizes less, potential cure with resection higher)

LAUNDRY DETERGENT POD INGESTION

- <u>Background</u>: 17,230 children were exposed to laundry detergent pods as reported to the U.S. poison control centers from 2012 to 2013; 1 confirmed death
- majority of cases <3 years old (73.5%)
- ingestion major route of exposure (79.5%); attributed to colorful, candylike designs
- <u>Pathophysiology</u>: water-soluble packets burst easily → large volume of viscous liquid (pH 6.8–11) exposed to oropharynx, esophagus, stomach; aspiration possible
- may develop profound lethargy due to higher concentrations of propylene glycol and ethoxylated alcohols
- <u>Presentation</u>: vomiting, coughing or choking, drowsiness or lethargy, nausea, stridor, wheezing, drooling, throat pain, foaming at the mouth, respiratory distress, seizures, hematemesis, dysphagia, pulmonary edema, bradycardia, metabolic acidosis
- <u>Dx</u>: establish airway if hypoxia, hypoventilation, aspiration, acid/base status, or inability to protect airway due to decline in mental status; obtain imaging; possible panendoscopy

- obtain CXR if respiratory distress
- panendoscopy indicated if severe GI symptoms ± airway involvement; if minimal injury → initiate PO intake, OK to discharge with follow-up if tolerates; if injury → manage specific injury and consider repeat endoscopy in 4 to 6 weeks
- <u>Tx</u>: supportive care and symptomatic management, majority improve with observation
- racemic epinephrine, IV steroids, albuterol for pulmonary symptoms
- IV fluids, NPO, swallowing evaluation, ± gastric compression or dilution/irrigation/wash, nasogastric or postpyloric feedings for GI symptoms
- some poison centers recommend avoiding dilution until absence of neurologic deterioration is determined due to risk of aspiration
- <u>Complications</u>: low likelihood of developing long-term esophageal sequelae (eg, strictures) based on current literature

SECTION

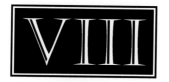

Surgery

CHAPTER

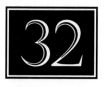

Laryngeal Laser Surgery

Haig Panossian and Peak Woo

LASER PHYSICS

- LASER—Light Amplification by Stimulated Emission of Radiation
- fundamental characteristics of laser beam
    1. Intensity: energy in focused, narrow beam
    2. Collimation: light waves parallel with minimal divergence and dissipation of energy
    3. Coherence: in phase spatially and temporally
    4. Monochromaticity: uniform wavelength
- Radiant exposure: relation of power density and time of laser use
- Power density: relationship between watts of laser energy delivered and area of tissue to which energy is delivered (W/cm^2)
- Fluence: radiant exposure especially relevant to pulsed lasers; optical energy delivered per unit area (J/cm^2)
- Lateral thermal energy spread: directly correlated to length of tissue exposure
- power density of laser directly correlated to watts and inversely to the square of spot size

LASER TISSUE INTERACTIONS

- Thermal relaxation time: time required for tissue to lose 50% of heat through diffusion
- Reflection: laser beam not absorbed, reflection off surgical instruments can cause inadvertent tissue damage
- Transmission: laser beam passes through tissue without being absorbed
- Absorption: each laser has characteristic chromophore that absorbs most of energy of beam
- Scatter/dispersion: partial absorption causing transmission to surrounding tissue
- Coagulation: low power density produces slow heating, increased spot size with low power (defocused beam)
- Vaporization: high-power density heats tissue quickly
- Cutting: photomechanical disruption due to extremely high power density

PROCEDURAL SAFETY

Operating Room (OR) Safety

- all OR staff aware of planned laser use and appropriately trained
- signs on outside of OR indicating that laser is in use

- all staff have proper safety eyewear (type differs for different wavelength)

Anesthesia Techniques

- catheter placed proximal to vocal folds if treating lesion/stenosis, which may impair passive exhalation and decreases risk of pneumothorax
- laser-safe endotracheal tube (may be coated with reflective material and/or have a proximal and distal cuff)
    1. oxygen levels lowered prior to laser use to less than 30% FiO_2

Jet Ventilation

- intermittent positive-pressure ventilation delivered through catheter
- laser use during periods of apnea
- catheter placed distal to lesion avoids quivering of vocal folds while oxygen delivered
    1. <u>Manual:</u> low frequency (10–16 insufflations per minute) through large-bore catheter
    2. <u>High frequency:</u> 100 to 300 insufflations per minute at low pressure (3 bars); Venturi effect produced through Hunsacker jet tube
- constant communication between surgeon and anesthesiologist

Patient Safety

- wet gauze or towel over patient's eyes, wet towels draped around laryngoscope so that patient's skin is not exposed
- prepare 60 mL Toomey syringe filled with saline and attached to red rubber catheter in case of airway fire
- wet cottonoids placed distal to target area to prevent damage from errant beam except during jet ventilation or in cases performed under apnea
- smoke suctioned via built-in evacuation port in laryngoscope or suction placed in oropharynx or in laryngoscope
- laser only activated on command from surgeon

Airway Fire

- Criteria
    1. ignition source (laser and heat above ignition temperature)
    2. medium (carbonized tissue, endotracheal tube, cottonoid)
    3. oxygen source to sustain combustion (blow-by, endotracheal tube, jet ventilation, distal lung reserve)

- Management
    1. prompt recognition: flash, plume of smoke
    2. turn off oxygen
    3. remove endotracheal tube
    4. extinguish with prepared saline

COMMONLY USED LASERS IN LARYNGEAL SURGERY

CO_2 Laser

- first reported series on CO_2 laser in 12 patients by Strong and Jako in 1972
- current workhorse in laryngeal surgery
- wavelength; color; chromophore: 10,600 nm; infrared (invisible); water
- Delivery systems: articulated arm connected to micromanipulator coupled to microscope lens (uses a red helium-neon laser aiming beam); flexible fiber
- cone-shaped impact with area of charring at center, then area of tissue desiccation and outer layer of edema
- Spot size: 100 to 150 microns
- Laser modes:
    ○ Continuous: power source keeps active medium in excited state; stable energy and intensity
        1. typically 4 to 6 watts
        2. useful for malignant tumors, as energy will spread to deeper tissue and help coagulate associated vessels and lymphatics
        3. coagulation of varix and vessels: milliwatts mode allows for 3 to 500 m watts at 100 micron spot size
        4. beam should be moved rapidly to avoid buildup of tissue char and deeper spread of thermal damage
    ○ Pulsed: intermittent power source provides sudden bursts of energy to active medium, delivers high energy in each pulse with no energy in between
        1. settings: 2 to 4 watts, 0.05- to 0.1-second pulse
        2. accurate and deep **cutting** effect with less thermal damage (and less coagulation) than continuous mode
        3. useful for benign nonvascular vocal fold lesions
- Automated pattern generators: innovation that uses surgeon's tracing to automate laser cut at greater speed than human operator; goal to minimize thermal effect and char
- Clinical application: division of web, synechiae; cricoarytenoid ankylosis (aryteηoidectomy), posterior glottic stenosis (transverse

cordotomy), premalignant and malignant neoplasia, cricopharyngeal myotomy, Zenker's diverticulectomy

Nd:YAG (Neodymium:Yttrium-Aluminum-Garnet)

- wavelength; color; chromophore: 1060 nm; near infrared
- delivery systems: fiberoptic fiber
- high degree of scatter with large spot size, small cutting effect, and substantial charring
- significant thermal effect; can cause voice damage through evaporation of lamina propria

KTP Laser (Potassium-Titanyl-Phosphate)

- wavelength; color; chromophore: 532 nm; green; oxyhemoglobin
- crystal doubles the frequency of a Nd:YAG laser (1060 nm)
- Delivery systems: fiberoptic fiber
- Spot size: 200 nm
- pulsed mode optimal for photocoagulation with a "near touch" technique to produce vascular effect without resulting adjacent tissue stiffness
- touch and nontouch techniques used for both thermal and photothermal effect
- well suited for office-based surgery; fiber placed through channeled flexible laryngoscope
- Typical settings: 15 ms pulse width, 500 to 750 mJ/pulse, 2 Hz repetition rate using 0.4 mm fiber resulting in fluence of 20 to 80 J/cm^2
- lower power for treatment of vascular lesions
- vary pulse duration to treat tissues with different thermal relaxation coefficients
- Clinical applications: vascular lesions, respiratory papilloma, dysplasia

Pulsed-Dye Laser (PDL)

- wavelength; chromophore: 585 nm; hemoglobin
- Delivery systems: fiberoptic fiber
- spot size 1 to 2 mm
- pulse duration nonadjustable, limited to 400 microsecond exposure
- Typical settings: 5 J/pulse, 1 Hz repetition rate resulting in fluence 19 to 76 J/cm^2
- Clinical applications: granuloma, vascular ectasias, Reinke's edema
- required frequent upkeep; largely replaced by use of KTP laser

Diode-Based Laser

- wavelength; color: 445 nm, blue
- <u>Delivery systems</u>: fiberoptic fiber
- pending U.S. Food and Drug Administration approval for use; newly introduced (2018) in Europe
- <u>Photoangiolytic effect</u>: high absorption in black and red spectrum
- cutting effect when used with close-to-contact method (less than 1 mm distance to target tissue)
- <u>Clinical applications</u>: currently under investigation, likely to replace KTP as primary office-based laser

CHAPTER

Voice Surgery

Haig Panossian, Mary J. Hawkshaw, and Robert T. Sataloff

DIRECT LARYNGOSCOPY

Laryngoscopes (Selected)

- <u>Jackson</u>: flat, removable blade
- <u>Holinger</u>: modified Jackson without removable blade, useful in cases of difficult exposure; small interior diameter does not permit stereoscopic vision
- <u>Dedo</u>: improved view of anterior commissure with stereoscopic vision; can use for subglottic work
- <u>Lindholm</u>: fits in vallecula, used in combination with Benjamin light clip
- <u>Sataloff</u>: triangular distal end to allow for exposure of anterior commissure and stereoscopic vision, built-in light carriers and suction port; five different sizes
- <u>Ossoff-Pilling</u>: distal end is reproduction of Holinger, but proximal end is large enough to allow for stereoscopic vision

Suspension Systems

- Lewy
- Boston University "Gallows"
- Bouchayer

Operating Microscope

- 400 mm or longer objective lens to allow for use with long instruments

Patient Positioning

- <u>Sniffing position</u>: neck flexed and head extended, with occiput supported
- protect teeth with toothguard (or wet gauze over palate if edentulous)

Anesthesia Concerns

- laser safety (addressed in Chapter 32)
- <u>Endotracheal tube</u>: as small as allowable (generally, 5.0), placed by skilled anesthesiologist
- <u>Jet ventilation</u>: with Hunsacker Mon-Jet catheter, placed above or below vocal folds
  1. can be placed by laryngologist to deliver oxygen when needed and removed to allow for increased working room

2. must be careful to avoid placing past areas of stenosis; expiration must be unobstructed to avoid development of pneumothorax

MICROSURGICAL TECHNIQUES

- have evolved as understanding of vocal fold anatomy has improved
- Microflap: (1) superficial mucosal incision made on superior surface, (2) blunt dissection used to elevate mucosa from lesion, (3) pathologic tissue excised, and (4) mucosa reapproximated
- now abandoned for small, benign lesions such as cysts in favor of mini-microflap
- Mini-microflap (Figure 33–1): (1) mucosal incision made directly overlying (superficial to) lesion at junction of vocal fold mass and normal tissue; (2) blunt dissection used to separate mass from residual superficial lamina propria when present, reflecting mass medially, then excised with overlying mucosa or by retaining small inferiorly based flap of mucosa; (3) healing by secondary intention
- submucosal resection with preservation of all epithelium preferred in some cases, when possible
- Hemostasis: submucosal injection of vasoconstrictor (epinephrine 1:10,000)—used when injection will not distort lesion and obscure borders of pathology (eg, small vocal fold cysts), or topical application of 1:1000 epinephrine-soaked cottonoids

Management of Vocal Fold Hemorrhage and Varicosities

- most hemorrhages resolve spontaneously, consider surgical evacuation of bulky hematoma persisting 48 to 72 hours
- varicosities or ectasias at risk for hemorrhage may be treated with vascular laser (usually KTP, see Chapter 32 for further details), or by resection
- larger varicosities may be treated with surgical excision of vessel with vascular knife

Management of Reinke's Edema

- incision along superior surface of vocal fold, and use fine suction to remove edema
- reapproximate mucosa; can trim redundant mucosa conservatively if necessary
- controversial whether to treat bilateral or to stage procedure—senior author (RTS) advises unilateral surgery in most cases, with second side staged if necessary

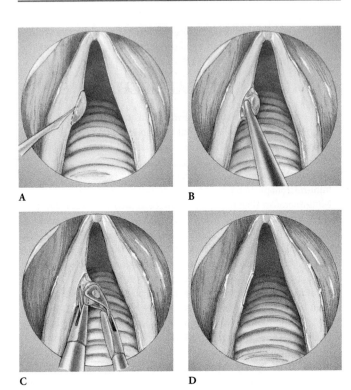

A

B

C   D

FIGURE 33–1. A. In elevating a mini-microflap, an incision is made with a straight knife at the junction of the mass and normal tissue. Small vertical anterior and posterior incisions may be added at the margins of the mass if necessary, usually using a straight scissors. **B.** The mass is separated by blunt dissection, splitting the superficial layer of the lamina propria and preserving it as much as possible. This dissection can be performed with a spatula, blunt ball dissector (illustrated), or scissors (as illustrated in **A**). **C.** The lesion is stabilized and a scissors (straight or curved) is used to excise the lesion, preserving as much adjacent mucosa as possible. The lesion itself acts as a tissue expander, and it is often possible to create an inferiorly based mini-microflap. **D.** The mini-microflap is replaced over the surgical defect, establishing primary closure and acting as a biological dressing. Used with permission from Sataloff et al., *Professional Voice: The Science and Art of Clinical Care* (4th ed.). San Diego, CA: Plural Publishing; 2017.

Management of Granulomas

- initial management usually nonsurgical with aggressive reflux therapy, steroids, voice therapy
- <u>Chemical tenotomy</u>: botulinum toxin injection to lateral cricoarytenoid (LCA) muscle can be used as adjunct to decrease phonatory trauma

- if large and/or recurrent, surgical excision may be indicated with botulinum toxin as adjunct
- jet ventilation or intermittent apnea may be preferred to avoid endotracheal tube obstructing or traumatizing lesion
- use of vasoconstrictor injection may help to delineate border of lesion and control bleeding
- use microsurgical principles to excise lesion with cold instruments; take care not to violate perichondrium of arytenoid cartilage
- laser may be used to excise and/or cauterize base of lesion with caution; may cause burn leading to recurrence
- injection of corticosteroid into base of resected lesion and/or botulinum toxin to bilateral LCAs performed at conclusion of surgery, or a week or more pre-op

Management of Papilloma

- surgical treatment may vary depending if patient is adult or has juvenile-onset papilloma
- avoid jet ventilation to prevent distal seeding of papilloma
- after exposure and suspension, use 0° and 70° endoscope to examine for papilloma in ventricle, anterior commissure, and infraglottis
- use cold instruments and microflap technique to separate lesions from underlying tissue, including vocal ligament
- if lesions are bilateral and near anterior commissure, treat unilateral and stage procedure to avoid creating laryngeal web
- can use powered instruments (ie, microdebrider) for bulky lesions, even on vibratory margin
- debulk large supraglottic lesions with 4.0 mm/tricut angle-tip laryngeal blade at 3000 to 5000 rpm
- limit trauma to mucosa with 3.5 mm angle-tip skimmer blade at 500 rpm
- can use KTP or CO_2 laser, taking care not to cause muscle injury with CO_2 laser
- Cidofovir: inhibits viral DNA polymerase
  1. use in larynx is off-label; concentration range 5 to 15 mg/mL
  2. inject submucosally prior to excision and/or following resection
- Bevacizumab (Avastin): vascular endothelial growth factor (VEGF) inhibitor; prevents angiogenesis
  1. inject submucosally and use KTP angiolytic laser to resect lesions
  2. may improve disease control and lengthen interval between procedures

Vocal Fold Scar/Sulcus/Web Surgery
(See Chapters 9 and 12)

MANAGEMENT OF VOCAL FOLD PARESIS/PARALYSIS

Injection Medialization Laryngoplasty

- often initial step, especially if awaiting possible recovery of vocal fold function
- may be performed under general anesthesia in operating room (OR) or local anesthesia in office, with exceptions
- injection of material into paraglottic space just lateral to vocalis muscle to medialize vocal fold
- Short-term injectables: saline, voice gel, Gelfoam; used as trial injection prior to longer-term injection or framework surgery
- Intermediate-term injectables: hyaluronic acid
- Long-term injectables: AlloDerm, calcium hydroxyapatite; usually performed in OR under general anesthesia via suspension laryngoscopy and transoral injection—less margin for error with longer-lasting materials
- Permanent injectables: Teflon, autologous fat

Injectables

- Saline: duration 1 to 10 days
- Bovine gelatin/Gelfoam: duration 4 to 6 weeks; mixed with saline for injection
- Carboxymethylcellulose (CMC)/voice gel: duration 5 to 8 months; 25- to 27G needle
- Hyaluronic acid: average duration of 4 months, improvement of voice quality of up to 12 months reported
- Micronized AlloDerm/Cymetra (Allergan, Irvine, California): duration 6 to 12 months
- Calcium hydroxylapatite (CaHA): microspheres added to CMC gels to prolong effect; duration 12 to 18 months; complications including severe vocal fold stiffness and granulation tissue have been reported
- Polytetrafluoroethylene/Teflon (Chemours, Wilmington, Delaware): no longer used due to formation of foreign-body inflammatory granulomas and other complications
- Autologous fat
  1. general anesthesia
  2. abdominal fat harvested with liposuction, irrigated gently with saline, and then loaded into 18G needle loaded on Brünings syringe
  3. injection performed using suspension laryngoscopy

4. requires overcorrection by 30% to 40% to account for expected resorption (3–4 months)
5. overcorrection mandates that only one vocal fold be treated fully to avoid airway compromise

Laryngeal Framework Surgery

Type I Thyroplasty

- popularized by Isshiki et al
- performed with local anesthesia under conscious sedation to allow for phonation and optimal positioning of implant
    1. preoperative IV steroid ± antibiotics (surgeon preference, weak evidence)
    2. thyroid cartilage exposed and outer perichondrium elevated and retracted
    3. thyrotomy window marked with 3-mm inferior strut (to prevent breakage of cartilage), with anterior border approximately 7 mm (females) or 9 mm (males) from midline
    4. implants can be wedge-shaped silicone (preformed Montgomery system or hand-carved Silastic block) or strips of expanded polytetrafluoroethylene (Gore-Tex; W.L Gore, Newark, Delaware)
    5. use flexible bronchoscope after implant placed to confirm that mucosa remains intact without implant extrusion and to evaluate position of implant and edema; may be used during surgery, helpful especially in difficult cases
    6. can perform bilateral implants as long as airway edema is minimal after initial side
- Complications: intraoperative or postoperative extrusion of implant, shifted implant with inadequate or excessive medialization, excessive anterior or inferior placement leading to strained phonation, hemorrhage with hematoma along vibratory margin and subsequent stiffness, infection (rare), airway obstruction (rare)

Arytenoid Adduction/Rotation and Arytenoidopexy

- indicated to correct posterior glottic gap; common in high vagal injury
- arytenoid adduction recreates tension in direction of LCA muscle— often performed in conjunction with type I thyroplasty under local anesthesia
    1. expose posterior margin of thyroid cartilage and free piriform sinus mucosa

2. create posterior thyroid cartilage window to expose muscular process of arytenoid
3. 4-0 nylon suture(s) placed through muscular process
4. ends of suture passed through thyroid ala in direction of LCA and tied on external cartilage; may require drilled guide holes if cartilage ossified

- arytenoidopexy pulls arytenoid cartilage against the cricoid cartilage near midline and stretches vocal fold
    1. expose posterior thyroid cartilage and release inferior constrictor muscle from thyroid lamina
    2. identify cricoid cartilage at cricothyroid joint and separate joint with scissors
    3. release piriform sinus and divide LCA and PCA muscles from muscular process
    4. dissect PCA muscle from posterior cricoid cartilage
    5. place 3-0 or 4-0 Prolene suture through posterior cricoid cartilage and through cricoarytenoid joint, then wrap around anterolateral arytenoid and back again through joint and cricoid cartilage, tie on posterior face
    6. check that vocal process position is adequate at habitual speaking pitch; may require additional sutures to adjust

Laryngeal Reinnervation Techniques (*See* Chapter 18)

- focus on maintaining muscle tone and prevent atrophy and fibrosis
- synkinesis is abnormal laryngeal innervation that occurs from regenerating axons cross-innervating adductors and abductors
- can result in motion impairment, spasticity, or tonic adduction or abduction
- neuromuscular pedicle introduced by Tucker for selective reinnervation of PCA
    1. implant cuff of omohyoid with intact motor branch from ansa cervicalis over PCA
    2. rates of success have varied
- ansa cervicalis to RLN nerve transfer introduced by Crumley with goal to provide dynamic adduction in unilateral vocal fold paralysis
    1. uses branch of ansa to sternothyroid and anastomoses to RLN distal to lesion
    2. can prevent synkinesis by providing neural input to promote tone and bulk, stabilize arytenoid (unopposed cricothyroid activity pulls cartilage anteriorly)
    3. success rates may be higher in pediatric and younger patients
- laryngeal pacing can be implanted in PCA with set rate of stimulation; active area of research that shows promise

IN-OFFICE PROCEDURES

- usually tolerated well by patients with adequate topical anesthesia
- useful in cases in which general anesthesia should be avoided for medical comorbidity or patient convenience
- anesthesia techniques vary by surgeon, but general recommendation is for decongestant spray and local anesthesia (atomized topical 4% lidocaine) of nasal cavity, followed by topical lidocaine or cetacaine to tonsillar pillars, pharynx and base of tongue, then topical 4% lidocaine administered via transoral curved cannula, catheter threaded through channel of flexible laryngoscope (if available), or transtracheal injection
- flexible laryngoscope provides visualization of larynx during procedure
- electromyogram (EMG)-coupled needles can assist in localization of target muscle and confirm needle placement when injection is transcervical
- channeled flexible laryngoscope allows for passage of laser fibers, flexible instruments such as biopsy forceps
- curved instruments available for transoral biopsies, resection of lesions, and other indications

Injection Laryngoplasty Approaches

- one of most common indications for an in-office procedure
- have assistant hold flexible (or rigid) laryngoscope in position once larynx in view
- Transoral approach: via curved orotracheal injector
- transcutaneous approaches
- thyrohyoid membrane approach
  1. technically easier in men with prominent thyroid cartilage and acute thyrohyoid angle
  2. use 1.5″-length needle (gauge dependent on injectable material) with single or double bend and insert at superior thyroid notch
  3. visualize needle tip in supraglottis and direct toward injection site(s)
- transcartilaginous approach
  1. direct route to vocal fold through thyroid cartilage
  2. most successful in younger patients with nonossified cartilage
  3. needle tip may become obstructed while passing through cartilage
  4. insert straight needle approximately 5 mm lateral to midline and 3 to 4 mm above inferior border of cartilage until tip is visualized lateral to vocal ligament in middle to posterior third of membranous vocal fold

- cricothyroid membrane approach
  1. preferable for needle to remain submucosal and not enter airway prior to injection
  2. insert needle 5 to 10 mm lateral to midline and aim superiorly at approximately 30° to 40° until tip visualized lateral to vocal ligament; distances and angles depend on gender and needle position (against bottom of thyroid cartilage or on top of cricoid cartilage)

POSTOPERATIVE VOICE CARE

- <u>Voice rest</u>: recommendations vary by surgeon
- recommended up to a week following vibratory margin surgery to allow for re-mucosalization, can be less for framework surgery if postoperative examination shows no evidence of vibratory margin hemorrhage
- recent research has shown that fibroblast proliferation enhanced by vibration via voice use and may enhance wound healing, so prolonged voice rest may be counterproductive and promote stiffness
- <u>Steroids</u>: intraoperative use common to limit postoperative swelling; postoperative use varies among surgeons and is anecdotal
- <u>Antireflux medications</u>: proton pump inhibitors ± H2 blockers beneficial in patients with laryngopharyngeal reflux in perioperative period to avoid stomach content contact with healing mucosa
- <u>Voice therapy</u>: recommended perioperative to promote healthy vocal use and avoid phonotrauma once patient is brought off voice rest
- *see* Chapter 37 for further details

CHAPTER

34

Surgical Airway

Harleen Sethi, Justin Ross, Mary J. Hawkshaw, and Robert T. Sataloff

CRICOTHYROTOMY

Introduction

- preferred in airway emergencies due to its simplicity and speed if trained surgeon is unavailable to perform tracheotomy
- mnemonic for predictors of a difficult cricothyrotomy ("SHORT"): S: surgery; H: hematoma; O: obesity; R: radiation (burn or other distortion); T: tumor
- Relevant anatomy: cricothyroid membrane extends from the inferior border of the thyroid cartilage to the superior cricoid rim; composed of fibroelastic tissue

Indications

- emergency airway when intubation and ventilation have failed or intubation is contraindicated
- failure to maintain oxygenation through less invasive means (ie, bag-mask ventilation)

Contraindications

- Absolute: endotracheal intubation can be performed safely; transection of trachea; severely fractured laryngeal cartilages; obstruction at or below the cricothyroid membrane
- Relative: children <10 to 12 years old (tracheotomy or percutaneous needle cricothyrotomy and subsequent jet ventilation after are preferable); bleeding diathesis; massive neck edema or swelling; acute laryngeal disease

Technique Pearls

- immobilize superior cornua of thyroid cartilage with the thumb and third finger of the nondominant hand while the forefinger palpates the cricothyroid membrane
- make the incision in the inferior aspect of the cricothyroid membrane to avoid superiorly based vessels
- aim scalpel caudally during horizontal incision to avoid vocal fold injury

Complications

- Intraoperative: incorrect tube placement, bleeding, esophageal or mediastinal perforation, thyroid injury
- Perioperative: aspiration, subcutaneous emphysema, pneumomediastinum, vocal fold or laryngeal injury
- Long term: subglottic stenosis, dysphonia, dysphagia, infection

Postoperative Management

- may be decannulated directly from cricothyrotomy if <24 hours required and in some other cases
- after patient has been stabilized, the cricothyrotomy should be converted to a formal tracheotomy ideally within 72 hours
- appropriate ventilator settings, sedation should be considered for the patient

PERCUTANEOUS NEEDLE CRICOTHYROIDOTOMY

Introduction

- technique preferred over surgical cricothyrotomy for failed airway in infants and children <10 to 12 years old due to the small caliber of the cricothyroid membrane and difficulty of safely inserting a tracheotomy tube
- Indications: rescue airway in infants and children <12 years of age when tracheotomy is not possible; obstruction above the level of the cricothyroid membrane; temporary measure until definitive airway can be established
- Contraindications: same as surgical cricothyrotomy
- a definitive airway should be established within 45 minutes to avoid hypoventilation

Complications

- <u>Intraoperative</u>: hemorrhage, hypoxia, posterior tracheal perforation, bleeding, air embolism, airway barotrauma, subcutaneous and mediastinal emphysema, needle displacement, kinking of catheter
- <u>Postoperative</u>: pneumothorax, aspiration, vocal fold or laryngeal injury
- <u>Long term</u>: tracheal and subglottic stenosis, infection, persistent stoma, tracheomalacia, tracheoesophageal fistula, tube obstruction, dysphonia, dysphagia

OPEN TRACHEOTOMY

Introduction

- elective or emergent surgical formation of a temporary opening in the trachea
- leading indication during the latter half of the 20th century was prolonged mechanical ventilation especially in intensive care unit (ICU) settings
- used to administer positive-pressure ventilation, to provide a patent airway, and to provide access to the lower respiratory tract for airway clearance

Terminology

- **Tracheotomy**: derived from Greek words "tracheia arteria" meaning "to cut" and used to describe a temporary opening in the anterior tracheal wall
- **Tracheostomy**: derived from the Greek ending "stoma," meaning "to finish with an opening or mouth," which is used in scenarios in which the trachea is brought to the skin and sewn place to create a permanent opening (eg, during laryngectomy)
- **Decannulation**: process of removing tracheotomy tube once no longer needed

Relevant Anatomy/Landmarks

- **Cricoid cartilage**: complete ring of cartilage around the trachea located inferior to thyroid cartilage at the level of C6
- **Strap muscles**: sternohyoid, sternothyroid, thyrohyoid, omohyoid
- **Innominate artery**: crosses anterior to the trachea from left to right
- **Thyroid isthmus**: lies across the second and fourth tracheal rings

- in children, the larynx is located more cephalad than in adults
- in a newborn airway, epiglottis and soft palate approximate, allowing for simultaneous swallowing and nasal breathing

Indications

Adult

- <u>Prolonged mechanical ventilation</u>: respiratory disease, neuromuscular disease, depressed mental status (Glasgow Coma Scale <8)
- pulmonary toilet
- surgical access
- <u>Airway obstruction</u>: epiglottitis/supraglottitis, neoplasia, bilateral vocal fold paralysis, angioedema, foreign body, blunt/penetrating trauma, obstructive sleep apnea, glottic stenosis or subglottic stenosis

Pediatric

- <u>Cardiopulmonary</u>: bronchopulmonary dysplasia, congenital heart disease, pneumonia, pulmonary hypertension, restrictive lung disease
- <u>Craniofacial malformations</u>: Apert syndrome, CHARGE syndrome*, micrognathia, oculo-auriculo-vertebral syndrome, Pierre-Robin sequence
- <u>Neurologic</u>: Arnold-Chiari malformation, brain tumor, cervical spine injury, central hypoventilation or apneic, encephalopathy, neuromuscular, obstructive hydrocephalus, seizure disorder, traumatic brain injury
- <u>Trauma</u>: maxillofacial fractures, laryngotracheal trauma, laryngomalacia
- <u>Upper airway obstruction</u>: laryngeal web or cyst, neoplasm, subglottic hemangioma, subglottic stenosis, tracheoesophageal fistula, tracheomalacia, vocal fold paralysis
- *CHARGE = Coloboma of the eye, Heart defects, Atresia of the choanae, Retardation of growth and/or development, Genital and/or urinary abnormalities, and Ear abnormalities and deafness

Relative Contraindications

- situation in which endotracheal intubation can be achieved safely
- short-lived airway obstruction (eg, epiglottitis, angioedema)
- uncontrolled coagulopathy
- inability to access trachea (ie, severe neck burn, obstructive tumor or necrotic tissue due to radiation or chemotherapy)

Technique Pearls

Emergency Tracheotomy

- do not waste time on prep or cautery
- stay midline
- in difficult cases, locate airway with an 18-gauge needle on a 10-mL syringe placed through trachea below thyroid isthmus and incise vertically above and below
- when inserting the tracheotomy tube, the tip should be held at 90° to the trachea and rotated to lie parallel as it is completely inserted
- cautery should be avoided due to fire risk in the presence of >30% FiO_2
- if available, inject additional lidocaine in the paratracheal tissue prior to incising trachea

Elective Surgical Tracheotomy

- beginning with a horizontal or small vertical incision at the second tracheal ring is recommended for optimal cosmesis
- when dissecting deep cervical fascia, be cognizant of the anterior jugular veins and branches
- tracheal incision type is based on surgeon preference and can include vertical, horizontal, H-shaped, cruciate, Bjork flap (recommended by senior author, RTS), etc
- in older patients, tracheal rings will be calcified, and heavy scissors may be used to incise necessary portion of anterior tracheal rings

Complications

- Intraoperative: hemorrhage, pneumothorax, pneumomediastinum, airway fire, intraoperative tracheoesophageal fistula, postobstructive pulmonary edema
- Postoperative: tube obstruction, dislodged tracheotomy tube, postoperative hemorrhage, wound infection, subcutaneous emphysema, accidental decannulation
- Late: granulation tissue, tracheoesophageal fistula, tracheoinnominate artery fistula, tracheal stenosis, tracheal necrosis, tracheomalacia, tracheocutaneous fistula, depressed scar

TRACHEOTOMY CARE AND MANAGEMENT OPTIONS

Tracheotomy Tube Care

- humidified air and saline drops to reduce tracheal crusting and mucus plugs
- frequent wound care
- keep skin under inferior flange dry
- acute tube occlusion is typically caused by mucous plugging → remove inner cannula and attempt suctioning.
- peristomal granuloma is a frequent cause of bleeding during tube manipulation → tx with silver nitrate cautery or excision (if large)

Tube Options

- cuffed versus cuffless
- reusable versus disposable versus no inner cannula
- fenestrated versus nonfenestrated
- polyvinyl chloride (PVC) versus silicone versus polyurethane versus metal (Jackson)
- angled versus curved

Sizing (See Table 34–1)

- dimensions of tracheotomy tubes are given by their inner diameter, outer diameter, length, and curvature

Cuffs, Caps, Feeding, and Speaking

- cuff pressure should be maintained at less than capillary pressure (<26 cm H_2O or 20 mm Hg) to avoid pressure necrosis, including subglottic stenosis, tracheal-innominate artery erosion, or tracheomalacia
- cuff should be kept inflated for at least 1 day postoperatively to reduce aspiration
- occlusive cap placement prevents air flow through the tube and requires breathing around tube via mouth and nose
- in spontaneously breathing patients, occluding tube with a cap or finger facilitates speech and swallowing
- one-way valves (eg, Passy-Muir) allow airflow through tracheotomy tube during inspiration; during expiration valve closes, and air flows through vocal folds

TABLE 34–1. Common Tracheotomy Tube Sizes

Inner Diameter (mm)	Outer Diameter (mm)	Length (mm)
Shiley Single-Cannula Tube (SCT)		
6.0	8.3	67
7.0	9.6	80
8.0	10.9	89
9.0	12.1	99
10.0	13.3	105
Shiley Double-Cannula Tube (same as Jackson)		
5.0 (6.7 mm without inner cannula)	9.4	62
6.4 (8.1 mm without inner cannula)	10.8	74
7.6 (9.1 mm without inner cannula)	12.2	79
8.9 (10.7 mm without inner cannula)	13.8	79
Portex Flex Disposable Inner Cannula (DIC)		
6.0	8.2	64
7.0	9.6	70
8.0	10.9	74
9.0	12.3	80
10.0	13.7	80
Bivona Mid-Range Aire-Cuff		
6.0	8.8	67
7.0	10.0	80
8.0	11.0	89
9.0	12.3	99
10.0	13.3	105

TABLE 34-1. *continued*

Inner Diameter (mm)	Outer Diameter (mm)	Length (mm)
Shiley XLT Proximal Extension		
5.0	9.6	90 (20 mm proximal, 37 mm radial, 33 mm distal)
6.0	11.0	95 (23 mm proximal, 38 mm radial, 34 mm distal)
7.0	12.3	100 (27 mm proximal, 39 mm radial, 34 mm distal)
8.0	13.3	105 (30 mm proximal, 40 mm radial, 35 mm distal)
Shiley XLT Distal Extension		
5.0	9.6	90 (5 mm proximal, 37 mm radial, 48 mm distal)
6.0	11.0	95 (8 mm proximal, 38 mm radial, 49 mm distal)
7.0	12.3	100 (12 mm proximal, 39 mm radial, 49 mm distal)
8.0	13.3	105 (15 mm proximal, 40 mm radial, 50 mm distal)
Rusch Ultra TracheoFlex with adjustable flange		
7.0	10.4	63
8.0	11.4	99
9.0	12.4	117
10.0	13.4	117
11.0	14.4	116
Bivona Mid-Range Aire-Cuf Adjustable Neck Flange		
6.0	9.2	110
7.0	10.6	120
8.0	11.7	130
9.0	12.9	140

- contraindications to capping or one-way speaking valves
    1. Relative: unconscious or comatose patients, thick secretions
    2. Absolute: inflated tracheotomy tube cuff, foam-cuffed tracheotomy tube, severe upper airway obstruction

Immediate Postoperative Care

Patients and Caregivers

- education should be provided to both parties prior to performing an elective tracheotomy, when possible
- should receive a checklist of emergency supplies prior to discharge that is near the patient at all times
- skill set of both parties should be evaluated prior to discharge to assess competency of tracheotomy care procedures
- once stoma is mature, patients or caretakers may perform tube changes

All Patients

- all supplies required to replace a tracheotomy tube should be at bedside or within reach
- Essential supplies: replacement tracheotomy tube of the same size, one of a smaller size, appropriate-sized obturator, flexible suction tubing and suction apparatus, scissors, gloves, replacement ties, water-based lubricant, endotracheal tube
- bag valve mask should ideally be kept at bedside
- should deflate cuff when mechanical ventilation is no longer required
- perform first tube change on day 5 to 7; if inserted percutaneously, wait until day 10 to ensure maturation of the tract

Emergency Situations

- Mature stoma: replace tube with the same size or a size smaller (if stenosed), observation alone is appropriate in select circumstances in which patient is able to oxygenate and ventilate with minimal effort (may circumvent formal decannulation protocol)
- Immature stoma (<5–7 days): stay sutures or a Bjork flap can improve ability to recannulate in emergency situations; stay sutures unnecessary if Bjork flap used, but the former is recommended in children
    1. If stay sutures available: pull stoma close to skin surface prior to replacement of dislodged
    2. If no stay sutures are present: reinsert tube normally (if possible) or over a bougie

3. <u>If no tracheotomy tube is available</u>: stomal intubation with an endotracheal tube
- if unable to establish airway via stoma → attempt oral intubation
- patient must know how to self-remove cap in case the tube is ever erroneously capped with the cuff inflated

Long-Term Considerations

- <u>Adult</u>: effect on speech, swallowing, capping/types
- <u>Pediatric</u>: long-term complications (tracheal infections, tracheal stenosis, speech delays), social stigma and lifestyle modifications, financial burden

DECANNULATION

Decannulation Criteria

- there is a lack of clinical evidence supporting specific criteria
- intact mental status, ability to protect airway (intact cough reflex), patent airway, and no requirement for ventilatory support are the usual minimum standards
- presence of coordinated swallowing is beneficial, but unnecessary if patient is able to protect airway and has access for enteral nutrition
- no aspiration events that would preclude decannulation
- patients with chronic neuromuscular disease may not tolerate long-term decannulation
- spontaneous capped breathing trial of at least 24 to 48 hours is advised by most clinicians
- stomal maintenance devices can be used for patients who cannot be decannulated

Decannulation Preparation

- <u>Flexible laryngoscopy</u>: presence of one mobile vocal fold or patent glottis
- <u>Bronchoscopy</u>: rule out suprastomal granuloma, tracheomalacia, lesion
- discussion with family about care needs and discharge preparation
- children >2 years of age require a daytime capping trial → if successful, other options include capped sleep study, capped exercise test, and nighttime in-hospital capping trial
- in children <2 years of age or a child who fails capping trial, decannulation needs to be individualized

Decannulation Protocol

Assessing Adult Decannulation Readiness

- indications for tracheotomy placement have resolved or improved substantially
- patient tolerates a capping trial without stridor
- fiberoptic laryngoscopy confirms airway patency to the level of the glottis and immediate subglottis
- patient has an adequate level of consciousness and laryngopharyngeal function to protect the lower airway from aspiration
- patient has an effective cough while tracheotomy tube is capped
- all procedures that require general endotracheal anesthesia in the near future have been completed

Adult Decannulation Protocol

- remove the tracheotomy tube
- clean and cover the site with a dry semi- or fully occlusive dressing, or adhesive tape
- instruct the patient to apply pressure over the dressing with fingers when talking or coughing
- change dressing daily and as needed if moist with secretions until the site has healed
- monitor for decannulation failure

Assessing Pediatric Decannulation Readiness

- flexible or rigid bronchoscopic evaluation of the airway in the operating room while spontaneously breathing is important for young children
- gently finger-occlude the stoma and observe the patency and dynamics of the airway as the patient breathes
- specific observations within the airway should be made including areas of obstruction, stenotic segments, dynamic collapse, and at least one mobile vocal fold
- peristomal granulomas should be removed via laser, cautery, or cold knife technique

Pediatric Decannulation Protocol

- if patent airway confirmed in operating room, can decannulate immediately or in 24 hours per clinician preference
- capping and downsizing remain controversial and are not universally implemented

- apply occlusive dressing as in an adult
- monitor overnight in a pediatric ICU and discharge following day

PERCUTANEOUS TRACHEOTOMY

Introduction

- minimally invasive technique resulting in decreased time, financial burden, and stress to a critically ill patient as compared to open tracheotomy
- Toye and Weinstein first described via the Seldinger technique in 1969
- Ciaglia introduced the dilational percutaneous technique in 1985, and it consequently became more customary in the ICU setting

Indications

- adult intubated ICU patients
- obstruction of upper respiratory tract
- prolonged mechanical ventilation in respiratory failure
- need for improving pulmonary toilet
- severe sleep apnea

Contraindications

- <u>Absolute</u>: obstructing neck mass or thyromegaly, high innominate artery, pediatric patients (<8 years old)
- <u>Relative</u>: PEEP >20 cm H_2O, coagulopathy (ie, INR >1.5, platelets <50,000), underlying soft tissue infection or abscess, unprotected airway, access during airway emergency

Technique Pearls

- slight overdilation and leaving the single dilator in situ for 10 to 15 seconds facilitates placement of tracheotomy tube
- potential areas of resistance during tracheotomy tube insertion: interface between the loading dilator and tracheotomy tube and upon balloon insertion

Complications (Early and Late)

- <u>Intraoperative</u>: desaturation, bleeding, infection, accidental extubation, posterior wall injury, false passage, pneumothorax,

pneumomediastinum, subcutaneous emphysema, accidental
decannulation
- <u>Perioperative</u>: infection
- <u>Postoperative</u>: O_2 desaturation, hypotension, tachycardia,
pneumothorax, pneumomediastinum

Comparison With Open Tracheotomy

- the percutaneous method is simple, fast, and minimally invasive,
which leads to less stress to the patient compared with surgical
tracheotomy
- using bronchoscopy to guide percutaneous tracheotomy provides
the advantage of visualizing tracheal mucosal injury, tracheal wall
abnormalities, and vocal fold and subglottic injury present prior to
tracheotomy
- decreased operative time and postoperative infections, but no
difference in bleeding or mortality rate
- open tracheotomy is preferable in more difficult surgical anatomy

SECTION

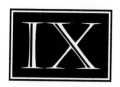

IX

Swallowing Disorders

SECTION

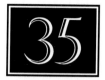

Dysphagia

Jonathan Aaron Harounian and Nausheen Jamal

INTRODUCTION

- <u>Dysphagia</u>: sensation of food being delayed in its normal passage from mouth to stomach
- approximately 20% incidence
- occurs in all age groups but prevalence increases with age
- associated with reduction in quality of life, anxiety, depression, loss of self-esteem, isolation, and loss of pleasure of eating

PHASES OF NORMAL SWALLOWING

Oral Phase

- under voluntary control
- can be bypassed or modified (such as via reduced food consistency, as with liquids; syringing food to back of mouth; holding head back so that gravity carries food to pharynx)
- subdivided into preparatory phase (preparation of food bolus) and transit phase (transport of food bolus to pharynx); requires
  1. lip closure to maintain oral competency and hold food in mouth anteriorly
  2. tension in labial and buccal musculature to close lateral and anterior sulci
  3. rotary motion of jaw for chewing and of tongue (most crucial element) to position food on teeth during mastication
  4. forward bulging of soft palate to seal oral cavity
  5. propulsion of food bolus into dorsum of tongue

Pharyngeal Phase

- under reflexive/involuntary control
- cannot be bypassed—airway protection occurs during this phase
- dynamic separation of alimentary and ventilatory streams

Pharyngeal Deglutition

- velopharyngeal closure via palatal and pharyngeal muscle contraction to prevent nasal regurgitation
  1. levator veli palatini (cranial nerve [CN] X) to lift soft palate
  2. palatopharyngeus (CN X) and superior pharyngeal constrictor (CN X) to constrict pharynx
- propulsion of food bolus from base of tongue (BOT) retraction to pharynx

- airway protection via laryngeal elevation and closure
  1. Elevation: contraction of strap muscles for upward and forward displacement of hyoid/larynx under BOT
  2. Closure (three sphincters): (1) epiglottis and aryepiglottic folds; (2) false vocal folds; (3) true vocal folds (most important)
- pharyngeal contraction/shortening to propel bolus through pharynx and prevent residual food
- relaxation of cricopharyngeus and anterosuperior displacement of larynx helps open upper esophageal sphincter (UES)
- passage of bolus into cervical esophagus

Esophageal Stage (See Chapter 36)

EVALUATION OF DYSPHAGIA

History

- location of symptoms
- Character: solid and/or liquid dysphagia, gradual/abrupt, progressive/stable/intermittent, duration, modifying factors, context of onset
- Associated signs/symptoms: odynophagia, aspiration, cough, regurgitation, halitosis, weight loss, globus, voice changes, gagging, choking, pneumonia, weight loss, otalgia, weakness, fatigue, depression, mental status changes, drooling, heartburn, chest pain, malnutrition, dehydration
- Pertinent factors: diet, lifestyle, reflux, trauma, caustic ingestion, foreign body, head and neck malignancy, radiation therapy, neurological disease, autoimmune disorder, age, hormonal imbalance
- prior workup/interventions
- involvement of other disciplines as needed (gastroenterology [GI], pulmonology, neurology, speech-language pathology, etc)

Examination

Introduction

- complete head and neck examination
- full neurologic examination
- indirect mirror and/or endoscopic examination of the larynx
- assessment of voice
- validated surveys/questionnaires: EAT-10 (Eating Assessment Tool–10), MDADI (MD Anderson Dysphagia Inventory),

SWAL-QOL (Swallow Quality of Life), SSQ (Sydney Swallowing Questionnaire)
- assessment of swallowing

Bedside Evaluation

- performed by speech-language pathologist and/or otolaryngologist
- perceptual evaluation of facial, oral cavity, pharyngeal, laryngeal and respiratory control without visualization of swallow structures in addition to patient's ability to follow directions
- food administered to patient in various textures, and subjective signs/clues used to detect penetration/aspiration
- throat clearing, cough, "wet" voice/gurgling, eyes watering, secretion management suggest penetration/aspiration
- inexpensive, fast/convenient, no radiation exposure, no transportation required
- not sensitive for silent penetration and aspiration episodes
- most helpful in determining need for additional instrumental assessment

Functional Endoscopic Evaluation of Swallowing (FEES) with Sensory Testing (FEESST)

- performed by otolaryngologist and/or speech-language pathologist
- assesses pharyngeal dysphagia, laryngeal function, treatment strategies, handling of secretions, penetration/aspiration (before or after swallow)
- does not evaluate oral or esophageal phases directly, although indirect assessment possible
- no radiation
- accurate anatomical information
- limited ability to detect penetration/aspiration during the swallow as pharynx contracts and closes against scope (blind spot)
- primarily able to assess penetration/aspiration before and after the swallow
- better able to detect micropenetration and aspiration as compared to MBSS
- ability to introduce therapeutic strategies (postural adjustments and swallowing maneuvers) if impaired swallow is demonstrated; unlike MBSS, does not increase radiation exposure
- unlike MBSS, useful in biofeedback to teach complicated behavioral strategies to patients to assure safer, more efficient swallow

Videofluoroscopy and Modified Barium Swallow Study (VFS, VFSS, MBS, MBSS)

- performed by speech-language pathologist + radiologist, otolaryngologist
- only available procedure that allows direct observation of aerodigestive tract during all stages of deglutition from oral preparatory stage to lower esophageal sphincter
- patient sits upright in normal eating position
- identifies presence of aspiration during swallow of any food consistency, assesses speed of swallow, and defines immediate oropharyngeal motility disorders
- ability to introduce therapeutic strategies (postural adjustments and swallowing maneuvers) during study to improve swallow and restore oral intake
- purpose of study is to restore or retain oral intake, not just evaluate or stop the patient from eating

Barium Swallow Study/Esophagram

- <u>Diagnostician</u>: radiologist, otolaryngologist, gastroenterologist
- assessment of esophageal dysphagia—for liquids only (does not assess solid dysphagia)
- inexpensive, noninvasive
- contrast study to assess for primarily structural/luminal abnormalities or issues with motility
- performed supine in order to eliminate gravity to isolate evaluation of peristalsis

Esophagoscopy

- performed by gastroenterologist or otolaryngologist
- otolaryngologists typically perform this procedure awake (as transnasal esophagoscopy) or under general anesthesia (rigid or flexible transoral approach)
- gastroenterologists typically perform this procedure under sedation with a large-bore scope as a transoral approach
- useful in assessing for structural abnormalities; less utility in assessing for functional abnormalities

Manometry and pH-Impedance Testing

- performed and interpreted by gastroenterologist and/or otolaryngologist

- assesses esophageal motility disorders and adequacy of function of upper and lower esophageal sphincters typically via transnasal catheter
- events grouped into acidic, weakly acidic, or nonacidic reflux
- only liquid motility disorders tested; performed supine or upright using 10 sips of water
- assesses proximal versus distal, and supine versus upright reflux events
- symptom correlation (using Reflux Symptom Index)
- assesses stasis, intraesophageal versus extraesophageal reflux

ETIOLOGY AND TREATMENT

Zenker's Diverticulum

- pseudo diverticulum of esophageal mucosa through Killian's triangle (inferior to thyropharyngeus m. and superior to cricopharyngeus m.), posterior midline or left-sided
- <u>History</u>: older male (in 60s), progressive dysphagia (initially transient), history of aspiration, halitosis, cough, throat gurgling, and regurgitation of undigested food
- <u>Exam</u>: typically no obvious abnormalities; may have audible regurgitation sounds, emaciation, dehydration, possible Boyce sign— swelling in neck that gurgles on palpation due to air passage from the sac rostrally
- <u>Dx</u>: contrast esophagram, FEES (esophagopharyngeal reflux/ regurgitation after swallow), transnasal esophagoscopy (TNE)
- <u>Tx</u>: endoscopic diverticulotomy with endoscopic stapler, CO_2 laser, LigaSure or Harmonic; transcervical open diverticulectomy

Killian-Jamieson Diverticulum

- true diverticulum inferior to transverse fibers of cricopharyngeus and lateral to longitudinal muscle of esophagus (Killian-Jamieson space); typically smaller and more rare than Zenker's
- History: similar presenting symptoms as Zenker's but more often asymptomatic
- Dx: contrast esophagram (antero-lateral and more commonly left-sided)
- Tx: transcervical excision, consider nerve monitoring as RLN crosses Killian-Jamieson space and may be at risk of injury

Cricopharyngeal Dysfunction and Spasm

- <u>History</u>: dysphagia localized to cervical esophagus (nonspecific), globus sensation, choking, exacerbated by stress, reflux

- <u>Dx</u>: contrast esophagram (cricopharyngeal bar with or without functional obstruction), FEES (esophagopharyngeal reflux/regurgitation after swallow), manometry with elevated UES pressure (most accurate)
- <u>Tx</u>: UES dilation, botulinum toxin injection, open/endoscopic cricopharyngeal myotomy, reflux control

Laryngopharyngeal Reflux (LPR)
(See Chapter 22)

- <u>History</u>: globus, hoarseness, throat clearing, cough, choking, halitosis, rarely heartburn, others; sometimes, only dysphagia
- <u>Exam</u>: postcricoid edema/erythema, interarytenoid pachydermia/erythema, Reinke's edema
- <u>Dx</u>: history and physical (H&P) in addition to response to empiric treatment, 24-hour pH impedance monitoring (gold standard)
- <u>Tx</u>: lifestyle modifications (smoking cessation, weight loss, avoid eating before lying supine if nocturnal reflux occurs, avoid caffeine, chocolate, fried food, alcohol, onions, spicy and acidic foods, elevate head of bed); medical (H2 blocker, proton pump inhibitor), surgical (fundoplication)

Esophageal Dysmotility and Obstruction

- <u>History</u>: often presents as thoracic dysphagia (food-sticking-in-chest sensation) but may present as cervical dysphagia (nonspecific symptoms), chest pressure/pain, cough, heartburn, weight loss
- <u>Exam</u>: nonspecific but may have pooling of secretions in pyriform sinuses on laryngoscopy
- <u>Dx</u>: esophagram, pH/impedance testing, esophagoscopy, FEES (presence of esophagopharyngeal reflux/regurgitation after swallowed bolus disappears below hypopharynx)
- <u>Tx</u>: reflux management, GI referral, general surgery referral in select cases

Head and Neck Malignancies

- <u>History</u>: significant smoking/alcohol use, weight loss, trismus, hemoptysis, dysphonia, progressive dysphagia, throat/neck pain, voice change, otalgia
- <u>Exam</u>: neck mass; oral cavity, oropharyngeal, or laryngeal lesion/mass
- <u>Tx</u>: surgery, radiation and/or chemotherapy, dysphagia therapy during and after treatment

Head and Neck Malignancy
Posttreatment Dysphagia

Post-Radiotherapy/Chemoradiation Dysphagia

- short-term edema and long-term fibrosis/stenosis (~6 months); synergistic effect with concurrent chemotherapy
- <u>Exam</u>: physical obstruction, functional deficits (laryngeal elevation, pharyngeal contraction)
- <u>Dx</u>: laryngoscopy, FEES, esophagoscopy/TNE, esophagram, MBSS
- <u>Tx</u>: pharyngeal and/or esophageal dilation, swallow therapy, gastrostomy or alternative feeding route for enteral nutrition

Postsurgical Dysphagia

- depends on anatomical resection (tongue, posterior oral cavity, pharynx, larynx)
- <u>Dx</u>: endoscopic evaluation (laryngoscopy, esophagoscopy), MBSS, esophagram
- <u>Tx</u>: swallow therapy before, during, and after treatment; surgical dilation

Presbyphagia

- older adults have increased lingual atrophy/fatty infiltration, and decreased strength, endurance, and mobility and pharyngeal muscles
- swallowing is slower due to a delay in pharyngeal swallow response and decreased pharyngeal sensation to stimuli
- increased pooling of secretions due to decreased swallow frequency
- <u>Dx</u>: H&P, MBSS, FEES
- <u>Tx</u>: swallow therapy, prosthetic devices

Neuromyogenic

Stroke/Traumatic Brain Injury or Neuropathy

- <u>History</u>: focal neurologic deficit, aspiration pneumonia, cranial/central or peripheral neuropathy
- <u>Exam</u>: mainly affects oral competency with incomplete oral clearance, premature spillage, decreased laryngeal sensation, pharyngeal weakness, dysarthria
- <u>Dx</u>: FEES ± sensory testing (FEESST), MBSS laryngoscopy/videostroboscopy to assess vocal fold mobility
- <u>Tx</u>: swallow therapy, dietary/lifestyle modifications, injection laryngoplasty/medialization thyroplasty, if indicated

Cranial Nerve Palsy/Paralysis

- <u>History</u>: dysphonia, globus, choking, aspiration pneumonia
- <u>Exam</u>: vocal fold paresis/paralysis, reduced medial pharyngeal constriction, tongue weakness/atrophy with or without fasciculations
- <u>Dx</u>: videostroboscopy, FEES, FEESST
- <u>Tx</u>: swallow therapy, injection laryngoplasty/medialization thyroplasty (for vocal fold paresis or paralysis)

Extrapyramidal Syndrome (Parkinson's Disease, Parkinsonism)

- <u>History</u>: resting hand/head tremor, bradykinesia, rigidity, ataxia
- <u>Exam</u>: oral stage deficits, xerostomia from high levodopa dosage, soft monotone voice, occasional voice tremor
- <u>Dx</u>: FEES, MBSS
- <u>Tx</u>: treatment of extrapyramidal syndrome, swallow therapy

SWALLOW REHABILITATION STRATEGIES

- <u>Effortful swallow</u>: patient squeezes all throat and neck muscle to improve BOT contact to posterior pharyngeal wall → increases pharyngeal clearance
- <u>Masako technique</u>: patient holds tip of tongue between teeth during swallow → increased BOT strength and bolus transit through pharynx
- <u>Mendelsohn maneuver</u>: manual anterosuperior displacement of larynx → prolong UES opening
- <u>Supraglottic swallow</u>: patient holds breath before swallow and voluntarily coughs after swallow; followed by an additional swallow to clear any residuals
- <u>Change size of bolus</u>: easier to manage small bites/sips than large ones
- <u>Change food consistency</u>: higher rate of penetration/aspiration with liquids (especially thin liquids); thicker consistencies easier to manage but poorly accepted by patients—commonly leads to dehydration
- <u>Postural changes</u>: (1) head rotation to side of weaker pharyngeal function → increases pyriform sinus/lateral channel clearance; (2) chin tuck → facilitates vallecular clearance
- <u>Cyclical ingestion</u>: alternating ingestion of solids and liquids → increases solid bolus clearance from pharynx

CHAPTER

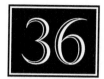

36

Esophageal Motility, Stenosis and Achalasia

Andrew E. Lee, Jennifer M. Schwartz, Katherine L. Tsavaris, and Asyia Ahmad

ESOPHAGEAL ANATOMY

Gross Anatomy

- the esophagus originates at the cricopharyngeus muscle in the neck at the level of C6
- it descends within the neck along the posterior aspect of the trachea until tracheal bifurcation
- the esophagus lays rear to the left main-stem bronchus and left atrium in the posterior mediastinum
- the proximal aorta and arch are anterior to esophagus; the descending aorta courses laterally and then posteriorly behind the esophagus
- the esophagus enters the abdominal cavity via the diaphragmatic hiatus at the level of T10 and terminates at the esophagogastric junction (EGJ)
- average length: 18 to 26 cm
- the proximal 5% to 30% of the esophagus is composed of skeletal muscle and the distal 50% to 60% of the distal esophagus is composed of smooth muscle; between the skeletal and smooth muscle there is a transition zone of indeterminate length

Sphincters

- two high-pressure sphincters exist at either end to prevent reflux: the upper esophageal sphincter (UES) and lower esophageal sphincter (LES)
- unlike the LES, the UES is created by a band of skeletal muscle (cricopharyngeus muscle) bowed around the esophagus
- when contracted the cricopharyngeus muscle acts as a "sling" around of the esophagus
- the LES is a high-pressure area composed of (1) thickening of the muscularis externa circular smooth muscle layer, (2) diaphragmatic crural muscles, and (3) muscular component from the gastric cardia

Microscopic Anatomy

- four distinct layers of the esophagus exist (listed in order of closest to the lumen): mucosa, submucosa, muscularis externa, adventitia
- the mucosa consists of epithelium, lamina propria, and the muscularis mucosa
- the epithelium of the esophagus is nonkeratinized, stratified squamous epithelium
  1. serves as a mechanical barrier of protection

    2. metaplasia of the epithelium may occur with repeated insult (eg, gastroesophageal reflux disease [GERD])

- the lamina propria is composed of supportive connective tissue and contains blood vessels and inflammatory cells
- the function of the muscularis mucosa has not been fully understood
- the submucosa is a connective tissue layer, which contains blood and lymph vessels, mucus-secreting glands, and nerves
- a plexus of nerves within the submucosa (Meissner's plexus) innervates the muscularis mucosa
- the muscularis externa is composed of an outer longitudinal and inner circular muscle layer, with slight overlap existing between the two layers
- there is slight overlap between the two layers
- between the muscle layers is a tissue bed that contains neurons called Auerbach's plexus
- Auerbach's plexus is composed of postganglionic parasympathetic fibers that receive neural input from the vagus to coordinate esophageal peristalsis
- disruption of the Auerbach's plexus causes disruption in the coordination of peristalsis and leads to motility disorders
- the adventitia is the outermost connective tissue covering
- the esophagus lacks a serosa

COORDINATION OF SWALLOWING

- three phases of swallowing: oral, pharyngeal, and esophageal

Oral Phase

- occurs after mastication when the decision to swallow has been made
- the proximal aspect of the tongue is placed firmly against the hard palate
- a food bolus laying in the central crease of the tongue is directed posteriorly by the action of the intrinsic muscles of the tongue and genioglossus
- the dorsum of the tongue contracts against the hard palate pushing the bolus into the posterior oropharynx

Pharyngeal Phase

- consists of many coordinated movements that occur nearly simultaneously

1. the levator veli palatini, tensor veli palatini, and palatoglossus muscles lift and tighten the soft palate and uvula to wall of the nasopharynx from the oropharynx
2. the styloid, styloglossus, stylopharyngeus, palatoglossus, and posterior belly of the digastric raise the larynx
3. the geniohyoid, mylohyoid, anterior belly of the digastric and thyrohyoid muscles contract to pull the larynx forward
4. the combined upward and anterior movement of the larynx opens the UES
5. the epiglottis covers the larynx to prevent aspiration
6. the UES relaxes almost simultaneously as the larynx is raised
7. once the food bolus passes into the esophagus through an open UES the pharyngeal phase ends

- at baseline, continual stimulation of the cricopharyngeus muscle via motor neurons keep the UES contracted
- decreased firing of the motor neurons relaxes the cricopharyngeus muscle and relaxes the UES
- relaxing of the UES must occur prior to opening of the UES

Esophageal Phase

- swallowing stimulates afferent sensory nerves in the larynx and pharynx to travel to the medulla; vagal efferents then carry output to proximal striated muscle groups of the esophagus
- vagal nerves release acetylcholine (ACh) on nicotinic receptors of motor end plates, thereby initiating contraction
- consecutive activation of motor end plates causes peristaltic contraction toward the distal esophagus
- peristaltic waves stimulated by a swallow are termed *primary peristaltic contractions*; these waves transverse the entire length of the esophagus
- peristaltic waves can also be induced by local stretch when sensed by afferent nerves within the esophageal wall
- peristaltic waves stimulated by focal stretch of the wall are called *secondary peristaltic contractions*; these waves travel only from the point of distention toward the distal esophagus
- additionally, tertiary waves can occur with swallowing or spontaneously and are nonperistaltic in nature
- smooth muscle activation of the esophagus is more complex than striated muscle activation
- it requires synchronous coordinated relaxation and contraction of outer longitudinal and inner circular muscles
- this coordination is orchestrated by inhibitory neurons and excitatory neurons within the Auerbach's plexus

- the main stimulatory neurotransmitter is ACh; the main inhibitory neurotransmitter is nitric oxide (NO)
- contraction of proximal smooth muscle segments and relaxation of distal smooth muscle segments in relation to a food bolus helps to move the food bolus distally
- contraction of the outer longitudinal muscle works to shorten the muscle segment moving the food bolus toward the stomach
- contraction of a slightly overlapping area of circular muscle occurs to force the food bolus into the next muscle segment
- the food bolus is pushed distally with successive contractions of the smooth muscle layers until it reaches just proximal to the LES
- additionally, smooth muscle contraction of the mid to distal esophagus is also indirectly influenced via vagal stimulation synapsing on Auerbach's plexus

Relaxation of the LES Sphincter

- the LES tone is a result of the tonic property of the smooth muscle itself as well as the neural input of stimulatory and inhibitory neurons
- normal tone: 10 to 40 mm Hg
- LES relaxation is triggered by:
    1. stretch of the proximal side of the EGJ by a food bolus sensed by afferent fibers
    2. inhibitory neuronal activation releasing inhibitory neurotransmitters, more specifically NO and vasoactive intestinal peptide (VIP)
- sphincter sufficiency is also supplemented by the right crus of the diaphragmatic hiatus and the angle at which the esophagus enters the stomach
- muscular, hormonal, and neuronal factors contribute to physiologic control of LES relaxation and contraction
- LES relaxation allows the LES to open and for a food bolus to enter the stomach
- once a food bolus has passed, the LES contracts to prevent reflux of gastric materials

HIGH-RESOLUTION ESOPHAGEAL MANOMETRY

- small, flexible tube is passed through nasal cavity and into patient's stomach
- pressure sensors spaced at 1-cm intervals
- sensors detect pressure in multiple different directions
- records the contractions of the esophageal muscles during deglutition

Integrated Relaxation Pressure (IRP)

- mean pressure during the 4 seconds of maximal EGJ relaxation in the 10-second window beginning at upper esophageal relaxation
    1. an assessment of the EGJ relaxation with wet swallows
    2. normal value is <15 mm Hg
    3. elevated levels indicate that the EGJ is not relaxing appropriately with wet swallows

Contractile Deceleration Point (CDP)

- inflection point along the 30 mm Hg isobaric contour at which propagation velocity slows; CDP must be localized within 3 cm of the proximal margin of the LES
    1. location on manometric tracing where velocity of the peristaltic pressure wave begins to slow as it moves toward the EGJ
    2. landmark used to calculate distal latency

Distal Latency (DL)

- interval of time between upper esophageal sphincter relaxation (swallow) and CDP
    1. an assessment of premature esophageal body contractions
    2. normal is ≥4.5 seconds
    3. <4.5 seconds indicates esophageal spasm

Distal Contractile Integral (DCI)
(See Table 36–1)

- product of amplitude, duration, and length (measured in mm Hg*s*cm) of the distal esophageal contraction
    1. an assessment of esophageal body peristaltic pressure

ESOPHAGEAL MOTILITY DISORDERS

Achalasia

Epidemiology

- incidence of approximately 1 in 100,000 per year in United States but may be underestimated
- <u>Bimodal distribution</u>: large peak around age 70 with smaller peak around age 30

TABLE 36–1. Distal Contractile Integral Is a Measure of Contractile Vigor

Distal Contractile Integral Classification	Value (mm Hg*s*cm)
Failed	<100
Weak	100–450
Ineffective	0–450
Normal	450–8000
Hypercontractile	>8000

Source: Adapted from Kahrilas PJ, Bredenoord AJ, Fox M, et al. The Chicago Classification of Esophageal Motility Disorders, v3.0. *Neurogastroenterol Motil.* 2015;27(2):160–161.

- may present at any age but increased risk with age
- equal gender distribution and no racial predilection

Pathophysiology

- inflammatory, neurodegenerative condition of the esophagus
- loss of postganglionic inhibitory neurons of the myenteric plexus leads to a decrease in inhibitory transmitter (NO, VIP) concentration, leading to a lack of LES relaxation and causing chest pain and dysphagia
- excitatory neurons remain intact in early disease
- loss of excitatory neurons containing acetylcholine occur in the later stages of achalasia leading to flaccid esophageal paralysis and nocturnal regurgitation

Causes

- idiopathic
- Infectious: herpes simplex virus, measles virus
- Pseudo-achalasia: related to tumors or illnesses that infiltrate the myenteric plexus; represents 5% of achalasia cases, and 50% of those cases are due to an adenocarcinoma of the gastroesophageal junction
- other causes of pseudo-achalasia include:
  1. pancreatic cancer
  2. hepatocellular cancer
  3. lung cancer

    4. amyloidosis

    5. sarcoidosis

    6. pancreatic cyst

- paraneoplastic:
    1. small cell lung cancer (Anti-Hu antibodies)
    2. non-Hodgkin's lymphoma
    3. ovarian cancer
- **Chagas disease**: endemic disease of central Brazil, Venezuela, and northern Argentina caused by protozoan *Trypanosoma cruzi* passed by the Reduviid (kissing) bug:
    1. causes destruction of autonomic ganglion cells throughout the body, including the gastrointestinal (GI), cardiac, and respiratory tracts
    2. abnormal esophageal peristalsis is first detected after 50% of ganglion cell destruction, and esophageal dilatation occurs after 90% destruction
- **Allgrove's disease**: known as "Triple-A Syndrome"—**A**chalasia, **A**lacrima (insufficient tear production), **A**drenocorticotropic hormone deficiency
    1. autosomal recessive disorder that presents in childhood
    2. alacrima and hypoglycemia are the earliest manifestations
- **Obstetric achalasia**: rarely can affect pregnant patients
- **Post-sleeve achalasia**: patients that have dysphagia after surgery should undergo an upper endoscopy to rule out mechanical causes; manometry can be performed for further evaluation
- **Parkinson's achalasia**: Lewy bodies (intracytoplasmic eosinophilic inclusion bodies) can be found within myenteric plexus in these patients

Types of Achalasia

Type I (Classic Achalasia)

- characterized by incomplete LES relaxation
- aperistalsis and absence of esophageal pressurization
- represent 55% of achalasia cases
- responds to both pneumatic dilation and surgical or endoscopic myotomy
- high-resolution esophageal manometry findings:
    1. elevated mean integrated relaxation pressure (IRP) >15 mm Hg
    2. 100% failed peristalsis—distal contractile integral (DCI) <100 mm Hg
    3. distal latency (DL) <4.5 seconds with DCI <450 mm Hg*s*cm

Type II (Achalasia With Compression)

- characterized by incomplete LES relaxation, aperistalsis and panesophageal pressurization in at least 20% of swallows
- represent 40% of achalasia cases
- carries a positive predictive value for responsiveness to therapy, and is the subtype with the highest response to pneumatic balloon dilatation and Heller's myotomy
- high-resolution esophageal manometry findings:
  1. elevated mean IRP (>15 mm Hg)
  2. 100% failed peristalsis (DCI <100 mm Hg)
  3. panesophageal pressurization with at least 20% of swallows

Type III (Spastic Achalasia)

- characterized by incomplete LES relaxation and premature contractions (DL <4.5 seconds) in at least 20% of swallows
- represent 5% of achalasia cases
- carries a negative predictive value for response to pneumatic dilatation
- surgical or endoscopic myotomy are the therapies of choice
- high-resolution esophageal manometry findings:
  1. elevated mean IRP (>15 mm Hg)
  2. no normal peristalsis
  3. premature contractions with DCI >450 mm Hg*s*cm for ≥20% of swallows

Presentation

- solid and liquid dysphagia and chest pain are early symptoms
- nocturnal regurgitation of undigested food and weight loss are late symptoms
- chest pain may improve or disappear with time
- other symptoms include heartburn, nocturnal cough, choking, hiccups, and aspiration
- many describe eating as a strenuous activity that is worsened if food is rapidly consumed and may complain of halitosis
- weight loss can be seen in cases of pseudo-achalasia
- rarely, patients have airway compromise secondary to a dilated esophagus compressing on the trachea

Complications

- aspiration pneumonia is common

- squamous cell carcinoma is a rare complication and is likely secondary to high levels of nitrosamines produced by bacterial overgrowth in a stagnant esophagus
- higher risk of adenocarcinoma compared to the general population
- no current evidence to support primary screening for cancer
- untreated and advanced disease may lead to megaesophagus, requiring an esophagectomy

Diagnosis

- chest x-ray, barium esophagram, computed tomography (CT)/ magnetic resonance imaging (MRI), upper endoscopy, high-resolution esophageal manometry

Chest X-Ray

- may show air-fluid level within the esophagus
- reveals pneumonia, masses, or deviated airway

Barium Esophagram

- evaluates esophageal phase of swallowing
- will often show a dilated esophagus with distal tapering referred to as the **"bird's beak"**
- inability of swallowed air to pass into stomach leads to **lack of gastric air bubble**
- megaesophagus in late disease

CT/MRI

- demonstrates dilated liquid/food filled esophageal with thickening of esophageal wall
- may be considered to rule out underlying malignancy

Upper Endoscopy

- often normal in early stages of achalasia
- puckered LES and dilated esophagus in later stages
- may see stasis esophagitis or candida colonization in the obstructed esophagus
- resistance through LES should raise suspicion of achalasia
- helpful in excluding secondary causes of achalasia such as gastric carcinoma

High-Resolution Esophageal Manometry

- gold standard test
- hypertensive LES that fail to relax with deglutition, pressurization of esophagus, no progressive peristalsis

Treatment

- medical management such as proton-pump inhibitors (PPIs), calcium-channel blockers, and nitrates are recommended for those who cannot undergo surgical or endoscopic therapies
- lifestyle management should be a part of every patient's regimen

Lifestyle Management

- eat foods very slowly, and chew thoroughly, wash down meals with plenty of water, and avoid eating near bedtime

Calcium-Channel Blockers

- <u>Mechanism</u>: causes relaxation via inhibition of calcium entry into excitable cells
- <u>Medications</u>: nifedipine
- should be taken 30 minutes prior to meals for best response
- response rates highly varied: 0% to 75%
- <u>Adverse effects</u>: hypotension, dizziness, weakness, headache, nausea, abdominal pain, diarrhea, constipation, lower extremity swelling, flushing of the skin, skin rash, anaphylaxis

Nitrates

- <u>Mechanism</u>: direct relaxant effect on esophagus
- <u>Medications</u>: isosorbide dinitrate
- should be taken 15 minutes prior to meals for best response
- response rates varied: 53% to 87%
- <u>Adverse effects</u>: hypotension, dizziness, weakness, headache, weakness, flushing skin, anaphylaxis
- contraindicated with concurrent use of Sildenafil

Botulinum Toxin Injection

- injection into the LES muscle performed during endoscopy, leading to symptom relief in approximately two-thirds of patients for 3 months to 1 year

- botulinum toxin targets excitatory neurons in the LES, causing relaxation
- can be done repetitively, but there is a loss of response over time with subsequent injections
- reserved for patients who cannot undergo other surgical/endoscopic options
- one-fifth of patients may experience chest pain after procedure

Pneumatic Balloon Dilation

- deflated balloon advanced via guidewire and fluoroscopic support to the LES, and inflated to tear the muscularis propria
- approximately 60% response rate after one dilation; increased response rate after consecutive dilations
- often advised to have postendoscopic upper GI series to rule out perforation
- perforation occurs in up to 1% to 5% of pneumatic balloon dilations, and present with chest pain
- other common post-op symptoms: GERD, bleeding

Heller Myotomy

- laparoscopic procedure to separate the LES muscles from the serosal layer
- often coupled with a Dor (or anterior) fundoplication due to high incidence of iatrogenic GERD
- relieves symptoms in up to 90% of patients
- symptoms are gone in about 75% of patients 10 years after operation

Peroral Endoscopic Myotomy (POEM)

- use electrical scalpel through endoscope to make incision in esophageal lining to create a tunnel between the inner lining and outer muscular layer of esophagus
- high incidence of postoperative GERD
- shorter hospital stays postoperatively

OTHER MOTILITY DISORDERS

Esophagogastric Junction Outflow Obstruction

- <u>Epidemiology</u>: estimated prevalence of 16/1000 among those with suspected achalasia

- <u>Pathophysiology</u>: impaired LES relaxation with preserved peristalsis on high-resolution esophageal manometry
- <u>Etiology</u>: may be an initial presentation of achalasia, or due to distal stricturing from chronic reflux, tight Nissen fundoplication site; often found as an incidental finding
- <u>Presentation</u>: can be asymptomatic, or present with dysphagia, atypical chest pain, regurgitation
- <u>Dx</u>: high-resolution esophageal manometry
  1. elevated mean IRP (>15 mm Hg) with high intrabolus pressure
  2. sufficient peristalsis with a DL >4.5 seconds
- <u>Tx</u>: no treatment if patient is asymptomatic; treatments depend on etiology and severity of symptoms; Sildenafil can be considered; other treatments include pneumatic balloon dilation, Botox injection or Heller's myotomy

Distal Esophageal Spasm

- <u>Epidemiology</u>: prevalence between 3% and 9% in those with symptoms of dysphagia; mean age of diagnosis of 60 years; has a slight female predominance
- <u>Pathophysiology</u>: deficiency of nitric oxide in esophageal smooth muscle leads to unopposed activation of cholinergic neurons, causing intermittent, simultaneous nonperistaltic contractions
- <u>Presentation</u>: intermittent dysphagia and odynophagia to solids and liquids, heartburn, chest pain, weight loss (uncommon)
- may mimic a myocardial infarction, and cardiac sources of chest pain must be ruled out prior to esophageal workup
- symptoms typically occur in the evening and nighttimes, and are exacerbated by times of physical or emotional stress, and ingestion of cold liquids
- <u>Dx</u>: high-resolution esophageal manometry (HREM) is considered the gold standard; barium esophagram may help in diagnosis
  1. HREM shows premature contractions (distal latency <4.5 seconds) in at least 20% of swallows with a normal integrated relaxation pressure
  2. DES may be missed on HREM as spasm is only an intermittent disturbance
  3. barium esophagram shows the classic "corkscrew" pattern and may not record DES given its intermittent nature
  4. barium esophagram can detect anatomic abnormalities such as diverticula
- <u>Tx</u>: PPI, nitrates, phosphodiesterase-5 (PDE-5) inhibitors, calcium-channel blockers (CCBs), tricyclic antidepressants (TCAs), botulinum toxin; role of surgery remains controversial because of the lack of outcome studies

1. high-dose PPIs should be considered in all patients
2. nitrates (isosorbide dinitrate) help decrease contraction duration but not contraction amplitude
3. PDE5 inhibitors (Sildenafil) cause decrease in esophageal contraction amplitude via nitric oxide release in the smooth muscle cells
4. CCBs (nifedipine, diltiazem) cause smooth muscle relaxation
5. TCAs (amitriptyline, imipramine) can help relieve DES-associated chest pain but benefits may take up to 8 weeks to work; associated with sedation, dizziness, constipation, and QTc prolongation.

Hypercontractile Esophagus (Jackhammer Esophagus)

- <u>Pathophysiology</u>: likely secondary to excessive cholinergic activity or myocyte hypertrophy
- <u>Presentation</u>: intermittent chest pain and dysphagia
- <u>Dx</u>: high-resolution esophageal manometry is the gold standard, showing a distal contractile integral (DCI) >8000 mm Hg*s*cm in at least 20% of swallows with a normal distal latency and normal IRP; esophageal pH monitoring is recommended given its relationship with GERD
- <u>Tx</u>: PPIs are first-line therapy; nitrates and CCBs appear to reduce LES pressure and contraction amplitude

Scleroderma Esophagus (Progressive Systemic Sclerosis)

Epidemiology

- 20 cases per million per year in the United States
- most commonly seen in Caucasian females between 45 and 60 years of age
- more aggressive disease seen in African Americans and Native Americans
- the esophagus is affected in up to 90% of those with scleroderma who have had esophageal evaluations

Pathophysiology

- autoimmune disorder characterized by small vessel vasculitis, excess tissue fibrosis, and smooth muscle atrophy

- causes aperistalsis of the lower two-thirds of the esophagus and a low-pressure LES
- systemic sclerosis is associated with the **Anti-Scl-70** and **Anti-RNA Polymerase III** antibodies
- there is a limited variant known as **CREST** syndrome, which is associated with the **Anti-Centromere** antibody

Systemic SSx

- hardening of skin is hallmark sign
- other SSx: Raynaud's phenomenon (usually the earliest sign), pulmonary fibrosis, pulmonary arterial hypertension, pericarditis, hypertensive renal crisis, fatigue, weight loss
- **CREST syndrome** (limited disease): **C**alcinosis, **R**aynaud's phenomenon, **E**sophageal dysmotility, **S**clerodactyly, **T**elangiectasias

Esophageal and Oral SSx

- decreased oral aperture, difficulty chewing, difficulty performing routine dental care such as brushing teeth and flossing
- decreased salivary production can lead to periodontal disease
- severe heartburn, dysphagia to solids and liquids, chest pain, candida esophagitis
- malabsorption may occur secondary to bacterial overgrowth, leading to dyspepsia and epigastric abdominal pain

Diagnosis

- HREM: normal UES pressure, aperistalsis of the distal two-thirds of esophagus with preservation of peristalsis in the proximal third of the esophagus, and low or absent LES pressure
- Barium swallow: dilated, flaccid esophagus similar to achalasia

Treatment

- acid suppression with PPI and lifestyle changes
- calcium-channel blockers for Raynaud's phenomenon.
- antireflux surgery may exacerbate dysphagia if a tight fundoplication is created
- GERD behavior management: (1) small, nonfatty meals; (2) avoid recumbent position at least 2 hours after eating; (3) elevate the head of bed to at least 6 inches; (4) avoid tight-fitting clothing; (5) avoid agents that decrease LES pressure such as caffeine, tobacco, alcohol, mints, chocolate, garlic, onions, calcium channel blockers, β-adrenergics

- <u>Complications</u>: erosive esophagitis, ulcerations, recurrent strictures, Barrett's esophagus, adenocarcinoma

Ineffective Esophageal Motility

- <u>Pathophysiology</u>: most often secondary to uncontrolled gastric reflux
- <u>Presentation</u>: dysphagia, heartburn, or atypical chest pain due to GERD
- <u>Dx</u>: high-resolution esophageal manometry shows a normal IRP with ≥50% ineffective swallows (weak or failed)
    1. <u>Weak</u>: DCI 100 to 450 mm Hg*cm*s
    2. <u>Failed</u>: DCI <100 mm Hg*cm*s
- <u>Tx</u>: acid-suppression and GERD behavior management

Fragmented Peristalsis

- <u>Pathophysiology</u>: commonly seen in patients with severe GERD and respiratory symptoms
- <u>Presentation</u>: dysphagia, heartburn, or atypical chest pain due to GERD
- <u>Dx</u>: high-resolution esophageal manometry
    1. >5 cm peristaltic breaks in >50% of wet swallows
    2. 30% of more wet swallows with distal amplitudes of <30 mm Hg
- <u>Tx</u>: acid-suppression and GERD behavior management

STRUCTURAL DISORDERS OF THE ESOPHAGUS

Esophageal Strictures

Introduction

- **simple strictures:** defined as short (<2 cm), focal, and straight, with a diameter ≥12 cm
- **complex strictures:** defined as long (>2 cm), tortuous, and angulated, with a narrow diameter <12 cm
- lesion is typically located at the level of or distal to the point where the patient localizes the dysphagia
- <u>Presentation</u>: solid food dysphagia, with intermittent symptoms occurring when the esophageal lumen is ≤20 mm, and continuous symptoms present when lumen is ≤13 mm
- benign strictures are caused by inflammatory states that promote collagen and fibrous tissue deposition

- malignant strictures result from intrinsic luminal tumor growth or extrinsic esophageal compression

Diagnosing Esophageal Strictures

- **endoscopy** is the best diagnostic tool for esophageal strictures, as it allows for direct visualization of the esophagus; premalignant or malignant conditions can be evaluated, and therapeutic intervention can be performed, if necessary
- **barium swallow** can also diagnose strictures; however, this imaging modality should only be used first if there is suspicion for concurrent hypopharyngeal pathology, such as the presence of a ring, web, or diverticulum

Treatment of Esophageal Strictures

- **endoscopic dilation** is the mainstay of treatment
- endoscopy allows for evaluation for presence of Barrett's esophagus or esophagitis and allows for therapeutic intervention with dilation
- goal of dilation is to increase the luminal diameter to ≥12 to 14 mm, which typically results in immediate improvement of dysphagia
- types of dilators include **bougie-type** and **balloon dilators**
- there is no literature to support a difference between bougie-type and balloon dilation
- risk of esophageal perforation is increased with complex strictures
- high-risk populations for endoscopic dilation:
    1. acute or incompletely healed esophageal perforation
    2. malignant strictures
    3. severe pulmonary or cardiac disease or bleeding disorders
    4. pharyngeal or cervical deformity, recent surgery, large thoracic aneurysm
    5. eosinophilic esophagitis, pemphigus vulgaris, and epidermolysis bullosa-induced strictures
    6. food impaction

ETIOLOGIES OF BENIGN STRICTURES

Peptic Strictures

- occur in 7% to 23% of patients with untreated reflux esophagitis; however, 25% have no antecedent symptoms
- more common in Caucasian men
- typically located at squamocolumnar junction, <1 cm in length

- increased prevalence in patients with structural disorders, such as an incompetent LES, presence of hiatal hernia, or a diaphragmatic defect (right crus)
- <u>Presentation</u>: insidious onset of solid food dysphagia, many may have antecedent heartburn
- history alone can diagnose approximately 80% of cases
- impaired esophageal motility delays esophageal clearance and plays a role in stricture formation
- <u>Pathogenesis</u>: inflammation associated with gastroesophageal reflux extends through all layers of the esophageal wall, causing connective tissue deposition and subsequent formation of fibrosis, scarring, shortening and loss of muscle compliance, leading to stricture formation
- <u>Dx</u>: endoscopy; barium swallow may also be used
  1. endoscopy offers direct visualization of the esophagus for diagnosis, allowing for simultaneous therapeutic intervention, if necessary
  2. barium swallow should be performed first only if there is a concern for hypopharyngeal pathology, such as the presence of a Zenker's diverticulum or cricopharyngeal bar
- <u>Tx</u>: acid suppression with PPI, endoscopic dilation, or intralesional steroid injection in refractory strictures
- treatment with PPIs decrease the need for repeated dilations to approximately 30%

Pill-Induced Strictures

- injury occurs just above where the esophagus physiologically narrows: at the tracheal bifurcation, above the LES and above other strictures
- <u>Pathogenesis</u>: ingested tablets or capsules lodge in the esophagus, subsequently releasing undiluted contents directly into the esophageal mucosa, leading to caustic injury of the mucosa; injury may be caused directly by concentrated medication, which can be caustic, or by interaction with refluxed gastric contents; alkali ingestion leads to liquefactive necrosis causing an inflammatory response with scar formation, and may alter pressure and motility and promote acid reflux, whereas acid ingestion induces coagulation necrosis and eschar formation
- sustained-release formulations are more likely to cause stricture formation
- medications commonly known to cause injury include ferrous sulfate, tetracyclines (specifically doxycycline), phenytoin, bisphosphonates (specifically alendronate), potassium chloride and aspirin
  1. ferrous sulfate and doxycycline cause acidic injury

2. phenytoin and alendronate cause alkaline injury; alendronate is the most commonly reported cause of serious pill-induced esophageal injury
3. potassium chloride causes local tissue hyperosmolarity
4. aspirin causes intracellular damage

-   <u>Presentation</u>: presents with sudden onset of odynophagia or retrosternal pain; slowly progressive painless dysphagia is uncommon, but more commonly observed with alendronate, quinidine, or potassium chloride
-   complications include hemorrhage, esophageal perforation, mediastinitis, and fibrotic stricture formation
-   <u>Dx</u>: demonstration of typical symptoms may be enough to make diagnosis; however, endoscopy is indicated with gradual onset of symptoms, presence of severe symptoms, persistent symptoms 1 week after discontinuation of culprit medication or in immunocompromised patients
-   <u>Tx</u>: avoidance of further mucosal injury and discontinuation of culprit medication; endoscopic dilation may be used
-   <u>Prevention</u>:
    1. patients should drink at least 4 oz. (120 mL) of fluid with ingestion of any pill and at least 8 oz. with pills known to cause injury
    2. patients should remain upright for at least 10 minutes after ingestion of any pill and at least 30 minutes with pills known to cause esophageal injury
    3. pills known to cause esophageal injury should be avoided in bedridden patients, as well as in patients with known esophageal compression, stricture, or dysmotility

Radiation-Induced Strictures

-   late sequelae of radiation therapy for esophageal cancer, lung cancer, lymphoma
-   variable time interval between radiation therapy and development of stricture, ranging from months to years
-   <u>Pathophysiology</u>: radiation causes subepithelial fibrosis, thickening of the esophageal wall and stenosis
-   factors that contribute to the development of strictures: dose and frequency of radiation, field size, fractionation, concomitant treatment with chemotherapy
-   <u>Dx</u>: endoscopy for direct visualization of mucosa
-   <u>Tx</u>: strictures tend to be refractory to endoscopic dilation; intralesional steroid injection used with refractory strictures

Caustic Strictures

- corrosive agents comprise a wide range of chemicals that lead to significant tissue damage
- in adults, these injuries are most commonly observed with suicide attempts
- severity of the injury depends on the pH of ingested substance, whether it is a solid or liquid, duration of exposure, and quantity ingested
- <u>Pathophysiology</u>: tissue damage occurs within seconds of ingestion of strong corrosive agent; within the first 24 hours, hemorrhage, thrombosis, and inflammation ensue
- <u>Presentation</u>: dysphagia, odynophagia, and drooling
- stricture formation is by far the most common late complication of corrosive injury, with prediction of development of stricture formation based on initial endoscopy or CT
- low-grade injuries (grades 1–2a) rarely cause stricture formation
- stricture formation is seen in up to 80% of patients with high-grade burns (grade 3b)
- <u>Dx</u>: endoscopy within 3 to 48 hours of injury allows for assessment of extent and severity of caustic injury; can be safely repeated within 3 weeks without increasing risk of perforation
  1. endoscopy lacks the ability to accurately predict the depth of necrosis, better demonstrated on CT scan
- endoscopic grading using the **Zargar Classification**
  1. grade 0 = normal
  2. grade 1 = edema and hyperemia of the mucosa
  3. grade 2a = superficial localized ulcerations, friability, and blisters
  4. grade 2b = circumferential and deep ulcerations
  5. grade 3a = multiple and deep ulcerations and small scattered areas of necrosis
  6. grade 3b = extensive necrosis
- <u>Tx</u>: endoscopic dilation is the first-line treatment option, which can be attempted safely after healing of acute injury, typically between 3 and 6 weeks after injury.
  1. approximately half of dilations are successful, as most caustic strictures tend to be refractory to dilation
  2. emergency surgery is required when transmural necrosis of the GI tract is observed

Anastomotic Strictures

- postoperative strictures may develop after esophagectomy and esophagogastrostomy or total gastrectomy

- incidence of stricture formation ranges from 5% to 46%
- operative factors such as type of anastomosis, presence of anastomotic leakage, and intraoperative blood loss all contribute to likelihood of stricture formation
- high rate of recurrence, due to underlying fibrosis and ischemia
- <u>Presentation</u>: dysphagia with inability to pass endoscope
- <u>Dx</u>: endoscopy
- <u>Tx</u>: strictures tend to be refractory to dilation
  1. adding intralesional steroid injection to dilation has not been found to be effective
  2. electrocautery needle-knife incision in refractory cases was successful with short strictures (<1 cm) after a single treatment and longer strictures after approximately 3 sessions

Epidermolysis Bullosa

- inherited bullous disease, which includes many distinct phenotypic subtypes
- dystrophic epidermolysis bullosa most commonly involves the esophagus
- characterized by marked fragility of epithelial tissue, manifesting with blister formation and nonhealing wounds following minor trauma
- repeated insult to the mucosa eventually leads to fibrosis and esophageal stricture formation
- <u>Presentation</u>: odynophagia and dysphagia
- <u>Tx</u>: dilation must be performed with extreme caution due to the fragility of the mucosa with increased risk of perforation
  1. balloon-type dilators offer an advantage due to their radial dilating force, which decreases risk of mucosal damage

Lichen Planus

- chronic skin disorder of unknown etiology and high relapse rate that presents with recurrent, pruritic papular eruptions that coalesce into rough scaly patches
- commonly affects flexor surfaces of the wrists, legs, and trunk, but can also affect the glans penis, and oral, anal, and vaginal mucosa
- oral lichen planus is common, and present in >50% of patients who have skin manifestations, typically presents as nonerosive lesions in the buccal mucosa
- affects the upper and mid-esophagus, sparing the GE junction (atypical for reflux esophagitis)
- esophageal lichen planus is a rare cause of esophageal stricture

- <u>Dx</u>: endoscopy with biopsy
  1. endoscopy demonstrates presence of lacy white papules, erosions, desquamation, and stenosis
  2. direct immunofluorescence reveals globular IgM deposits at the junction of the squamous epithelium and lamina propria

Pemphigus Vulgaris

- acquired antibody-mediated bullous disease that usually presents in the fourth to sixth decades of life
- autoantibodies against desmogleins 1 and 3
- presents with flaccid blisters that easily rupture (+ Nikolsky sign)
- oral lesions tend to appear the earliest, before presenting on the skin
- patients commonly present with dysphagia, odynophagia, or retrosternal burning
- esophageal lesions may appear similar to skin lesions, as flaccid blisters or erosions, or they can present as red longitudinal lines along the entire esophagus
- <u>Dx</u>: endoscopy with biopsy
  1. endoscopic biopsy specimens must include the entire esophageal mucosa and basement membrane, which demonstrates suprabasilar cleavage
  2. direct and indirect immunofluorescence shows intracellular immunoreactants along the border of keratinocytes in the epidermis
- <u>Tx</u>: moderate-to-high-dose corticosteroids; endoscopic dilation may be performed for severe esophageal disease, but must be done with caution to avoid injury as mucosa is fragile and highly susceptible to mucosal tearing

Eosinophilic Esophagitis (EoE)

- more common in men <50 years old who have history of asthma, atopy, or allergic rhinitis
- observed in patients with severe GERD and Schatzki's ring
- <u>Pathophysiology</u>: not completely understood, but most likely driven by a combination of genetic, immunologic, and environmental factors. Current research postulates that an impaired immunologic response to common antigens triggers the inflammatory cascade, causing the uncontrolled activation of eosinophils and the release of cytokines, mast cells, and basophils.
- <u>Presentation</u>: typically presents with recurrent food impactions and dysphagia with solid foods

- <u>Dx</u>: endoscopy with biopsy demonstrating >15 eosinophils/HPF
    1. findings on endoscopy include ringed esophagus with or without strictures, a small-caliber esophagus, linear furrowing, erythema, edema, eosinophilic microabscesses, granularity, and nodularity
    2. however, the esophagus may also appear normal on EGD
- <u>Tx</u>: PPI therapy, symptom diary, allergy testing, swallowed fluticasone, montelukast, steroids (budesonide); endoscopic dilation performed if significant esophagitis present after removal of food bolus; patient education
    1. patient should be placed on PPI for 2 to 4 weeks prior to performing endoscopic dilation
    2. dilation may be contraindicated in patients who have high esophageal impactions associated with a stricture, as high risk of esophageal perforation due to overtube injury
    3. counsel patient to eat slowly, adequately chew food, and avoid foods that may cause impaction

Herpes Simplex Virus (HSV)

- more commonly caused by HSV-1, but can also be seen with HSV-2
- causes small discrete vesicular or bullous lesions with erythematous base, with a predilection for the mid and distal esophagus
- vesicular lesions progress to form "volcano ulcers," which are punched-out circumscribed ulcers with raised edges
- ulcer may become confluent and form an esophageal stricture, however, this is an infrequently observed complication
- esophageal infections are primarily seen in individuals with HIV, cancer patients with granulocytopenia, and organ transplant patients; rarely can be seen in immunocompetent patients
- <u>Presentation</u>: odynophagia is the most common presenting symptom, occurring in over 76% of patients; dysphagia, substernal chest pain
- <u>Dx</u>: EGD with biopsy obtained from ulcer edge
- <u>Pathology</u>: red or amphophilic intranuclear inclusions with a peripheral rim of chromatin
- <u>Tx</u>: acyclovir

Cytomegalovirus (CMV)

- causes erosion, erythema, and serpiginous/shallow ulcers in the mid or distal esophagus
- complications of esophageal infection include stricture formation; however, this is an infrequently observed finding

- esophageal infections are primarily seen in individuals with HIV, cancer patients with granulocytopenia, and organ transplant patients; rarely can be seen in immunocompetent patients
- <u>Presentation</u>: odynophagia, dysphagia, substernal chest pain
- <u>Dx</u>: EGD with multiple biopsies taken from ulcer bed
  1. biopsy demonstrates intranuclear and cytoplasmic inclusion bodies with peripheral clearing, giving an "owl's eye" appearance
- <u>Tx</u>: ganciclovir

Other Rare Postinfectious Causes of Esophageal Strictures

- tuberculosis
- *Candida albicans*
- syphilis
- histoplasmosis

Post-Sclerotherapy

- sclerotherapy can be used to control actively bleeding esophageal varices; however, it is associated with a variety of local and systemic complications
- causes significant tissue necrosis, which can result in ulceration, resulting in bleeding or stricture formation, observed in up to 40% of cases
- alternatively, variceal band ligation has a significantly lower incidence of complications compared to sclerotherapy
- variceal injection-induced strictures lead to significant morbidity in up to 50% of cases and require repeated treatment with dilation therapy

Photodynamic Therapy (PDT)

- PDT is an older endoscopic treatment for Barrett's esophagus with high-grade dysplasia and early esophageal cancer
- the most common adverse effect is esophageal stricture formation
- the exact mechanism of injury is unknown, but it is likely an inflammatory reaction that induces fibrosis with subsequent stricture formation
- patients typically present with dysphagia approximately 3 weeks after PDT
- strictures are more likely to occur if endoscopic mucosal resection is performed prior to PDT, prior history of esophageal stricture, or multiple treatments of the same esophageal segment

- <u>Tx</u>: endoscopic dilation; esophageal stenting in refractory strictures using self-expanding plastic and metal stents (SEMS, SEPS)
- most post-PDT strictures are complex, requiring multiple dilations with high rates of recurrence

Post-Radiofrequency Ablation (RFA)

- RFA is a treatment modality used to eradicate dysplasia and intestinal metaplasia in patients with dysplastic Barrett's esophagus (BE)
- most efficient treatment modality and standard of care for patients with BE
- utilizes thermal injury to induce cellular damage
- studies have shown that 78% of patients will achieve complete remission of intestinal metaplasia, and 91% will achieve complete remission of dysplasia after approximately 2 to 3 treatments with RFA
- most commonly observed adverse event is esophageal stricture formation, with 5.1% of patients developing strictures after treatment with RFA; however, incidence of stricture increases to 13.3% when RFA is combined with EMR
- no significant difference in postablative stricture formation between ultra-long-segment BE and long-segment BE
- <u>Tx</u>: endoscopic dilation

Refractory Strictures

- strictures that are unable to be dilated to a diameter of 14 mm over 5 sessions at 2-week intervals
- complex strictures are more difficult to treat and tend to be refractory or recur, despite dilation therapy
- **Intralesional injection of steroids**: indicated with refractory strictures; may reduce inflammation and subsequent fibrosis, preventing stricture recurrence; combination therapy with acid suppression may diminish the need for repeat dilations with peptic strictures and radiation-induced strictures
- **Self-expanding metal stents (SEMS)**: long-term success observed when used for postradiation strictures; complications include stent migration and hyperplastic tissue formation
- **Self-expanding plastic stents (SEPS)**: decreased risk of hyperplastic tissue overgrowth, but high rate of stent migration observed with proximal and distal strictures
- **Needle-knife incision**: high success rate when used for anastomotic strictures; low incidence of esophageal perforation

SCHATZKI RING

- a concentric submucosal fibrotic thickening most commonly found at the squamocolumnar junction; also known as the "lower esophageal ring" or "B ring"
- associated with the presence of hiatal hernia, suggesting acid exposure as an underlying etiology
- <u>Presentation</u>: intermittent dysphagia to solids or food impaction
- continuous or persistent symptoms occur when the esophageal lumen becomes ≤12 mm
- <u>Dx</u>: barium esophagram with solid bolus challenge
- <u>Tx</u>: most are asymptomatic and do not require treatment; symptomatic rings can be treated with mechanical dilation; endoscopic incision or thermal ablation may be used for rings refractory to dilation
  1. dilation performed using an 18- to 20-mm dilator; does not require gradual dilation

ESOPHAGEAL WEBS

- thin membrane of mucosal and submucosal tissue that can cause a protrusion or partial obstruction into the esophageal lumen
- etiology unknown, but hypothesized to be remnants of incomplete vacuolation of esophageal epithelium
- most commonly seen in Caucasian females
- <u>Presentation</u>: typically asymptomatic, but may present with dysphagia to solids, pica, nasopharyngeal reflux, aspiration
- associated diseases/syndromes include Plummer-Vinson syndrome, cicatricial pemphigoid, epidermolysis bullosa, graft versus host disease
- <u>Dx</u>: barium swallow
- <u>Tx</u>: mild symptoms can often be alleviated by lifestyle modifications; endoscopic dilation is almost always effective if treatment is indicated

ESOPHAGEAL DIVERTICULUM

Traction Diverticula

- typically seen in the lower third of the esophagus
- periesophageal inflammation leads to fibrosis and adhesion formation due to traction against the esophageal wall, creating a true diverticulum
- associated with mediastinal lymphadenitis, tuberculosis, silicosis

Pulsion Diverticula

- mucosal outpouching formed by increased intraluminal pressure against a weakened esophageal wall, creating a false diverticulum
- account for the majority of diverticula
- associated with nutcracker esophagus, diffuse esophageal spasm, a hypertensive LES
- midesophageal and epiphrenic diverticula are typically incidental findings, but may be associated with hypertensive LES
- <u>Presentation</u>: when symptomatic, may present with dysphagia, regurgitation of food, weight loss, heartburn, chronic cough, aspiration, and chest pain
- traction diverticula often lack esophageal symptoms, presenting more often with pulmonary complaints
- <u>Dx</u>: best evaluated by barium radiography, endoscopy can also be used; CXR or CT Chest can help support diagnosis
- <u>Tx</u>: targeted at treating the underlying etiology
  1. if dilation is necessary, it should be performed over a guidewire with fluoroscopy to decrease risk of perforation
  2. surgery is rarely indicated

ESOPHAGEAL MALIGNANCIES

Introduction

- squamous cell carcinoma predominates worldwide and in developing countries; however, adenocarcinoma predominates in the United States
- overall, poor prognosis due to lack of symptoms in early course and thus are diagnosed late in the course, when the cancer has metastasized
- when symptomatic, presents with progressive dysphagia for solids and then for liquids, with associated weight loss
- screening and surveillance has offered tremendous opportunities for early intervention, improving the cure rate and decreased morbidity associated with treatment

Squamous Cell Carcinoma (SCC)

- <u>Epidemiology</u>: SCC is the most common type of esophageal carcinoma worldwide, most commonly seen in men, with African Americans being disproportionately affected
- arises in the mid or upper two-thirds of esophagus

- risk factors include tobacco, alcohol, diets deficient in vitamins A, C, and E, zinc, folate, and selenium
- <u>Predisposing conditions</u>: achalasia, Plummer-Vinson syndrome, tylosis, caustic injury
- <u>Pathogenesis</u>: chronic inflammation leading to regeneration of squamous mucosa, with dysplastic changes occurring over decades
- <u>Dx</u>: endoscopic biopsy, CT scan of the chest and abdomen, endoscopic ultrasound (EUS), positron-emission tomography (PET) scan
- <u>Tx</u>: endoscopic mucosal resection if tumor limited to mucosa; in most cases neoadjuvant chemoradiotherapy typically followed by complete surgical resection is the mainstay of treatment for locally advanced cancer in surgically eligible patients

Adenocarcinoma

- <u>Epidemiology</u>: adenocarcinoma is more common in the United States, with incidence rates nearly doubling, from 35% to 61% over the last 30 years, attributed to the decline of SCC, but also the rise in obesity and related conditions; increased incidence in Caucasian males
- arises in lower third or distal esophagus
- <u>Pathogenesis</u>: healing erosive esophagitis leads to metaplastic changes of normal squamous epithelium to columnar epithelium with goblet cells in the distal esophagus, a process known as intestinal metaplasia
- adenocarcinoma is associated with GERD and Barrett's esophagus (BE); among all patients with GERD, only 10% to 15% are found to have Barrett's esophagus
    1. risk factors associated with the development of BE include long-standing GERD, male gender, central obesity, and age >50 years
    2. BE on endoscopy demonstrates extension of salmon-colored mucosa ≥1 cm proximal to the GE junction with biopsy confirmation
    3. surveillance of BE is used to identify individuals at risk for progression to esophageal adenocarcinoma: BE without dysplasia requires repeat EGD every 3 to 5 years; BE with low-grade dysplasia can be treated with endoscopy therapy or alternatively, repeat EGD every 12 months; BE with high-grade dysplasia should be managed with endoscopic therapy at time of diagnosis
- <u>Dx</u>: endoscopic biopsy, CT scan of the chest and abdomen, EUS, PET scan
- <u>Tx</u>: endoscopic mucosal resection or esophagectomy if tumor limited to mucosa; neoadjuvant chemotherapy or chemoradiotherapy followed by esophagectomy

EXTRINSIC STRUCTURAL DISORDERS OF THE ESOPHAGUS

Osteophytes

- hypertrophic spurs of the cervical vertebrae can cause compression of the esophagus, most commonly observed at the levels of C5–C7
- most commonly seen in males >50 years old
- <u>Presentation</u>: difficulty swallowing solid foods, with occasional odynophagia, globus-like sensation, cough, hoarseness, and an urge to clear the throat
- <u>Dx</u>: barium swallow with lateral views
- <u>Tx</u>: dietary modification and reassurance; refractory cases may require surgical excision of osteophytes

Dysphagia Lusoria

- compression of the esophagus caused by an aberrant right subclavian artery; the right subclavian artery arises as the last branch of the aortic arch, coursing behind the esophagus to supply blood to the right arm resulting in dysphagia
- extrinsic compression of the esophagus due to a tortuous or aneurysmal aorta due to age-related changes
- typically observed in elderly and hypertensive females
- <u>Dx</u>: barium radiography has a classic appearance of a diagonal impression at the fourth thoracic vertebrae; endoscopy may reveal stenosis, kinking of the esophagus, or band-like pulsatile extrinsic compression

Malignancy

- lymphoma
- mediastinal lymphadenopathy
- gastric carcinoma

SECTION

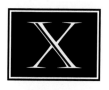

Therapy

CHAPTER

37

Voice Therapy

Bridget A. Rose and Justin Ross

SPEECH AND VOICE EVALUATION
Speech-Language Pathologist

- initial speech evaluation and follow-up therapy are performed by an American Speech-Language-Hearing Association (ASHA) certified and state licensed Speech-Language Pathologist (SLP)
- a therapist who has a background in professional voice use such as singing and/or acting may improve the quality to therapeutic intervention
- special diagnostic and intervention strategies are often used because of unusual vocal demands on professional voice users

Evaluation

- includes the initial objective and subjective measures, in-depth patient history, and a therapeutic trial
- objective and subjective evaluations are generally done by speech-language pathologists
- <u>Subjective measurements</u>: include perceptual assessment of voice and physical manifestations during **reading task** (eg, The Rainbow Passage) and within **conversational** speech, as well as patient questionnaires
- <u>Objective measurements</u>: include acoustic and aerodynamic measurements (eg, s/z ratio; sustained phonation times), **Paragraph reading** (eg, The Rainbow Passage), **CAPE-V** (Consensus Auditory-Perceptual Evaluation of Voice), **GRBAS** (grade, roughness, breathiness, asthenia, strain) Voice Rating Scale
- <u>Patient questionnaires</u>: **VRQOL** (Voice Related Quality of Life), **PVRQOL** (Pediatric version), **VHI-10** (Voice Handicap Index-10)
- external laryngeal palpation to assess tension and to help inform patients of anatomy landmarks and teach massage technique
- assessment of the presence of neurolaryngologic disorders such as tremor, abductor spasmodic dysphonia (serial 60s), adductor spasmodic dysphonia (serial 80s), dysarthria/imprecise or weak articulation (diadochokinesis)

Voice Use History

- determine phonotrauma/vocal misuse behaviors, such as sudden yelling or continuous loud voice use within work, home, and social settings
- length of time spent voicing, loud volume use, yelling

- extent of voice training
- daily vocal load (hours)
- vocal amplification for occupational voice use
- modifications made to voice use

VOICE THERAPY

Introduction

- <u>Therapeutic goals</u>: to produce optimal functionality within daily and specialized voice applications
- includes optimizing and rebalancing components of phonation (respiration, phonation, resonance)
- review of laryngeal anatomy, patient pathology, and postural alignment
- employ therapy trials to assess effort level, stimulability, and self-awareness
- emphasize carryover into everyday speech and professional functionality
- certain daily maintenance tasks (ie, vocal warm-up and cool down) may be encouraged following discharge from therapy
- a short course to review habitual vocal use may be re-prescribed if patient demonstrates new pathology or reduced proficiency during physician follow-up
- professional voice user population often requires maximum occupational voice (eg, coaches, athletic instructors, teachers, singers, actors, television and radio talents, voice-over talent, speech-language pathologists and physicians)

Indirect Therapy

- vocal hygiene and daily behavior with either positive or negative consequences discussed with patients including benefits of:
    1. appropriate hydration (based on age, activity level)
    2. elimination of smoking, vaping, and tobacco chewing
    3. soft cough and elimination of harsh throat clearing
    4. reduction of loud voice use
    5. adequate sleep, good nutrition, reduction of stress
    6. speaking in appropriate pitch ranges
    7. use of amplification
- long-term vocal preservation via use of proper techniques within work and social environments to increase ease of phonation with reduced vocal strain and fatigue

Direct Therapy

- sequential pattern of increased awareness and identification of habitual vocal traits, acquisition of new techniques, and subsequent carryover of efficient, effective phonation into habitual, functional use
- follow-up sessions usually weekly or biweekly
- length of rehabilitation: short course (eg, 1–2 sessions) to allow for immediate release of functional vocal tension; full course (6–8, 8–12 sessions) pre- and postoperatively

Pre- and Postoperative Therapy

- preoperative therapy imparts realistic view of postoperative outcomes, including awareness of desired vocal quality and vocal tone focus/placement
- may increase success rate of postoperative carryover technique for greater surgical outcomes
- sessions may range from 4 to 6 preoperative and 6 to 8 postoperative sessions depending on upcoming procedure schedule

Therapeutic Techniques

Masking

- diagnostic and therapeutic task used for functional/psychogenic dysphonia
- patient sits within an audio booth and decibel levels are increased while the patient reads a passage aloud
- patients may initiate spontaneous speech as they try to "listen" to their own vocal production at higher volume as their voices are "masked"

Confidential Voice Therapy

- <u>Tasks</u>: focus on breathy, soft/gentle, resonant production of speech → reduces hyperfunction, (eg, muscle tension dysphonia) and/or may improve vocal fold pathology (eg, polyp).
- reduce rate and loudness before rebuilding strength and intensity without compensatory tension

Resonant Voice Therapy (RVT) and Lessac-Madsen Resonant Voice Treatment (LMRVT)

- related therapies with resonant voicing therapy as basis for more formalized sequence of tasks

- Tasks: stretching and breathing maneuvers, voiced and unvoiced consonants, sequential progression from consonant-vowel (CV) combinations to conversational speech
- focus on a strong "anterior tone focus" that increases patient awareness of the voice resonating more generally within the oral cavity, while simultaneously allowing the patient to feel phonatory vibrations on his or her lips, tongue, and facial bones

Semioccluded Vocal Tract (SOVT) Exercises

- improves vocal fold efficiency via downstream occlusion
- increases supraglottal pressure and reduces transglottal pressure
- decreased vocal effort is emphasized while gradually increasing sound pressure levels and anterior tone focus/resonance *without increasing probability of high impact* contact of the vocal folds
- Tasks: straw phonation, lip or tongue out trills, cup bubble with water tasks, bilabial fricatives, unvoiced to voiced consonant speech, etc

Vocal Function Exercises

- can be utilized in conjunction with other therapies and allow for improved stamina, strength, and flexibility of phonation
- used for hyper- and hypofunctional patients
- Tasks: timed sustained pitches (C-D-E-F-G) and optimal stretching and contracting pitch glides within a 6-week protocol, twice daily until plateau is reached
- tapering protocol is available

Accent Method

- approach to improve synchronized use of respiration, phonation, resonance, and articulation for improved vocal quality and tone focus
- developed by Sven Smith in 1930s
- Tasks: combines efficient abdominal breathing training, use of prosodic speech elements (intonation stresses, intonation, volume variation), articulation, gestures, and rhythm → allows carryover into spontaneous continuous speech
- used more extensively in Europe than in the United States

Lee Silverman Voice Treatment Program (LSVT)™

- generally used in patients diagnosed with Parkinson's disease
- Program protocols:
  1. LSVT: 4 weeks (traditional every day, 4 days a week for a total of 16 sessions)

  2. LSVT-X: 8 weeks, twice weekly
  3. LSVT-BIG: supplemental
- modifies respiratory, laryngeal, and resonance subsystems of speech by targeting phonatory "effort" and increased SPL dB for carryover into everyday function
- requires professional certification

Circumlaryngeal Massage

- massage of the larynx and neck musculature to decrease tension and pain
- performed at home by patient ≥1/day recommended
- many report a comfortable "stretching" sensation during clinician-led massage
- often first line of therapy for patients with severe muscle tension dysphonia

Tongue Protrusion ("Tongue Out") Speech

- tasks that increase patient awareness of tongue base tension and its release during alternating tongue in and out of mouth during speech
- may also increase ease of movement/flexibility during speech

Abdominal/Diaphragmatic Breathing

- goal is to optimize breath control, increasing support and efficient use of airflow during speech and within specific styles of singing
- isolated tasks are employed initially to increase awareness of body movement during gentle, cyclical breathing (inhalation + exhalation = 1 cycle) and its connection to voice within several physical positions (supine, sitting, and standing)
- breathing pattern is observed and enhanced sequentially: structured tasks → spontaneous speech → reading → habitual conversational speech

Inhalation Phonation

- utilized if patient demonstrates severe muscle tension dysphonia (eg, functional dysphonia)
- may be trialed with patients who can speak during inhalation, then transfer fluent speech into exhalation
- challenging task to teach and master, may be a good first step to help segue to further tasks

Chant Speech (Chant to Speech)

- 3-step sequence to allow for increased energy, breath support, and subsequent improved resonant vocal quality
  1. utterance fully chanted on one pitch
  2. utterance chanted on one word and the rest spoken
  3. utterance fully spoken - the established energy support, increased resonance, and continuous airflow should carry over from chant to speech

VOICE THERAPY FOR SPECIFIC ETIOLOGIES

Spasmodic Dysphonia (SD)

- pre- and posttreatment therapy can be beneficial for patients who opt for surgical procedure or botulinum toxin (Botox) injections
- voice therapy especially beneficial for adductor SD (ADSD) patients
- course of pre- and posttherapy Botox injections is often helpful
- <u>Techniques</u>: gentle abdominal/diaphragmatic breathing patterns, ease of onset voicing and shorter phrase production, flow phonation and resonant voice therapy techniques for carryover effect into functional voice use
- release of muscle tension around larynx through circumlaryngeal massage

Essential Tremor

- generally presents during prolonged vowel phonation as a 4- to 6-Hz rhythmic cycle
- often demonstrate vocal breaks, strain, and struggling during speech
- may be mistaken for ADSD initially, trial therapy may help differentiate
- treatment allows clinician to "shape" the voice and allow tremor to be less conspicuous
- <u>Techniques</u>: ease of onsets, "staccato-like" voicing with the use of shortened duration of phrase length to approximately 5 syllables
- <u>Sequential tasks</u>: single syllable words → multisyllabic utterances incorporating patients' unique styles → conversation with emphasis on deliberate pauses for inhalation

Paradoxical Vocal Fold Motion (PVFM)

- there are several modifications of this technique that clinicians can choose to allow patients to adapt and eventually gain control over PFVM
- used for high-performance athletes regardless of age
- Techniques:
    1. abdominal breathing awareness/efficiency
    2. "rescue strategies" that move from sequential use of nasal "sniff" alternating with exhalation
    3. relaxed "open" throat tasks for increased oropharyngeal space
    4. use of "rhythmic walk" and breathing patterns to "pace" breath
    5. clinician can modify techniques for application in different sports

Transgenderism

- patients transitioning from male to female and female to male
- individual and/or group therapy options may be available
- SLP will address vocal pitch inflection, vocal quality, and vocal tone placement
- address linguistic and social differences in communication between genders, including; prosody, word choice, posture, gestures, and syntax
- Typical tasks may include: resonant voice therapy and vocal function exercises
- modifications in therapy can be dependent on changes in hormonal therapy
- refer to **WPATH**: World Professional Association for Transgender Health

Alaryngeal Speech (Postlaryngectomy)

- pre- and postsurgical counseling are essential to the special needs of a tracheotomy patient
- Therapy may address: decreased swallowing function, need for and use of alternative communication devices, care of alternative communication devices, support system before and after surgery

Electrolarynx

- electrical device that induces oropharyngeal mucosal vibration, allowing for voicing at a single or range of frequencies with preserved articulatory ability
- exhalation during this type of alaryngeal speech is unnecessary

- Used in several ways:
    1. **Transcervical**: placed against neck
    2. **Transoral**: sound delivered to mouth via tube,
    3. **Intraoral**: remote controlled build into upper orthodonture of patient

Tracheoesophageal Puncture (TEP) and Prosthesis/Valve

- a one-way, prosthesis valve is inserted into puncture, and patient can inhale and exhale as he or she uses finger to occlude the tracheostoma
- requires practice to coordinate release of airflow
- ~80% will master this technique
- Tracheostoma valve can be used also as a hands-free alternative to finger placement
- devices include duckbill style, indwelling prosthesis, low-pressure/low-resistance valve

Esophageal Speech

- patient "swallows" small amount of air then passes it back through the neopharynx
- rapid movement of air used to create words with tongue, lips, teeth, and palate
- Techniques: injection (using positive air pressure) and inhalation (using negative air pressure)
- difficult to master (~20% of patients)

SINGING VOICE AS A REHABILITATIVE INTERVENTION

Introduction

- singing voice specialists (SVSs) are experienced singing teachers specifically trained by medical professionals; background in vocal anatomy, objective/subjective measurements and pathologies is necessary
- beneficial if a licensed speech-language pathologist is also an experienced singer, but this is rare
- singing technique not considered medical "therapy," and it is currently illegal for a singing teacher to practice "voice therapy" in the United States

- SVS should not replace the patient's current voice teacher if patient currently studies; they may be included in rehabilitation after resolution of acute pathology
- singing voice habilitation can improve a nonsinger's rehabilitation outcomes
- members of the voice team should not assume that a professional or avocational singer is familiar with vocal anatomy
- laryngologists with vocal pedagogy training may perform an initial short singing voice evaluations; usually this evaluation is performed by an SVS
- self-consciousness, nervousness, emotional, or psychological stress may limit accurate evaluation of voicing behaviors; usually resolves with increased comfort across multiple treatment sessions
- SVS evaluates *only* after they receive the full, comprehensive evaluation and diagnosis from the treating physician

Subjective Assessment for Professional/Avocational Singer

- assess range and voice category (eg, bass, baritone, tenor, mezzo-soprano, soprano) and timbre, address vocal category misclassifications
- document voice quality (eg, pressed, strained, strangled, hoarse, nasality, etc)
- Register: assess voice quality in all registers, and any passaggio instability; changes dependent on laryngeal muscular function and vocal fold shape
- Vibrato: evaluate rate, extent, regularity, and waveform; natural rate is 6 Hz, slower in men, generally unaffected by pitch and effort; pitch fluctuation (extent) typically one-half semitone above and below
- Tremolo: (prominent wobble) present in elderly singers with poor vocal condition and laryngeal muscular control, not a true vibrato

Singing Voice Physical Evaluation

- Posture/stance: balanced with weight forward, knees slightly bent, and relaxed neck, shoulders, and torso
- Breathing: primarily abdominal with submaximal chest expansion, nasal inhalation (warming and humidification), no use of accessory muscles, relaxed neck and chest musculature
- Common technical errors: excessive tension of neck, chin, and muscles of mastication, lower lip and tongue retraction, elevation of larynx with ascending pitch, lack of abdominal muscle contraction prior to sound production, reduced or extensive oropharyngeal space, lowered palate

- compensatory neck muscle tension, tongue retrusion, and supraglottic hyperfunction more common in the presence of vocal fold pathology

Goals for Singing Voice Sessions

- improve efficiency and effective use of voice via reduced hyperfunction, good technique, healthy musculature engagement, and coordination of respiratory, phonatory, resonance, and articulation
- individualized treatment plan based on their pathology or technical skills (ie, vocal fold adduction tasks not utilized to address hemorrhage)
- Classical music: needs relatively stable laryngeal position (no rise and fall with pitch movement)
- Contemporary commercial music: watch for excessively high-placed larynx
- understand medical limitations, prognosis, and duration of recovery that can last for many months
- appropriate technique is most important regardless of vocal quality
- ideal sound may not be the goal during singing voice habilitation because of compromised vocal folds

Singing Voice Tasks

- patients taught to sing "by what they feel" not just what they hear and to establish new habits
- first establish current comfortable vocal range
- initial sessions may focus on strengthening flexibility and efficiency of voicing
- vocal tasks with musical patterns: straw phonation, flow phonation/ semioccluded vocal tract tasks, lip trills, glides (as previously mentioned)
- messa di voce tasks (sustained single note) → increase and decrease volume and improve stamina
- glottal "fry" tasks allow for gentle vocal fold adduction in short duration → demonstrate improved voicing to patient with careful carryover to speech
- alternating "twang" or hypernasal tasks (nasal occlusion) with normal singing → improves tone quality and placement
- scales and songs can often be taught to a nonsinger if he or she demonstrates adequate pitch-matching ability and ease of phonation
- abdominal/diaphragmatic breathing cyclical pattern → efficient airflow and support

CHAPTER

Swallow Therapy

Tess T. Andrews

PATIENT EVALUATION

Considerations Prior to Treatment

- intensive therapy may be recommended depending on etiology of swallowing dysfunction
- compensatory strategies can ensure adequate function and safety of swallowing if patient expected to recover in short time
- consider prognosis to ensure patient can tolerate therapy
- patients with degenerative diseases may benefit from initial therapy, but disease progression with loss of neuromotor control or cognitive impairment can limit long-term effectiveness
- compensatory strategies often are initiated at the time of videofluoroscopy to facilitate improved swallowing function
- notable improvement following initiation of a compensatory strategy may obviate need for a full swallowing treatment plan
- more extensive therapy commonly required for severe swallow dysfunction, especially if compensatory strategies alone are not efficient
- cognitive status can have substantial negative impact on swallowing therapy
- swallow maneuvers often require complex direction following, whereas compensatory strategies require less
- evaluate baseline respiratory function: some exercises or maneuvers (supraglottic or super-supraglottic swallow) require a short period of airway closure and adequate respiratory function
- family and/or caregiver support/accountability is essential to successful treatment, especially in patients with memory impairment or cognitive decline
- plan of care will need to be modified to accommodate patients without support
- patient motivation is key factor for consistent improvement and treatment success
- patients who are dependent on feeding tube may find oral feeding effortful, which can complicate and increase duration of therapy

PLAN OF CARE

- compensatory strategies allow clinicians to test alterations in bolus control with the goal of improving swallow efficiency and safety
- utilized at time of initial assessment to examine whether patient is stimulable for therapeutic techniques

Postural Changes

- can improve swallowing safety depending on location of biomechanical impairment by redirecting the flow of bolus

Head Back

- used when there is inefficient anterior-posterior bolus transit within the oral cavity by the tongue
- with the assistance of gravity, the bolus can bypass the oral cavity, and the pharyngeal swallow can take over

Chin Tuck

- head is tucked, and the chin is touching or is close to the neck
- narrows entrance to laryngeal vestibule; decreased distance between posterior pharyngeal wall and base of tongue/epiglottis
- bolus remains in oral cavity longer
- reduced the risk of aspiration pre-swallow for patients who demonstrate difficulty containing the bolus posteriorly due to incomplete lingual-velar valving, resulting in premature posterior spillage

Head Turn

- head turn toward a damaged or weak side of the pharynx narrows damaged side so the bolus flows down the stronger side
- effective in unilateral pharyngeal wall weakness or a vocal fold paresis or paralysis
- can add chin tuck when there is reduced or incomplete laryngeal closure resulting in aspiration during a swallow
- narrows the entrance to the laryngeal vestibule and increases vocal fold adduction
- head turn in either direction can be utilized for cricopharyngeal (CP) muscle dysfunction causing residue in the pyriform sinuses after a swallow
- pulls cricoid cartilage away from the posterior pharyngeal wall reducing pressure on CP muscle

Head Tilt

- directs bolus flow toward stronger side to compensate for unilateral oral and pharyngeal impairment that causes residue within the oral cavity, oropharynx, and hypopharynx

Reclined Position

- effective in poor pharyngeal constriction, incomplete laryngeal closure, and reduced distention of the pharyngoesophageal segment (PES) during swallow attempts that result in aspiration both during and after a swallow
- allows gravity to assist the patient in keeping bolus material in the hypopharynx rather than falling forward into the laryngeal vestibule

Safe Intake Strategies

- modify a behavior, environment, assistance, and/or presentation of the bolus, instead of the actual food or liquid item
- Small bites or sips and slow rate to allow for better bolus management —recommended if the patient aspirates on a larger bolus or while swallowing consecutively
- **Subsequent swallows** used to clear oropharyngeal or hypopharyngeal residue to reduce the risk of aspiration post-swallow
- **Cyclical ingestion**: alternating liquids and solids to flush residue from the pharynx
- **Prophylactic cough**: intentional cough after swallowing to expel residue from trachea or laryngeal vestibule—utilized if patient consistently demonstrates penetration or aspiration and has adequate pulmonary clearance
- **Avoid consecutive sips** (ie, single sips at a time): patients may aspirate only across consecutive sips of thin liquid, therefore avoiding this type of drinking is beneficial
- **Avoid straws**: can lead to more frequent penetration and aspiration

Diet Modification

- accounts for biomechanical impairments to improve safety and efficiency of swallow
- implemented if compensatory strategies and maneuvers alone are insufficient
- alteration of **liquids** indicated when:
  1. delayed trigger of pharyngeal swallow results in aspiration before a swallow
  2. delayed laryngeal closure yields aspiration during a swallow
- alteration of **solids** indicated when:
  1. poor oral control of the bolus throughout manipulation
  2. poor dentition results in inability to masticate regular solids

3. pharyngeal weakness leads to oropharyngeal and hypopharyngeal residue after a swallow
4. reduced cricopharyngeal distention yields residue in the hypopharynx after a swallow
- <u>Alternative methods of nutrition and hydration</u>: use a nasogastric (NG), gastrostomy or percutaneous endoscopic gastrostomy (PEG) tube, or jejunostomy (J) tube in place due to inability consume liquids and solids by mouth safely

Diet Levels

- **Regular solids**: no alteration of solid textures; "regular diet"
- **Soft solids** ("mechanical soft"): softer consistencies, avoiding dry/dense textures (ie, breads/meat)
- **Moist mechanical soft solids**: slick textures; solids accompanied by sauces/gravies to allow for easier bolus transit
- **Pureed solids**: blended textures; if the texture requires mastication, it is not a true puree

Thin Liquids

- preferable when a thickened consistency with a given anatomical impairment will lead to increased residue
- **Anatomic impairments**:
   1. oral tongue dysfunction if pharyngeal swallow is functional
   2. reduced tongue base retraction
   3. reduced pharyngeal constriction
   4. reduced laryngeal elevation
   5. reduced pharyngoesophageal segment distention
- if residue adheres 50% or more higher than pyriform sinus height, risk of aspiration post-swallow increased 30×

Thickened (Nectar, Honey)

- oral tongue dysfunction
- delayed pharyngeal swallow initiation
- proceed with caution and consider quality of life prior to implementing, may not be appropriate for some patients
- aspiration of water alone poses limited health risk when appropriate oral hygiene is maintained
- often, aspirated water is more benign than thickened liquids and should always be considered first
- **Aspiration guidelines**:
   1. consume only water outside of mealtime

2. perform oral care prior to consumption of water
3. sit upright and use appropriate swallowing strategies

Dehydration

- **Frazier Free Water Protocol**: allowance of water to prevent dehydration and promote swallowing with use of meticulous oral hygiene prior to trials to minimize disuse atrophy of swallow mechanism
- **Effects of dehydration**: confusion and lethargy, constipation, renal failure, weight loss, fever, increased fall risk, urinary tract infections, delayed progression in therapy, and predisposition to bacterial colonization within the oral cavity and oropharynx

SWALLOW THERAPY

Oral Preparatory and Oral Phase

- Oral prep phase: process of ingesting liquids or solids and preparing them to be swallowed via the teeth and muscles of mastication; preparation of the bolus
- Oral phase: transport of food through the oral cavity via propulsion of the tongue posteriorly with the goal of triggering the pharyngeal swallow

Tongue Tip Raises

- hard palate is contacted with the blade of the tongue utilized to push the bolus posteriorly

Oral Sensory Therapy Techniques

- used to augment sensory input (ie, bolus taste, temperature, volume, and viscosity)
- utilized with swallow apraxia or reduced coordination of swallow, tactile agnosia, delayed initiation of the oral and/or pharyngeal swallow and reduced sensation within the oral cavity
- **Technique:**
  1. downward pressure of spoon against the tongue when presenting solids
  2. sour bolus
  3. cold bolus
  4. presenting a bolus that requires mastication
  5. larger volume bolus

Oral Motor Control Exercises

- using range of motion to improve movement of the lips, jaw, oral tongue, and tongue base

Lingual Range of Motion Exercises

- elevation (anteriorly, posteriorly), protrusion, lateralization
- range of motion utilizing resistance (with a tongue blade, spoon, popsicle stick, etc)

Inter-Incisal Opening Exercises

- ensure adequate ability to accept the bolus and masticate efficiently
- masseter massage, range of motion exercises, and passive stretching
- **Passive stretching**: thumb and index finger in between teeth and mouth in open posture to stretch the jaw

Pharyngeal Phase

- when the bolus moves through the pharynx and the airway is protected

Supraglottic Swallow

- closes vocal folds before and during swallow to aid airway protection
- <u>Technique</u>: hold breath → put liquid into mouth and continue to hold breath → swallow while holding breath → cough prophylactically following swallow

Super-Supraglottic Swallow

- closure of laryngeal inlet via approximation of arytenoid mucosa with the epiglottic petiole before and during swallow
- promotes early airway protection and extends time of laryngeal elevation
- <u>Technique</u>: inhale and hold breath tightly while bearing down → continue to bear down and swallow → cough prophylactically following swallow

Effortful Swallow

- increases tongue base retraction during pharyngeal swallow, thereby improving efficiency of bolus clearance from the oropharynx (ie, valleculae)
  1. swallow hard, squeezing the muscles of the throat

Mendelsohn Maneuver

- increases extent and duration of hyolaryngeal excursion, therefore improving airway protection and increasing cricopharyngeal opening
- <u>Technique</u>: swallow and have patient feel larynx lift up and back down → hold larynx in elevated position during swallow → continue to hold for a few seconds and then allow it to fall

Range of Motion Exercises

- laryngeal closure
- vocal fold adduction
- base of tongue
- laryngeal elevation

Sensory Therapy

- for delayed or absent pharyngeal swallow
- **Thermal-tactile stimulation**: stimulating the anterior faucial arches to trigger pharyngeal swallow and heighten oral awareness

Pharyngeal Constriction Exercises

- **Masako maneuver**: hold tip of tongue between the teeth and swallow simultaneously to pull the pharyngeal wall forward to make contact with the base of tongue

Esophageal Phase

- bolus is carried through the esophagus and into the stomach via peristalsis
- upper esophageal sphincter returns to its tonic resting state after the bolus passes the pharyngoesophageal segment to prevent bolus backflow or regurgitation
- hyoid, larynx, and pharynx also return to their original resting states
- predominantly managed with surgical intervention or medications—limited role for speech-language pathologist

Cricopharyngeal Dysfunction

- may limit laryngeal elevation resulting in reduced pressure for bolus transit
- <u>Treatment options</u>:
    1. esophagoscopy with balloon dilation

  2. cricopharyngeal Botox injection and myotomy
  3. compensatory maneuvers using a head rotation

Shaker Exercise

- facilitates hyolaryngeal excursion to assist in pharyngoesophageal segment distention
- typically used as a preventative exercise
- <u>Technique</u>: lie flat on the floor or a bed with no pillow → lift head and look toward toes → hold for approximately 10 seconds

INDEX

Note: Page numbers in **bold** reference non-text material.